Non-Hodgkin's Lymphomas: New Insights and Therapeutic Strategies

Guest Editor

BRUCE D. CHESON, MD

HEMATOLOGY/ONCOLOGY CLINICS OF NORTH AMERICA

www.hemonc.theclinics.com

October 2008 • Volume 22 • Number 5

SAUNDERS an imprint of ELSEVIER, Inc.

W.B. SAUNDERS COMPANY
A Division of Elsevier Inc.

1600 John F. Kennedy Blvd. ● Suite 1800 ● Philadelphia, PA 19103-2899

http://www.theclinics.com

HEMATOLOGY/ONCOLOGY CLINICS OF NORTH AMERICA Volume 22, Number 5
October 2008 ISSN 0889-8588, ISBN 13: 978-1-4160-5875-5, ISBN 10: 1-4160-5875-3

Editor: Kerry Holland

Hematology/Oncology Clinics (ISSN 0889-8588) is published bimonthly by Elsevier Inc., 360 Park Avenue South, New York, NY 10010-1710. Months of issue are February, April, June, August, October, and December. Business and Editorial Offices: 1600 John F. Kennedy Blvd., Suite 1800, Philadelphia, PA 19103-2899. Customer Service Office: 11830 Westline Industrial Drive, St. Louis, MO 63146. Periodicals postage paid at New York, NY and additional mailing offices. Subscription prices are $262.00 per year (US individuals), $392.00 per year (US institutions), $131.00 per year (US students), $297.00 per year (Canadian individuals), $470.00 per year (Canadian institutions), $166.00 per year (Canadian students), $332.00 per year (international individuals), $470.00 per year (international institutions), $166.00 per year (international students). International air speed delivery is included in all *Clinics* subscription prices. All prices are subject to change without notice. **POSTMASTER:** Send address changes to *Hematology/Oncology Clinics of North America*, 11830 Westline Industrial Drive, St. Louis, MO 63146. Customer Service (orders, claims, online, change of address): Elsevier Periodicals Customer Service, 11830 Westline Industrial Drive, St. Louis, MO 63146. Tel: 1-800-654-2452 (U.S. and Canada). Fax: 314-523-5170. E-mail: journalscustomerservice-usa@elsevier.com (for print support); journalsonlinesupport-usa@elsevier.com (for online support).

Reprints. For copies of 100 or more, of articles in this publication, please contact the Commercial Reprints Department, Elsevier Inc., 360 Park Avenue South, New York, New York 10010-1710; Tel.: 212-633-3813, Fax: 212-462-1935, E-mail: reprints@elsevier.com.

Hematology/Oncology Clinics of North America is covered in *MEDLINE/PubMed (Index Medicus), EMBASE/ Excerpta Medica, and BIOSIS.*

Printed in the United States of America.

Contributors

GUEST EDITOR

BRUCE D. CHESON, MD
Professor of Medicine, and Head of Hematology, Georgetown University Hospital, Lombardi Comprehensive Cancer Center, Washington, District of Columbia

AUTHORS

FRANCESCO BERTONI, MD
Vice-Head, Laboratory of Experimental Oncology, Research Division, Oncology Institute of Southern Switzerland, Ospedale San Giovanni, Switzerland

FRANCO CAVALLI, MD, FRCP
Director, Oncology Institute of Southern Switzerland, Ospedale San Giovanni, Switzerland

BRUCE D. CHESON, MD
Professor of Medicine, and Head of Hematology, Georgetown University Hospital, Lombardi Comprehensive Cancer Center, Washington, District of Columbia

JAEHYUK CHOI, MD, PhD
Department of Dermatology, Yale University School of Medicine, New Haven, Connecticut

MARTIN DREYLING, MD, PhD
Professor, Department of Medicine III, University of Munich, Hospital Grosshadern, Munich, Germany

REBECCA L. ELSTROM, MD
Assistant Professor of Medicine, Division of Hematology/Oncology, Weill Cornell Medical College, New York, New York

RICHARD I. FISHER, MD
Samuel Durand Professor of Medicine, University of Rochester; Director, James P. Wilmot Cancer Center, Rochester, New York

FRANCINE M. FOSS, MD
Professor of Medicine and Dermatology, Department of Medical Oncology, Yale University School of Medicine, New Haven, Connecticut

JONATHAN W. FRIEDBERG, MD
Associate Professor of Medicine, University of Rochester; Director of Hematological Malignancy Clinical Research, James P. Wilmot Cancer Center, Rochester, New York

RANDY D. GASCOYNE, MD
Clinical Professor of Pathology, Department of Pathology and Laboratory Medicine; and Research Director, Centre for Lymphoid Cancers, British Columbia Cancer Agency, Vancouver Cancer Center, Vancouver, British Columbia, Canada

DAVID J. GOOD, MD
Department of Pathology and Laboratory Medicine, British Columbia Cancer Agency, Vancouver Cancer Center, Vancouver, British Columbia, Canada

JOHN G. GRIBBEN, MD, DSc, FMedSci
Professor of Experimental Cancer Medicine, Centre for Experimental Cancer Medicine, Barts and The London School of Medicine, London, United Kingdom

ELENA M. HARTMANN, MD
Scientist, Institute of Pathology, University of Würzburg, Würzburg, Germany

SANDRA J. HORNING, MD
Professor of Medicine, Department of Medicine/Oncology, Stanford Cancer Center, Stanford, California

ANNA JOHNSTON, MBBS
Visiting Physician, Service d'Hématologie, Hospices Civils de Lyon, Lyon, France

MATKO KALAC
Herbert Irving Comprehensive Cancer Center, College of Physicians and Surgeons, The New York Presbyterian Hospital, Columbia University, New York, New York

YUKIKO KITAGAWA, MD
Research Associate, Herbert Irving Comprehensive Cancer Center, Columbia University, New York, New York

FREDERICK LANSIGAN, MD
Medical Oncology, Yale University School of Medicine, New Haven, Connecticut

JOHN P. LEONARD, MD
The Richard T. Silver Professor of Medicine, Division of Hematology/Oncology, Weill Cornell Medical College, New York, New York

PETER MARTIN, MD
Fellow, Division of Hematology/Oncology, Weill Cornell Medical College, New York, New York

OWEN A. O'CONNOR, MD, PhD
Associate Professor of Medicine and Director, Lymphoid Development and Malignancy Program, Herbert Irving Comprehensive Cancer Center, Chief of Lymphoma Service, College of Physicians and Surgeons, The New York Presbyterian Hospital, Columbia University, New York, New York

GERMAN OTT, MD
Professor of Pathology, Department of Clinical Pathology, Robert-Bosch-Krankenhaus, Stuttgart, Germany

LUCA PAOLUZZI, MD
Research Associate, Herbert Irving Comprehensive Cancer Center, Columbia University, New York, New York

STEFAN PEINERT, MD
Department of Haematology, Peter MacCallum Cancer Centre, East Melbourne, Victoria, Australia

ANDREAS ROSENWALD, MD
Associate Professor of Pathology, Institute of Pathology, University of Würzburg, Würzburg, Germany

GILLES SALLES, MD, PhD
Professor of Medicine, Service d'Hématologie, Hospices Civils de Lyon, Université Lyon-1, Lyon, France

CHRISTIAN SCHMIDT, MD
Professor, Department of Medicine III, University of Munich, Hospital Grosshadern, Munich, Germany

JOHN F. SEYMOUR, MB, BS, FRACP, PhD
Associate Professor of Medicine and Head, Department of Haematology, Peter MacCallum Cancer Centre, East Melbourne; University of Melbourne, Parkville, Victoria, Australia

ANASTASIOS STATHIS, MD
Research Division, Oncology Institute of Southern Switzerland, Ospedale San Giovanni, Switzerland

JOHN W. SWEETENHAM, MD
Professor of Medicine, Cleveland Clinic Taussig Cancer Institute, Cleveland, Ohio

DARYL TAN, MBBS, MRCP
Consultant, Department of Hematology, Singapore General Hospital, Singapore

JULIE M. VOSE, MD
Neumann M. and Mildred E. Harris Professor, and Chief, Section of Hematology/Oncology, Internal Medicine, University of Nebraska Medical Center, Omaha, Nebraska

DAVID WRENCH, MB, MRCP
Clinical Research Fellow, Centre for Medical Oncology, Barts and The London School of Medicine, London, United Kingdom

JASMINE ZAIN, MD
Assistant Professor of Medicine, Herbert Irving Comprehensive Cancer Center, College of Physicians and Surgeons, The New York Presbyterian Hospital, Columbia University, New York, New York

EMANUELE ZUCCA, MD
Privatdozent of Oncology/Haematology, University of Bern, Bern; Head of Lymphoma Unit, Research Division, Oncology Institute of Southern Switzerland, Ospedale San Giovanni, Switzerland

Contents

> This article provides an overview of the pathology and classification of non-Hodgkin lymphomas. Key histologic features are described for the common entities including both B-cell and T/NK-cell lineages. Additionally, details of the characteristic immunophenotypic findings, molecular genetic results, and common or clinically relevant cytogenetic alterations are described. Helpful tables are included that outline the key diagnostic features.

> This article summarizes molecular and genetic features of B-cell non-Hodgkin lymphoma and focuses on diffuse large B-cell lymphoma, Burkitt lymphoma, follicular lymphoma, and mantle cell lymphoma. In each of these entities, hallmark genetic aberrations, cytogenetic characteristics, and alterations of single genes that might be involved in the pathogenesis and molecular evolution of the tumor are described. Recent results from gene-expression profiling studies are incorporated that are relevant for the classification of lymphoma entities, the prediction of their clinical behavior, and the identification of deregulated signal-transduction pathways that might represent potential targets in future therapeutic approaches.

> Patients who have non-Hodgkin's lymphoma or Hodgkin lymphoma most often present for medical attention because of signs or symptoms referable to enlarged lymph nodes or other disease-related symptoms (such as fevers, night sweats or fatigue). Less often, enlarged lymph nodes or splenomegaly may be incidental findings during evaluation for other medical issues. Determination of the extent of disease and accurate assessment of responses are necessary for appropriate management. Newer technologies have improved the ability to evaluate patients and to conduct clinical trials, leading to more effective therapies. This article addresses the

Diffuse large B-cell lymphoma (DLBCL) remains a curable lymphoma, with improved outcome resulting in large part from the incorporation of rituximab in standard regimens. The disease is heterogeneous clinically, morphologically, and molecularly. Recent insights into the molecular heterogeneity of DLBCL are beginning to yield novel therapeutics with significant promise for key subsets of patients. Although cyclophosphamide, hydroxydaunorubicin, vincristine, and prednisone chemotherapy with rituximab remains a standard therapeutic approach for most patients who have DLBCL, it is anticipated that novel agents will be included in treatment regimens for many patients in the near future.

Mantle cell lymphoma is characterized clinically by an aggressive clinical course and is relatively resistant to conventional chemotherapies. When in its advanced stages, currently available immunochemotherapy regimens remain noncurative despite high initial response rates. In contrast, consolidating high-dose therapy with autologous stem cell retransfusion significantly extends progression-free survival of young patients. Currently, allogenic bone marrow transplantation represents the only therapy with the potential for a curative approach, although associated with a high rate of complications. New concepts of therapy are urgently warranted, including new molecular approaches, such as bortezomib, thalidomide, lenalidomide, and temsirolimus.

Highly aggressive lymphomas are relatively uncommon in adults, comprising approximately 4% to 5% of all non-Hodgkin lymphomas in the United States and Western Europe. The designation of "highly aggressive" is generally restricted to precursor T-cell and B-cell lymphoblastic lymphoma/leukemia and Burkitt's lymphoma/leukemia. Treatment strategies for lymphoblastic lymphoma and Burkitt's lymphoma include complex, highly intensive combination chemotherapy regimens, which may be curative. As with other subtypes of NHL, emerging data from gene-expression profiling and related techniques are helping to define these entities more precisely and identify potential new rational therapeutic targets.

immune mechanisms to target and kill tumors. Foremost among these has been the development of monoclonal antibodies. Currently, an array of novel therapeutics in development may improve outcomes further, including novel monoclonals and other agents that take advantage of or optimize immune system function in the treatment of lymphoma or that provide other mechanisms of antitumor activity.

David Wrench and John G. Gribben

Non-Hodgkin's lymphoma (NHL) includes a diverse set of conditions ranging from high-grade aggressive to more indolent low-grade disease. Hematopoietic stem cell transplantation (HSCT) has a valuable role in the management of these conditions and can provide long-term remission in selected cases. This article presents the current use of allogeneic and autologous HSCT in a number of subtypes of NHL.

THE CLINICS ARE NOW AVAILABLE ONLINE!

Access your subscription at:
www.theclinics.com

Preface

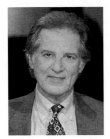

Bruce D. Cheson, MD
Guest Editor

Non-Hodgkin's lymphomas are a heterogeneous group of more than 60 entities that differ in morphology, genetics, immunology, clinical features, and outcome following therapy. Newer technologies, such as DNA microarray analyses, have demonstrated that tumors with a similar appearance under the microscope may have markedly distinct gene expression profiles, which are associated with a different clinical course. We also have learned that a lymphoma's microenvironment, characterized by lymphoma-associated macrophages, regulatory T cells, and a variety of cytokines, plays a major role in the behavior of lymphomas.

Importantly, over the past decade, major progress has been made in therapeutic approaches and the manner in which response to treatment is measured. The availability of clinically effective and well-tolerated monoclonal antibodies has improved the survival of patients who have indolent and aggressive lymphomas. Unfortunately, curative strategies remain elusive for indolent histologies and mantle cell lymphoma. New agents targeting novel pathways or influencing the host or tumor immunologic status are in clinical trials and may improve patient outcome. However, the optimal use of antibodies and other targeted agents remains to be defined. Staging and response assessment traditionally relied on physical examination and CT scans. The availability of metabolic imaging studies, especially 18F-fluoro-2-deoxy-D-glucose positron emission tomography, has the potential to alter staging, prognosis, and assessment of response. The larger role for this technology may be used in risk-directed therapeutic strategies leading to an improvement in patient outcome, by modifying therapy early in nonresponsive patients, or used to reduce treatment-related toxicities by limiting the amount of therapy required in responding patients. Traditional prognostic schemes are being revised to incorporate clinically relevant biomarkers with the goal of individualizing therapy.

Each of the authors of the various articles in the current *Hematology/Oncology Clinics of North America* has made major contributions to the understanding of non-Hodgkin's lymphomas and to the development of newer and more effective treatments. I hope this volume will convince the practicing hematologist/oncologist and

Hematol Oncol Clin N Am 22 (2008) xiii–xiv
doi:10.1016/j.hoc.2008.08.001
0889-8588/08/$ – see front matter © 2008 Elsevier Inc. All rights reserved.

hemonc.theclinics.com

the clinical researcher that enormous progress has been made in the treatment of non-Hodgkin's lymphomas. However, continued progress requires a dedication to high quality clinical research trials.

Bruce D. Cheson, MD
Georgetown University Hospital
Lombardi Comprehensive Cancer Center
3800 Reservoir Road NW
Washington, DC 20007, USA

E-mail address:
bdc4@georgetown.edu (B.D. Cheson)

Classification of Non-Hodgkin's Lymphoma

David J. Good, MD[a], Randy D. Gascoyne, MD[a,b],*

KEYWORDS

- Lymphoma • Classification • Pathology • Immunophenotype
- Molecular genetics • Cytogenetics

The classification of non-Hodgkin lymphoma has been a work in progress and has undergone many revisions to arrive at the current World Health Organization (WHO) classification used today. In North America, earlier classifications included the Rappaport classification[1] introduced in 1956 and the Lukes-Collins[2] classification introduced in 1974. The Working Formulation was published in 1982[3] and essentially replaced the previous classifications. The Working Formulation was a combination of the concepts and terms of the Rappaport classification, the Lukes-Collins classification, and the Kiel classification,[4] but it never was adopted as widely in Europe as in North America. The Kiel classification remained widely used throughout Europe, but the Working Formulation eventually became the predominant classification used in published research.

A high degree of inter- and intraobserver variability still existed in both diagnosis and subtyping of non-Hodgkin lymphoma.[5–8] This variability probably reflected the lack of widespread use of immunophenotyping, lack of access to cytogenetics, and the diverse definitions of lymphoma subtypes that were in use.

A proposal for a new approach to classify non-Hodgkin lymphomas was introduced in 1994, by a group of hematopathologists from Europe and the United States.[9] This proposal was more encompassing, taking into account the immunologic characteristics, genetic alterations, and the clinical characteristics of the disorders, instead of relying solely on the histopathologic features of the tumor cells. This classification system became known as the "Revised European-American Classification of Lymphoid Neoplasms" (REAL) classification.[10] Lymphomas could be diagnosed much more reproducibly than in previous systems, and the new clinical entities

[a] Department of Pathology and Laboratory Medicine, British Columbia Cancer Agency, Vancouver Cancer Center, 600 W 10th Avenue, Vancouver, BC V5Z 4E6, Canada
[b] Centre for Lymphoid Cancers, British Columbia Cancer Agency, Vancouver Cancer Center, Vancouver, BC, Canada
* Corresponding author.
E-mail address: rgascoyn@bccancer.bc.ca (R.D. Gascoyne).

Hematol Oncol Clin N Am 22 (2008) 781–805
doi:10.1016/j.hoc.2008.07.008
0889-8588/08/$ – see front matter © 2008 Elsevier Inc. All rights reserved.

proposed in the REAL classification were distinct. This approach subsequently was adopted as the WHO classification[11] and has become the standard approach for clinicians and investigators worldwide.

LYMPHOID TUMORS OF B-CELL LINEAGE
Precursor B-Cell Lymphoblastic Lymphoma

Precursor B-cell lymphoblastic lymphoma most often presents in the leukemic form, but it can have a lymphomatous presentation, frequently involving lymph nodes and skin. The cells have immature features including fine chromatin and scanty cytoplasm. The phenotype is that of an early-stage B-cell tumor with expression of Tdt, CD79a, CD10, and CD34. This entity can be difficult to distinguish from small round-cell tumors such as Ewing's sarcoma.[12] Therefore, a complete immunophenotype, including antibodies to CD99 and TdT and molecular diagnostic tests can prove useful.

Follicular Lymphoma

Follicular lymphoma (FL) is one of the most common non-Hodgkin lymphomas in the Western world, accounting for about 20% of all malignant lymphomas in adults.[13] The neoplastic cells are follicle center B cells, comprised of a mixture of centrocytes (small, nondividing B cells) and centroblasts (large, proliferating B cells) arranged into follicular structures (see **Fig. 1**). True neoplastic follicles have morphologic features that

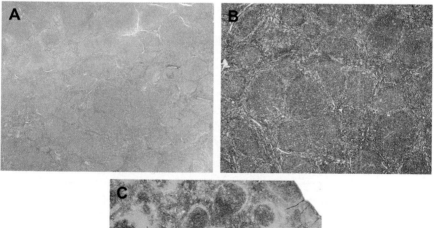
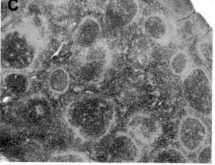

Fig. 1. (*A*) Low power appearance of follicular lymphoma (FL) with tightly clustered neoplastic lymphoid follicles. (*B*) Bcl-2 immunostain of a FL with intense staining of the malignant follicles. (*C*) CD10 stain shows staining of the follicle centers; absence of staining of the thin zone of marginal zone differentiation surrounding the follicles and numerous positive staining cells in the interfollicular area is a classic finding for FL.

help distinguish them from reactive follicles. They tend to be increased in number and closely packed, effacing the normal nodal architecture. These follicles are poorly defined, often lacking mantle zones as well as lacking polarization and the tingible body macrophages of reactive follicles. The malignant cells are not confined to the follicles and often spill over into the interfollicular areas.[14,15] This interfollicular infiltrate contains mainly centrocytes and is considered to be a dormant subpopulation of the tumor, whereas most of the proliferative activity occurs within the microenvironment of the follicle. The proportion of centroblasts and centrocytes varies from tumor to tumor, and it has been found that the proportion of centroblasts within the follicles of a FL can predict clinical outcome. This finding has led to the development of histologic grading systems to quantify objectively the number of centroblasts within follicles.[16–18] The WHO classification recommends evaluating 10 high-power fields (HPFs) and calculating the average number of centroblasts for one HPF.[19] This scheme has made grading of FL relatively reproducible but is not without problems. Core biopsies or small fragments of tissue obtained for lymphoma diagnosis may contain only a few neoplastic follicles, making formal grading impossible. Some tumors may have significant variability in the numbers of centroblasts present in different follicles. As well, with lack of experience, there may be morphologic difficulties in distinguishing centroblasts, large centrocytes, and/or follicular dendritic cells (FDCs).

FL may contain a diffuse component, an area of the lymph node lacking follicles and an FDC meshwork.[19,20] This component is not to be confused with the interfollicular component, which occupies the area between the neoplastic follicles. On occasion, the diffuse component can dominate, and a follicular component may not be identifiable. If the diffuse component contains more than 15 centroblasts per HPF, it is best classified as an area of diffuse large B-cell lymphoma (DLBCL). If the centroblast count is less than 15 per HPF, the term "diffuse follicle center cell lymphoma" is used, indicating the low-grade nature of the lymphoma.[19] Appropriate grading (grade 1 or 2) is used.

By immunohistochemistry, FL cells express pan–B-cell markers including CD20 and CD79a. Normal follicle center B-cell antigens such as CD10 and Bcl-6 frequently are expressed by the tumor cells, demonstrating a follicle center derivation. The typical immunophenotype is detailed in **Table 1**.

The genetic hallmark of FL is the t(14;18) translocation, seen in 80% to 90% of cases.[21,22] This translocation juxtaposes the *BCL2* gene on chromosome 18 with the immunoglobulin heavy-chain gene on chromosome 14,[23] leading to overexpression of the antiapoptotic protein Bcl-2 within the follicles.[24] The expression of Bcl-2 usually is reduced during the normal follicle center reaction, making reactive lymphoid follicles negative with this antibody. Therefore, expression of Bcl-2 by the neoplastic follicle center cells is used as a classic feature for diagnosis.

Mantle Cell Lymphoma

Mantle cell lymphoma (MCL) is a B-cell neoplasm arising from pregerminal center B cells that occupy the mantle zones surrounding the germinal center. The histologic appearance is that of a monomorphic population of small to medium-sized lymphocytes with irregular nuclear contours (**Fig. 2**).[25] A unique feature is the absence of scattered large centroblasts. Other commonly observed findings include admixed epithelioid histiocytes and fine perivascular sclerosis. Architecturally, three growth patterns are recognized: a true mantle zone pattern (7%), a nodular pattern mimicking FL (18%), and a diffuse pattern (75%). The cytologic features of MCL include two types, classic and blastoid.[25,26] The blastoid variant may present de novo or result from progression of the classic histology. The blastoid variant has a wide morphologic

Table 1
Key features of small B-cell lymphomas

Feature	FL	MCL	CLL/SLL	SMZL	MALT	LPL
Histology	Increased number of densely packed follicles Centrocytes and centroblasts	Monomorphic small lymphocytes with mitoses Scattered epithelioid histiocytes Perivascular sclerosis	Small round cells with clumped chromatin Growth centers	White pulp expansion Biphasic histology Moderately abundant clear cytoplasm	Small lymphocytes with abundant cytoplasm Monocytoid B cells Colonized follicles Lymphoepithelial lesions	Spectrum from small lymphocytes to mature plasma cells Primarily in bone marrow
Immunophenotype	CD10+ Bcl-2+ Bcl-6+	CD5+ CD23– FMC-7+ Cyclin-D1+	CD5+ CD23+ FMC-7– dim CD20 dim sIg	CD5– CD10– IgD+/– CD43–	CD5– CD10– CD43+/–	Lymphocytes: CD20+ CD10– CD5 (rarely positive) Plasma cells: CD138+
Molecular	t(14;18)	t(11;14)	Rare (14;19)	del 7q31-32	t(11;18), t(14;18) t(1;14), t(3;14), +3, other rare variants	Del 6q and 13q

Abbreviations: FL, follicular lymphoma; LPL, lymphoplasmacytic lymphoma; MALT, mucosa-associated lymphoid tissue lymphoma; MCL, mantle cell lymphoma; SLL/CLL, small lymphocytic lymphoma/chronic lymphocytic leukemia; SMZL, splenic marginal zone lymphoma.

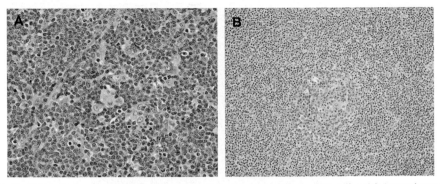

Fig. 2. (A) Typical morphology of mantle cell lymphoma with small B cells with irregular nuclei, scant cytoplasm, occasional mitoses, scattered epithelioid histiocytes and fine sclerosis around blood vessels. (B) Mantle cell lymphoma with a true mantle-zone pattern, whereby tumor cells surround a benign residual germinal center.

spectrum, some cases resembling lymphoblasts and others having a more heterogeneous morphology with larger cells, vesicular chromatin, and sometimes prominent nucleoli.[27]

MCL expresses the pan–B-cell markers CD20 and CD79a but is negative for the follicle center B-cell antigens CD10 and Bcl-6. The tumor cells characteristically are positive for the pan–T-cell antigen CD5. The hallmark of MCL is the overexpression of the cell-cycle regulator cyclin D1. Cyclin D1 is overexpressed as a consequence of t(11;14), which juxtaposes the cyclin D1 gene next to the immunoglobulin heavy-chain gene enhancer element.[28] The nuclear expression of cyclin D1 by immunohistochemical staining is diagnostic of MCL in the right histopathologic context. The underlying genetic abnormality also can be demonstrated in almost all cases of MCL by using cytogenetics and/or fluorescent in situ hybridization for t(11;14).

Small Lymphocytic Lymphoma/Chronic Lymphocytic Leukemia

Chronic lymphocytic leukemia (CLL) primarily involves the peripheral blood and bone marrow. Lymph nodes, however, frequently are involved and show a diffuse infiltrate of neoplastic lymphocytes that morphologically resemble the neoplastic cells in the peripheral blood and the bone marrow.[29] Tissue involvement may occur without an overt leukemic phase, leading to the term "small lymphocytic lymphoma" (SLL). SLL mainly involves lymph nodes and extranodal tissues and, to a lesser extent, peripheral blood and bone marrow. If a lymphocytosis in excess of 5×10^9/L is present at diagnosis, the disease is labeled CLL. These two entities now are considered a single disease with different tissue expressions.[29,30]

In the lymph node, SLL is comprised mainly of small lymphocytes (with round nuclei, clumped chromatin, and scant cytoplasm) with a smaller number of prolymphocytes and paraimmunoblasts. A characteristic feature is the concentration of prolymphocytes and paraimmunoblasts in small clusters, forming proliferation or growth centers (also called "pseudofollicular growth centers") (**Fig. 3**).[31] Occasionally, SLL can show plasmacytoid differentiation, and these patients may present with a serum monoclonal paraprotein, usually IgM.[31–34] Such cases have all the morphologic and immunophenotypic features of CLL and cannot be distinguished reliably; therefore cases previously identified as lymphoplasmacytoid lymphoma are included within the SLL/CLL category.

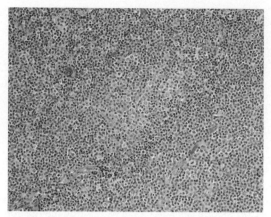

Fig. 3. Typical lymph node biopsy in a case of small lymphatic lymphoma with a diffuse infiltrate of small B cells and a growth center in the middle showing large numbers of pro-lymphocytes and paraimmunoblasts.

SLL/CLL cells express the pan–B-cell markers CD20 and CD79a and are characteristically positive for the pan–T-cell antigen CD5. The cells are also CD23 positive. By flow cytometry, they characteristically show dim expression of CD20 as well as dim expression of either kappa or lambda surface light chain.

Marginal Zone B-Cell Lymphoma

The WHO classification categorizes marginal zone lymphomas (MZL) into three different clinicopathologic entities: MZL of mucosa-associated lymphoid tissue (MALT), splenic MZL (SMZL), and nodal MZL (NMZL).[11] It originally was thought that these three entities share a common origin in the marginal zone cell, but they each have unique clinical and molecular characteristics and should be separated for diagnostic and therapeutic purposes.[35]

Extranodal Marginal Zone Lymphoma of Mucosa-Associated Lymphoid Tissue

Extranodal MZL of MALT, or MALT lymphoma, is a lymphoma often arising at mucosal sites (ie, gastrointestinal tract, salivary gland). Similar lymphomas, however, can be seen in extramucosal sites such as the skin and are thought to be within the spectrum of MALT lymphomas. This neoplasm is comprised of small to intermediate-size B cells, occasional transformed blasts, and plasma cells (**Fig. 4**). The architectural appearance, immunophenotype, and immunoglobulin gene mutation status of the MALT lymphomas strongly suggest that they are of true marginal zone/memory B-cell origin.

Splenic Marginal Zone Lymphoma

SMZL is an indolent B-cell lymphoma of the spleen characterized by a nodular lymphoid infiltrate located in white pulp with variable red pulp infiltration, marginal zone differentiation, and follicular replacement by neoplastic cells.[35] The white pulp nodules are composed of an inner central zone of small lymphocytes located in the mantle zone and replacing the germinal center and a peripheral zone of medium-sized cells with clear cytoplasm and scattered blasts, the marginal zone component. In the red pulp, both large and small cells can be present. Rare cases show an exclusive diffuse infiltration of the red pulp with white pulp atrophy.[36] Lymphoma cells may have

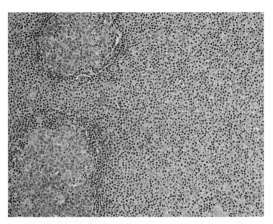

Fig. 4. A pulmonary mucosa-associated lymphoid tissue lymphoma shows two or three classic findings, including reactive follicles and an interfollicular infiltrate of small B cells with moderate amounts of clear cytoplasm. Typical lymphoepithelial lesions (the third component of typical mucosa-associated lymphoid tissue lymphomas) are not seen in this image.

variable degree of plasmacytic differentiation, including as a characteristic feature the presence of monoclonal plasma cells in the germinal center.

The clinical and morphologic features of SMZL overlap with another entity, splenic lymphoma with villous lymphocytes, characterized by splenomegaly and moderate lymphocytosis comprising small, abnormal lymphocytes with thin, short, unevenly distributed villi. Previous studies had concluded that splenic lymphoma with villous lymphocytes and SMZL are the same entity.[37] Very recent work suggests that a subset of these cases with characteristic peripheral blood lymphoid morphology including basophilic villous projections reveals predominantly splenic red pulp infiltration and a phenotype reminiscent of hairy cell leukemia variant and may represent a distinct entity.[38]

The tumor cells are positive for the B-cell antigens CD20 and CD79a, often showing cytoplasmic monotypic immunoglobulin and Bcl-2, but typically lack CD5, CD10, Bcl-6, CD23, CD43, and cyclin D1.

Nodal Marginal Zone Lymphoma

NMZL by definition presents with nodal disease without mucosal or splenic involvement.[39] Morphologically the infiltrate occupies the interfollicular area and/or the marginal zones of residual follicles. Unlike MALT lymphoma or SMZL, NMLZs are poorly characterized biologically, and several studies have questioned whether they represent a distinct clinicopathologic entity.[40,41] Some cases diagnosed as NMZL seem to be subclinical MALT lymphomas first presenting with nodal disease. Some other entities, such as FL with marked marginal zone differentiation and lymphoplasmacytic lymphomas (LPL) with nodal involvement, can mimic NMZL. Nevertheless, a number of cases remain that cannot be classified into other entities with marginal zone distribution.

Lymphoplasmacytic Lymphoma

LPL is a neoplasm mainly involving the bone marrow but also occasionally present in spleen and lymph nodes. LPL typically is not leukemic, distinguishing it from CLL. It is comprised of a morphologic spectrum of small lymphocytes, many with plasmacytoid morphology, and a significant component of mature plasma cells. This lymphoma often is associated with a serum monoclonal IgM paraprotein, and patients also may have hyperviscosity symptoms. In clinical practice, the terms "lymphoplasmacytic lymphoma" and "Waldenstrom's macroglobulinemia" often are used interchangeably. Other lymphomas, such as MALT lymphoma, SMZL, or CLL may present with an IgM paraprotein, however.[42]

In LPL the bone marrow demonstrates an interstitial and nodular infiltration by lymphoplasmacytic cells and mature plasma cells.[43] The plasma cells may contain cytoplasmic globules (Russell bodies) and intranuclear pseudoinclusions (Dutcher bodies). Nodal or extranodal infiltration by LPL can be very difficult to distinguish from NMZL or MALT lymphoma on morphologic grounds alone.

Immunophenotyping by flow cytometry or immunohistochemistry shows two distinct populations: lymphoplasmacytic cells staining for the B-cell marker CD20 but not for plasma cell markers and plasma cells staining for plasma cell markers such as CD138 or CD38 but lacking CD20. Demonstration of light-chain restriction in plasma cells is a finding that should be present to diagnose LPL. Markers associated with other low-grade lymphomas are usually absent, although rare cases can be CD5 positive.

Diffuse Large B-Cell Lymphoma

DLBCL is a malignant proliferation of large B cells with very heterogeneous morphology, phenotype, and molecular and clinical findings.[44,45] It may develop de novo or arise from a previous indolent lymphoma and may be predominantly nodal or may involve extranodal sites. The most common extranodal site is the gastrointestinal tract, but virtually any extranodal location can be seen.

Several morphologic variants of DLBCL (centroblastic, immunoblastic, anaplastic, plasmablastic, T-cell/histiocyte-rich, and anaplastic lymphoma kinase [ALK]-positive DLBCL) are included in the WHO classification.[46] The new WHO classification will recognize ALK-positive DLBCL as a distinct entity.

DLBCL typically effaces the normal lymph node architecture with a diffuse proliferation of large lymphoid cells (**Fig. 5**). The proliferation may involve the whole lymph node or may show partial involvement, sometimes in an interfollicular or sinusoidal

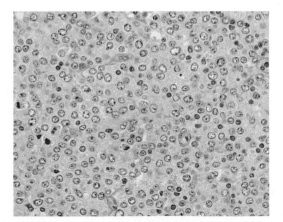

Fig. 5. A typical diffuse large B cell lymphoma.

pattern. The large lymphoid cells are heterogeneous in morphologic appearance. The most common is the centroblast, which has oval to irregular nuclei, vesicular chromatin, and two to four small membrane-bound nuclei. Immunoblasts have similar chromatin but have a single prominent, centrally located nucleolus. Rarely, the large lymphoid cells can have an anaplastic appearance with very irregular nuclei, occasionally resembling Reed-Sternberg cells. In the T-cell/histiocyte-rich variant of DLBCL, most of the tissue is comprised of small reactive T cells and histiocytes with fewer than 10% large malignant B cells, which can assume any of the morphologic appearances described here.

In the current WHO classification plasmablastic lymphoma (PBL) is listed as a rare variant of DLBCL. It often presents in the oral cavity in the setting of HIV infection and frequently is associated with latent Epstein-Barr virus (EBV) infection. The tumor cells have immunoblastic or plasmablastic features but do not show further plasmacytic differentiation. Immunophenotypically, PBL often lacks expression of CD20 and CD45 but shows expression of CD138.[47] This entity can be difficult to distinguish from poorly differentiated myeloma, but clinical findings and serum protein studies can be helpful. In 2008 the new WHO classification will list a spectrum of disorders under the rubric of PBL, including ALK-positive DLBCL, primary effusion lymphoma, and typical PBL as described earlier.[48] The DLBCL variants and subtypes are detailed in **Table 2**.

Regardless of the morphology, DLBCL expresses various pan–B-cell markers including CD19, CD20, and CD79a. Other immunophenotypic markers are variable. The germinal center B-cell markers CD10 and Bcl-6 are expressed in approximately 30% to 40% of cases and in 50% to 70% of cases, respectively.[49–51] Bcl-2 expression is seen in approximately 40% to 75% of cases.[52] CD5 is expressed in about 10% of cases and can be present either in de novo DLBCL or as a transformation (Richter's) from SLL/CLL.[53] The proliferation index, as measured by Ki-67 or MIB-1 staining, is usually high (40% to > 90%).

Burkitt's Lymphoma

Burkitt's lymphoma (BL) is described in the WHO classification as classic BL and two variants: BL with plasmacytoid differentiation and atypical Burkitt/Burkitt-like lymphoma.[54] The classic form shows a monomorphic proliferation of medium-sized cells with round nuclei and multiple small, centrally located basophilic nucleoli (**Fig. 6**). The cytoplasm is deeply basophilic and usually shows multiple vacuoles caused by the presence of lipid, often seen better in touch preparations or bone marrow aspirates. The mitotic rate is high with numerous admixed tingible body macrophages phagocytosing abundant apoptotic debris and creating a starry-sky pattern.[54] The tumor cells in BL with plasmacytoid differentiation show a more eccentrically placed nucleus and tend to occur in association with immunodeficiency. Burkitt-like lymphoma and BL with plasmacytoid differentiation tend to have greater nuclear pleomorphism than classic BL, and both tend to have a smaller number of more prominent nucleoli. The plasmacytoid variant has, in addition, monotypic cytoplasmic immunoglobulin. Atypical BL is morphologically similar to BL, but with more pleomorphism or large cells than classic BL and a proliferation fraction of more than 90%.

Regardless of subtype, BL typically expresses pan–B-cell antigens, including CD19, CD20, and CD79a, and co-expresses CD10 and Bcl-6 but not CD5, CD23, Bcl-2, CD138, or TdT. The proliferation fraction is nearly 100%.[54,55] The hallmark of BL is t(8;14), involving a recombination between the IG heavy chain locus and the MYC oncogene.

Table 2
Key features of DLBCL variants and subtypes

Feature	T-Cell/Histiocyte-Rich	ALK + DLBCL	Primary Mediastinal Large B-Cell Lymphoma	Intravascular Large B-Cell Lymphoma	Primary Effusion Lymphoma	Plasmablastic Lymphoma
Histology	Abundant reactive T cells ± histiocytes < 10% large neoplastic B cells Virtual absence of small B cells	Large cells with plasmablastic features May be confused with an epithelial neoplasm Sinus infiltration common	Large cells with moderate amount of clear cytoplasm Fine sclerosis	Large cells growing in the lumina of small blood vessels Can resemble centroblasts or immunoblasts	Plasmablastic or immunoblastic morphology Abundant basophilic cytoplasm	Plasmablastic or immunoblastic morphology without/with plasmacytic differentiation Often present in oral cavity and associated with HIV infection
Immunophenotype	CD20+ CD79a+	CD20– CD79a- CD45+ IgA+/– EMA+ CD138+ CD30– ALK+	CD20+ CD79a+ CD30+/– (weak) CD23+/– Surface Ig– CD15–	CD20+ CD79a+ CD5–/+	Loss of B cell surface markers CD3+ CD30+ CD138+ HHV-8+	CD20– CD79a–/+ CD45– CD138+ EBV+/– HHV8–/+
Molecular	*IGH* often not clonal because of limiting tumor cells	t(2;17)(p23;q23)	Gains of 2p GCB-type of DLBCL	Variable	Clonal *IGH*	Variable

Abbreviations: ALK, anaplastic lymphoma kinase; DLBCL, diffuse large B-cell lymphoma.

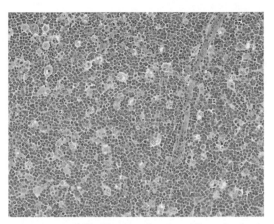

Fig. 6. Low power appearance of Burkitt lymphoma with a classic starry sky appearance caused by the presence of phagocytic histiocytes engulfing nuclear debris resulting from apoptopic cell death. Note the frequent mitoses.

LYMPHOID TUMORS OF T-CELL/NATURAL KILLER–CELL LINEAGE
Precursor T-Lymphoblastic Lymphoma/Leukemia

T-cell lymphoblastic lymphoma/leukemia (T-LBL/T-ALL) is a neoplasm thought to arise from malignant thymocytes.[56] It may involve primarily bone marrow and peripheral blood (T-ALL) or present with primary involvement of nodal or extranodal sites (T-LBL). These entities often are considered to represent a spectrum of a single disease because of histologic, immunophenotypic, cytogenetic and clinical similarities. Although frequently accompanied by a mediastinal mass and bulky adenopathy, T-ALL by definition is characterized by marrow involvement of more than 25%. In contrast, T-LBL is characterized most typically by a large anterior mediastinal mass with less than 25% marrow involvement. The lymphoblasts in T-ALL/LBL usually are of medium size with a high nuclear cytoplasmic ratio and immature or finely dispersed chromatin, typically without prominent nucleoli. Involved lymph nodes usually are completely effaced. The cells show a high mitotic rate and often a leukemic pattern of infiltration with associated crush artifact.

The immunophenotype of T-ALL/LBL is variable but is typically positive for Tdt and demonstrates one or more T-cell antigens including CD1a, CD2, CD3, CD4, CD5, CD7, and CD8. CD3 often is cytoplasmic and is considered lineage specific. CD4 and CD8 are often co-expressed. CD10 may be seen as well as the myeloid antigens CD13 and CD33.

T-Cell Prolymphocytic Leukemia

T-cell prolymphocytic leukemia (T-PLL) is a rare mature T-cell neoplasm of older adults occurring slightly more frequently in males. In the past, some of these cases were classified as T-cell CLL, but this term is no longer used; instead, such cases are recognized as the small-cell variant of T-PLL. The current WHO classification describes three morphologic variants of T-PLL: typical, small-cell, and cerebriform.[57] The diagnosis usually is made from a peripheral blood film, which shows mainly small to medium-sized lymphocytes, often with irregular nuclei and occasional small nucleoli and usually a very high white blood cell count (**Fig. 7**).[57,58]

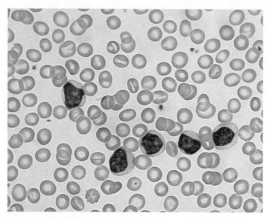

Fig. 7. Peripheral blood smear shows T-cell prolymphocitic lymphoma with medium-large lymphoid cells with easily recognizable nucleoli.

Immunophenotyping shows a mature T-cell phenotype with most cases being CD4 positive and CD8 negative. In approximately 25% of cases, CD4 and CD8 are co-expressed. A smaller percentage of cases are CD4 negative and CD8 positive.

T-Cell Large Granular Lymphocytic Leukemia

T-cell large granular lymphocytic leukemia (T-LGL) is a chronic clonal proliferation of cytotoxic T lymphocytes, often presenting with cytopenias, and may be accompanied by other autoimmune diseases. Normally, large granular lymphocytes comprise 5% to 15% of lymphocytes in the peripheral blood and can be increased transiently in reactive states and viral infections. T-LGL is diagnosed when there is a persistent (> 6 months) increase (> 2 × 10^9/L) in large granular lymphocytes with no clearly identified cause.[59] T-LGLs are intermediate to large in size with round to slightly irregular nuclei, mature chromatin, and increased amounts of pale cytoplasm (**Fig. 8**). Variable numbers of randomly distributed azurophilic granules can be seen in the cytoplasm. Bone marrow involvement by T-LGL disease often is subtle and

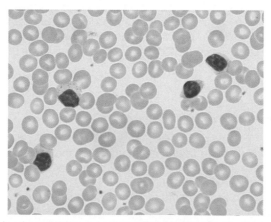

Fig. 8. Peripheral blood smear shows more mature lymphoid cells. Some contain fine azurophilic granules in their cytoplasm.

difficult to identify because the cells are morphologically similar to granulocytic or monocytic precursors.[60] There often is subtle interstitial infiltration of individual lymphocytes or small clusters. Reactive lymphoid aggregates composed of B and T cells may be present also.

Immunophenotypically, T-LGL cells express CD2, CD3, CD8, CD5, CD7, and CD57.[61] There is variable expression of CD56.

Aggressive Natural Killer–Cell Leukemia

Aggressive NK-cell leukemia is a rare disorder characterized by a proliferation of NK cells.[62] As with most leukemias, primarily blood and bone marrow are involved. The leukemic cells are very similar in appearance to large granular lymphocytes, although they may be slightly larger with more nuclear irregularity. The pattern of bone marrow involvement is variable, from extensive to subtle interstitial infiltration.

Immunophenotypically, NK cells are positive for CD2, CD56, and cytotoxic molecules. They are negative for surface CD3 and usually are negative for CD57.

Adult T-Cell Leukemia/Lymphoma

Adult T-cell leukemia/lymphoma is a mature T-cell neoplasm of post-thymic lymphocytes, linked to the human T-cell lymphotropic virus, HTLV-1. A leukemic picture in seen in approximately 65% of patients; the remaining have a lymphomatous form that involves lymph nodes and/or skin.[63] In the peripheral blood, the leukemic cells are pleomorphic, with the predominant cell being a medium-sized lymphocyte with condensed chromatin and a convoluted or polylobated nucleus often called a "flower cell." The bone marrow may or may not be involved, and the infiltration often is very subtle or patchy. The infiltration in the lymph nodes often is diffuse, with the paracortical area expanded by an infiltrate of lymphocytes of various sizes with various nuclear shapes. The histologic appearance may be indistinguishable from other peripheral T-cell lymphomas.[64]

The immunophenotype of the adult T-cell leukemia/lymphoma cell is that of an activated mature T lymphocyte. The cells express CD2, CD3, and CD5 and often are CD7-negative. The most common immunophenotypic profile is CD4 positive/CD8 negative, but cases in which cells co-express these two markers or express only CD8 have been described. A characteristic feature is the strong expression of CD25.

Mycosis Fungoides

Mycosis fungoides (MF) is one of the most common forms of cutaneous lymphoma, characterized by patches, plaques, and eventually tumor formation, typically occurring on sun-protected skin. Morphologically, MF shows a band-like infiltrate of atypical lymphocytes in the papillary dermis with areas of epidermotropism.[65,66] Only a small proportion of cases have collections of atypical lymphocytes in the epidermis, known as "Pautrier microabscesses." (**Fig. 9**) The epidermal lymphocytes often are surrounded by halos along the basal layer. The epidermis shows little spongiosis and vacuolar change.

Immunophenotypically, MF usually expresses the pan–T-cell markers CD2, CD3, and CD5, often with a loss of CD7.[67] Most cases have CD4-positive T cells, with only a small percentage of cases that have the same clinical course and histologic appearance expressing CD8.[68] The loss of pan–T-cell markers usually is a feature of disease progression and is rare in early-stage lesions.

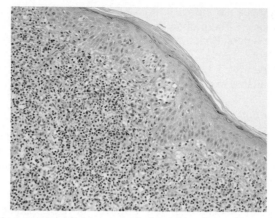

Fig. 9. Skin biopsy in a patient who has mycosis fungoides shows the typical epidermotropic infiltrate and Pautrier's microabscesses.

Sézary Syndrome

Sézary syndrome (SS) is a mature T-cell neoplasm characterized by widespread erythroderma, distinctive epidermotropic skin lesions, and circulating neoplastic cerebriform lymphocytes.[69] SS can arise as a primary disseminated leukemic disorder (primary SS) or can occur in a clinical setting of long-standing MF (secondary SS). The circulating neoplastic cells have distinctive cerebriform nuclear outlines with a high nuclear cytoplasmic ratio. At low magnification, these cells often appear darker than normal lymphocytes and have a wide range of nuclear size from small Sézary cells (known as "Lutzner cells") to large cells. Skin biopsies in SS may lack the characteristic epidermotropism, seen in MF, making the diagnosis difficult.[70]

The immunophenotype is very similar to MF and represents that of a mature T cell, classically CD4-positive. There may be complete or partial loss of CD7 or dim CD7 expression, with expression of pan–T-cell markers CD2, CD3, and CD5. Expression of CD8 is rarely seen.

Primary Cutaneous CD30-Positive T-Cell Lymphoproliferative Disorders

The term "primary cutaneous CD30-positive T-cell lymphoproliferative disorder" refers to a spectrum of related cutaneous lymphomas arising from CD30-positive T cells.[71] This category includes primary cutaneous anaplastic large-cell lymphoma (C-ALCL) and lymphomatoid papulosis (LyP). A histologic spectrum exists between these disorders, but in most cases, LyP and C-ALCL can be distinguished by the density and distribution of the large CD30-positive tumor cells. In C-ALCL, tumor cells typically are present in large clusters and sheets and extend into the subcutaneous tissue, often surrounding and infiltrating blood vessel walls.[72] The tumor cells are highly pleomorphic with occasional hallmark cells and Reed-Sternberg–like cells present. LyP lesions usually are wedge shaped with a dermal and perivascular infiltrate of atypical T cells, often with an inflammatory background of small lymphocytes, eosinophils, and neutrophils. Three histologic variants are described, based on cytology and the number of large cells.[73] By immunohistochemistry, the tumor cells in both disorders usually are positive for CD4 but negative for CD8. There is frequent loss of pan–T-cell markers. CD30 is expressed by the majority of cells in C-ALCL and by the large cells in LyP. ALK expression is highly associated with systemic ALCL and only rarely is present in C-ALCL. Approximately 50% to 75% of C-ALCL and LyP express one or more cytotoxic granule proteins (TIA-1, granzyme B, perforin).[74]

Extranodal Natural Killer/T-Cell Lymphoma, Nasal Type

Extranodal NK/T-cell lymphoma, nasal type, is a predominantly extranodal lymphoma with predilection for the nasal cavity, nasopharynx, palate, skin, soft tissue, gastrointestinal tract, and testis.[75]

The histologic appearance is very similar, irrespective of the site. Tumor cells vary in size, with most cases having medium to large cells with irregular nuclei. The characteristic histologic features are angioinvasion and angiodestruction with large zonal areas of necrosis. A heavy admixture of inflammatory cells may be present (**Fig. 10**).[76]

Most nasal-type NK/T-cell lymphomas are thought to be of true NK-cell origin and express CD2, CD7, cytoplasmic CD3, and CD56. Tumor cells also are positive for EBV. There is an absence of surface CD3 and CD5 expression and no evidence of clonal T-cell receptor (*TCR*) gene[76] rearrangements. The key findings in extranodal NK/T-cell lymphoma and other more common T-cell lymphomas are detailed in **Table 3**.

Enteropathy-Type T-Cell Lymphoma

Enteropathy-type T-cell lymphoma (ETL), also known as intestinal T-cell lymphoma and enteropathy-associated T-cell lymphoma, is a primary extranodal T-cell lymphoma thought to arise from intraepithelial T cells.[77] In the intestine, it forms an ulcerating mass in the mucosa that invades through the wall, often leading to perforation. ETL has been classified into two groups based on morphologic, immunophenotypic, and genetic data.[78,79] Approximately 80% of ETLs have pleomorphic and sometimes anaplastic tumor cells, are highly associated with celiac disease (in up to 70% of cases), and demonstrate enteropathy-type mucosal changes adjacent to the tumor (in 85% of cases). The other 20% of ETLs have a relatively monomorphic population of small to medium-sized tumor cells, rarely are associated with celiac disease, and less frequently show histologic evidence of enteropathy-type mucosal changes (50%).

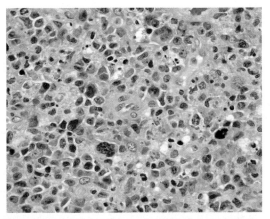

Fig. 10. A pleomorphic infiltrate of large neoplastic lymphoid cells in a patient who has a mid-facial mass. These cells expressed CD2, CD56, and latent Epstein-Barr virus, which is consistent with a diagnosis of nasal T/NK cell lymphoma.

Table 3
Key features of the most common T-cell lymphomas

Features	Extranodal NK/T-Cell Lymphoma, Nasal Type	Peripheral T-Cell Lymphoma, Unspecified	Angioimmunoblastic T-Cell Lymphoma	Systemic Anaplastic Large-Cell Lymphoma
Histology	Small to medium-sized atypical cells Angiocentric and/or angioinvasive growth May be admixture of inflammatory cells	Interfollicular expansion with heterogeneous cellular composition Atypical lymphocytes may be small to large Frequent inflammatory background Clusters of epithelioid histiocytes (Lennert's lymphoma)	Interfollicular expansion with regressed follicles Prominent post-capillary venules with arborization Clusters of lymphoid cells with clear cytoplasm Polymorphous cellular background May have large B-cell blasts	Monomorphic/pleomorphic cells Presence of hallmark cells (horseshoe- or wreath-shaped nucleus, prominent Golgi region) Propensity for lymph node sinus involvement Frequent mitoses
Immunophenotype	CD2+ CD56+ Surface CD3− Cytoplasmic CD3ε+ EBV+ Cytotoxic markers+	CD4 > CD8 Frequent loss of one of the pan–T-cell antigens (CD2, CD3, CD5, CD7)	CD3+ CD4+ CD8− CD10+ (T cells) CD21+ FDC meshworks EBV+ large B cells	CD30+ CD15− Bcl-2− EMA+ Loss of many T-cell antigens (eg, CD3) Cytotoxic markers+
Molecular	Gains of 2q, 15q, 17q, and 22q. Losses of 6q, 8p, 11q, 12q, and 13q	Gains of 7q22-31, 1q, 3p, 5p, and 8q2ter, losses of 6q22-24 and 10p13pter[97]	Trisomy 5, 21, and gains of 5q, 3q	t(2;5)(p23;q35) and variants

By immunohistochemistry, the pleomorphic variant commonly expresses CD3 and TIA1 but usually is negative for CD56, CD4, and CD5. CD8 is expressed in approximately 20% of cases. The monomorphic small-cell variant frequently expresses CD56 (> 90%) and CD8 (80%). It commonly expresses cytotoxic markers but is negative for CD4 and CD5.[78]

Hepatosplenic T-Cell Lymphoma

Hepatosplenic T-cell lymphoma is a rare, aggressive type of extranodal lymphoma derived from cytotoxic γδ T cells.[80,81] It is characterized by hepatosplenomegaly, bone marrow involvement, and peripheral blood cytopenias.

A distinctive pattern of infiltration is seen with tumor cells preferentially infiltrating the sinusoids of the splenic red pulp, liver, and bone marrow.[82] The malignant cells are medium-sized lymphoid cells with moderately clumped chromatin and a rim of pale cytoplasm.

A characteristic immunophenotype is seen with the cells being positive for CD2, CD3, and CD7 but negative for CD5, CD4, and CD8. They are positive for TCR-δ but negative for TCR-β F1. CD56 may be expressed. The cytotoxic granule-associated protein TIA-1 usually is positive, but perforin and granzyme B usually are negative. A small number of cases can have an αβ phenotype and are considered to be a variant.

Subcutaneous Panniculitis-Like T-Cell Lymphoma

Subcutaneous panniculitis-like T-cell lymphoma is a rare cytotoxic T-cell tumor involving subcutaneous tissue.[83,84] There is a subcutaneous infiltration of neoplastic lymphocytes that usually is lobular and rims the fat cells in a lacelike pattern. Areas of sheetlike growth are present in some cases. The lymphocytes vary from small to large and often infiltrate but do not destroy small blood vessels. Fat necrosis and single-cell apoptosis are common. Often histiocytes containing phagocytized cellular debris and red blood cells are present. Some cases may be associated with a systemic hemophagocytic syndrome.

The malignant cells in subcutaneous panniculitis-like T-cell lymphoma are most often CD8-positive cytotoxic lymphocytes expressing one or more cytotoxic granule proteins including TIA-1, granzyme B, and perforin and the αβ TCR. The tumor cells often are only focally CD56 positive but are negative for EBV.[85,86]

A small percentage of cases express the γδ TCR and have a more aggressive clinical course.[87] These cases now are recognized as a distinct entity and are given the term "cutaneous γδ T-cell lymphoma." The neoplastic cells have a similar subcutaneous infiltrative pattern but also show dermal extension. The presence of the γδ TCR can be demonstrated by immunohistochemistry either by direct staining or by the lack of staining for the αβ TCR.

Angioimmunoblastic T-Cell Lymphoma

Angioimmunoblastic T-cell lymphoma is a peripheral T-cell lymphoma associated with systemic disease.[87] Involved lymph nodes show a diffuse paracortical pattern of infiltration with some preservation of sinuses and prominent high endothelial venules, often in an arborizing pattern (**Fig. 11**). Regressed follicles are seen often. The infiltrate can vary from mainly lymphocytic to polymorphous, including eosinophils, histiocytes, plasma cells, and increased numbers of FDCs.[88,89] The diagnosis can be difficult to establish because only a small number of cases show atypia in small lymphocytes or have increased numbers of atypical medium-to-large cells, often with clear

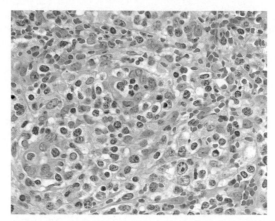

Fig. 11. A lymph node biopsy of a patient who has angioimmunoblastic T-cell lymphoma shows numerous atypical lymphocytes with clear cytoplasm and scattered small blood vessels.

cytoplasm. As well, not all cases have abnormal T-cell antigen loss by flow cytometric analysis or immunohistochemistry.

By immunohistochemistry, a mature T-cell phenotype is observed, usually with more CD4 than CD8 expression. FDC markers, such as CD21 and CD23, are helpful to highlight an FDC proliferation outside the residual follicles. Germinal center T-cell markers including CD10, bcl-6, and CXCL13 often are expressed by the T cells. CD20 may highlight scattered large B cells, which are often EBV positive, outside the follicles.[90]

Peripheral T-Cell Lymphoma, Unspecified

Peripheral T-cell lymphoma, unspecified, represents the largest group of T-cell lymphomas that have predominantly nodal involvement.[91] Often, there is generalized disease with involvement of bone marrow, liver, spleen, and, frequently, skin. Given the heterogeneity of this group, there is a broad morphologic spectrum.[92,93] Most cases show effacement of normal lymph-node architecture with a diffuse infiltration of medium- to large-sized lymphocytes. The cells often have pleomorphic nuclei with prominent nucleoli and admixed mitotic figures. Occasional Reed-Sternberg–like cells can be seen. Often, there is a mixed inflammatory background consisting of small lymphocytes, eosinophils, plasma cells, and histiocytes. Some histologic variants are recognized, including a T-zone variant and a lymphoepithelioid cell variant (also called "Lennert's lymphoma").

Immunophenotypically, most nodal peripheral T-cell lymphoma cases are CD4 positive and CD8 negative. Pan–T-cell antigens are expressed, but often there is aberrant loss of one or more. CD30 may be positive in large-cell variants, but cytotoxic granule-associated protein expression is rare. EBV expression may be seen in admixed B cells, but the tumor cells usually are negative.

Anaplastic Large-Cell Lymphoma

ALCL is a systemic T-cell lymphoma that affects both lymph nodes and extranodal sites including skin, bone, soft tissues, lung, and liver.[94] Involved lymph nodes may show a preferential paracortical or sinusoidal growth pattern with sparing of the B-cell areas.[95,96] The morphologic spectrum is broad; most cases have large

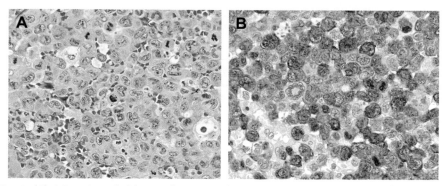

Fig. 12. (*A*) A lymph node biopsy of a young child who has anaplastic large-cell lymphoma demonstrating a pleomorphic infiltrate of large anaplastic T cells. (*B*) The same case stained with an antibody to anaplastic lymphoma kinase shows nuclear and cytoplasmic staining characteristics of the t(2;5) translocation.

monomorphic cells, and pleomorphic, small-cell, and lymphohistiocytic variants are less common. All cases typically contain hallmark cells, which are large cells with eccentric and horseshoe- or kidney-shaped nuclei, small nucleoli, and a paranuclear eosinophilic region (**Fig. 12**).

A key immunophenotypic finding is the strong, uniform membranous and/or Golgi CD30-staining pattern of tumor cells.[94–96] Most cases express one or more T-cell antigens. A smaller number have an apparent "null-cell" phenotype but often show a T-cell lineage at the genetic level. Most tumors also are epithelial membrane antigen positive. In the new WHO classification expected in 2008, ALK-positive cases will be distinguished from ALK-negative ALCL. The majority of ALK-positive cases harbor the t(2;5)/*NPM-ALK* translocation, which results in nuclear and cytoplasmic ALK protein expression. Variant translocations are recognized by their different ALK staining patterns.

REFERENCES

1. Hicks EB, Rappaport H, Winter WJ. Follicular lymphoma: a re-evaluation of its position in the scheme of malignant lymphoma, based on a survey of 253 cases. Cancer 1956;9(4):792–821.
2. Lukes RJ, Collins RD. Immunologic characterization of human malignant lymphomas. Cancer 1974;34(S8):1488–503.
3. National Cancer Institute sponsored study of classifications of non-Hodgkin's lymphomas: summary and description of a working formulation for clinical usage. The Non-Hodgkin's Lymphoma Pathologic Classification Project. Cancer 1982; 49(10):2112–35.
4. Lennert K, Stein H, Kaiserling E. Cytological and functional criteria for the classification of malignant lymphomata. Br J Cancer 1975;31(S2):29–43.
5. Kim H, Zelman RJ, Fox MA, et al. Pathology Panel for Lymphoma Clinical Studies: a comprehensive analysis of cases accumulated since its inception. J Natl Cancer Inst 1982;68(1):43–67.
6. Whitcomb CC, Crissman JD, Flint A, et al. Reproducibility in morphologic classification of non-Hodgkin's lymphomas using the Lukes-Collins system. The Southeastern Cancer Study Group experience. Am J Clin Pathol 1984;82(4):383–8.

7. NCI non-Hodgkin's Classification Project Writing Committee. Classification of non-Hodgkin's lymphomas. Reproducibility of major classification systems. Cancer 1985;55(1):91–5.
8. Dick F, VanLier S, Banks P, et al. Use of the working formulation for non-Hodgkin's lymphoma in epidemiologic studies: agreement between reported diagnoses and a panel of experienced pathologists. J Natl Cancer Inst 1987;78(6): 1137–44.
9. Harris NL, Jaffe ES, Stein H, et al. A revised European-American classification of lymphoid neoplasms: a proposal from the International Lymphoma Study Group. Blood 1994;84(5):1361–92.
10. Anon. A clinical evaluation of the International Lymphoma Study Group classification of non-Hodgkin's lymphoma. The Non-Hodgkin's Lymphoma Classification Project. Blood 1997;89(11):3909–18.
11. Jaffe ES, Harris NL, Stein H, editors. World Health Organization classification of tumors. Tumors of haematopoietic and lymphoid tissues. Lyon (France): IARC Press; 2001.
12. Ozdemirli M, Fanburg-Smith JC, Hartmann DP, et al. Differentiating lymphoblastic lymphoma and Ewing's sarcoma: lymphocyte markers and gene rearrangement. Mod Pathol. 2001;14(11):1175–82.
13. de Jong D. Molecular classification of follicular lymphoma: a cross talk of genetic and immunologic factors. J Clin Oncol 2005;23(26):6358–63.
14. Dogan A, Bagdi E, Munson P, et al. CD10 and BCL-6 expression in paraffin sections of normal lymphoid tissue and B-cell lymphomas. Am J Surg Pathol 2000;24(6):846–52.
15. Dogan A, Du MQ, Aiello A, et al. Follicular lymphomas contain a clonally linked but phenotypically distinct neoplastic B-cell population in the interfollicular zone. Blood 1998;91(12):4708–14.
16. Mann RB, Berard CW. Criteria for the cytologic subclassification of follicular lymphomas: a proposed alternative method. Hematol Oncol 1983;1(2):187–92.
17. Metter GE, Nathwani BN, Burke JS, et al. Morphological subclassification of follicular lymphoma: variability of diagnoses among hematopathologists, a collaborative study between the Repository Center and Pathology Panel for Lymphoma Clinical Studies. J Clin Oncol 1985;3(1):25–38.
18. Nathwani BN, Metter GE, Miller TP, et al. What should be the morphologic criteria for the subdivision of follicular lymphomas? Blood 1986;68(4):837–45.
19. Nathwani BN, Harris NL, Weisenburger DD, et al. Follicular lymphoma. In: Jaffe ES, Harris NL, Stein H, et al, editors. World Health Organisation classification of tumors. Tumors of haematopoietic and lymphoid tissues. Lyon (France): IARC Press; 2001. p. 162–7.
20. Hans CP, Weisenburger DD, Vose JM, et al. A significant diffuse component predicts for inferior survival in grade 3 follicular lymphoma, but cytologic subtypes do not predict survival. Blood 2003;101(6):2363–7.
21. Tilly H, Rossi A, Stamatoullas A, et al. Prognostic value of chromosomal abnormalities in follicular lymphoma. Blood 1994;84(4):1043–9.
22. Horsman DE, Gascoyne RD, Coupland RW, et al. Comparison of cytogenetic analysis, southern analysis, and polymerase chain reaction for the detection of t(14; 18) in follicular lymphoma. Am J Clin Pathol 1995;103(4):472–8.
23. Bakhshi A, Jensen JP, Goldman P, et al. Cloning the chromosomal breakpoint of t(14;18) human lymphomas: clustering around JH on chromosome 14 and near a transcriptional unit on 18. Cell 1985;41(3):899–906.

24. Lai R, Arber DA, Chang KL, et al. Frequency of bcl-2 expression in non-Hodgkin's lymphoma: a study of 778 cases with comparison of marginal zone lymphoma and monocytoid B-cell hyperplasia. Mod Pathol 1998;11(9):864–9.

25. Swerdlow SH, Berger F, Isaacson PG, et al. Mantle cell lymphoma. In: Jaffe ES, Harris NL, Stein H, et al, editors. World Health Organisation classification of tumors. Tumors of haematopoietic and lymphoid tissues. Lyon (France): IARC Press; 2001. p. 168–70.

26. Argatoff LH, Connors JM, Klasa RJ, et al. Mantle cell lymphoma: a clinicopathologic study of 80 cases. Blood 1997;89(6):2067–78.

27. Bosch F, Lopez-Guillermo A, Campo E, et al. Mantle cell lymphoma: presenting features, response to therapy, and prognostic factors. Cancer 1998;82(3): 567–75.

28. Rosenberg CL, Wong E, Petty EM, et al. PRAD1, a candidate BCL1 oncogene: mapping and expression in centrocytic lymphoma. Proc Natl Acad Sci U S A 1991;88(21):9638–42.

29. Braylan RC, Jaffe ES, Burbach JW, et al. Similarities of surface characteristics of neoplastic well-differentiated lymphocytes from solid tissues and from peripheral blood. Cancer Res 1976;36(5):1619–25.

30. Batata A, Shen B. Relationship between chronic lymphocytic leukemia and small lymphocytic lymphoma. A comparative study of membrane phenotypes in 270 cases. Cancer 1992;70(3):625–32.

31. Ben-Ezra J, Burke JS, Swartz WG, et al. Small lymphocytic lymphoma: a clinicopathologic analysis of 268 cases. Blood 1989;73(2):579–87.

32. Rozman C, Montserrat E, Vinolas N. Serum immunoglobulins in B-chronic lymphocytic leukemia. Natural history and prognostic significance. Cancer 1988;61(2):279–83.

33. Xu HJ, Roberts-Thomson PJ. Low molecular weight IgM in the sera of patients with chronic lymphocytic leukemia. Pathology 1993;25(1):52–6.

34. Yin CC, Lin P, Carney DA, et al. Chronic lymphocytic leukemia/ small lymphocytic lymphoma associated with IgM paraprotein. Am J Clin Pathol 2005;123(4): 594–602.

35. Mollejo M, Camacho FI, Algara P, et al. Nodal and splenic marginal zone B cell lymphomas. Hematol Oncol 2005;23(3-4):108–18.

36. Mollejo M, Algara P, Mateo MS, et al. Splenic small B-cell lymphoma with predominant red pulp involvement: a diffuse variant of splenic marginal zone lymphoma? Histopathology 2002;40(1):22–30.

37. Isaacson PG, Matutes E, Burke M, et al. The histopathology of splenic lymphoma with villous lymphocytes. Blood 1994;84(11):3828–34.

38. Traverse-Glehen A, Baseggio L, Callet-Bauchu E, et al. Splenic red pulp lymphoma with numerous basophilic lymphocytes: a distinct clinicopathologic and molecular entity? Blood 2008;111(4):2253–60.

39. Maes B, De Wolf-Peeters C. Marginal zone cell lymphoma—an update on recent advances. Histopathology 2002;40(2):117–26.

40. Campo E, Miquel R, Krenacs L, et al. Primary nodal marginal zone lymphomas of splenic and MALT type. Am J Surg Pathol 1999;23(1):59–68.

41. Camacho FI, Algara P, Mollejo M, et al. Nodal marginal zone lymphoma: a heterogeneous tumor: a comprehensive analysis of a series of 27 cases. Am J Surg Pathol 2003;27(6):762–71.

42. Lin P, Medeiros LJ. Lymphoplasmacytic lymphoma/Waldenstrom macroglobulinemia: an evolving concept. Adv Anat Pathol 2005;12(5):246–55.

43. Remstein ED, Hanson CA, Kyle RA, et al. Despite apparent morphologic and immunophenotypic heterogeneity, Waldenstrom's macroglobulinemia is consistently composed of cells along a morphologic continuum of small lymphocytes, plasmacytoid lymphocytes, and plasma cells. Semin Oncol 2003;30(2): 182–6.

44. De Paepe P, De Wolf-Peeters C. Diffuse large B cell lymphoma: a heterogeneous group of non-Hodgkin lymphomas comprising several distinct and clinicopathological entities. Leukemia 2007;21(1):37–43.

45. Pileri SA, Dirnhofer A, Went P, et al. Diffuse large B-cell lymphoma: one or more entities? Present controversies and possible tools for its subclassification. Histopathology 2002;41(6):482–509.

46. Gatter KC, Warnke RA. Diffuse large B cell lymphoma. In: Jaffe ES, Harris NL, Stein H, et al, editors. World Health Organisation classification of tumors. Tumors of haematopoietic and lymphoid tissues. Lyon (France): IARC Press; 2001. p. 171–4.

47. Delecluse HJ, Anagnostopoulos I, Dallenbach F, et al. Plasmablastic lymphomas of the oral cavity: a new entity associated with the human immunodeficiency virus infection. Blood 1997;89(4):1413–20.

48. Colomo L, Loong F, Rives S, et al. Diffuse large B cell lymphomas with plasmablastic differentiation represent a heterogeneous group of disease entities. Am J Surg Pathol 2004;28(6):736–47.

49. McCluggage WG, Catherwood M, Alexander HD, et al. Immunohistochemical expression of CD10 and t(14;18) chromosomal translocation may be indicators of follicle center cell origin in nodal diffuse large B-cell lymphoma. Histopathology 2002;41(5):414–20.

50. Pittaluga S, Ayoubi TA, Wlodarska I, et al. BCL-6 expression in reactive lymphoid tissue and in B-cell non-Hodgkin's lymphomas. J Pathol 1996;179(2):145–50.

51. Skinnider BF, Horsman DE, Dupuis B, et al. Bcl-6 and Bcl-2 protein expression in diffuse large B-cell lymphoma and follicular lymphoma: correlation with 3q27 and 18q21 chromosomal abnormalities. Hum Pathol 1999;30(7):803–8.

52. Gascoyne RD, Adomat SA, Krajewski S, et al. Prognostic significance of Bcl-2 protein expression and Bcl-2 gene rearrangement in diffuse aggressive non-Hodgkin's lymphoma. Blood 1997;90(1):244–51.

53. Matolcsy A, Inghirami G, Knowles DM. Molecular genetic demonstration of the diverse evolution of Richter's syndrome (chronic lymphocytic leukemia and subsequent large cell lymphoma). Blood 1994;83(5):1363–72.

54. Diebold J. Burkitt lymphoma. In: Jaffe ES, Harris NL, Stein H, et al, editors. World Health Organisation classification of tumors. Tumors of haematopoietic and lymphoid tissues. Lyon (France): IARC Press; 2001. p. 181–4.

55. McClure RF, Remstein ED, Macon WR, et al. Adult B-cell lymphomas with Burkitt-like morphology are phenotypically and genotypically heterogeneous with aggressive clinical behavior. Am J Surg Pathol 2005;29(12):1652–60.

56. Brunning RD, Borowitz M, Matutes E, et al. Precursor T lymphoblastic leukemia/ lymphoblastic lymphoma. In: Jaffe ES, Harris NL, Stein H, et al, editors. World Health Organisation classification of tumors. Tumors of haematopoietic and lymphoid tissues. Lyon (France): IARC Press; 2001. p. 115–7.

57. Catovsky D, Ralfkiaer E, Muller-Hermelink HK. T-cell prolymphocytic leukemia. In: Jaffe ES, Harris NL, Stein H, et al, editors. World Health Organisation classification of tumors. Tumors of haematopoietic and lymphoid tissues. Lyon (France): IARC Press; 2001. p. 195–6.

58. Valbuena JR, Herling M, Admirand JH, et al. T-cell prolymphocytic leukemia involving extramedullary sites. Am J Clin Pathol 2005;123(3):456–64.
59. Chan WC, Catovsky D, Foucar K, et al. T-cell large granular lymphocyte leukemia. In: Jaffe ES, Harris NL, Stein H, et al, editors. World Health Organisation classification of tumors. Tumors of haematopoietic and lymphoid tissues. Lyon (France): IARC Press; 2001. p. 197–8.
60. Morice WG, Kurtin PJ, Tefferi A, et al. Distinct bone marrow findings in T-cell granular lymphocytic leukemia revealed by paraffin section immunoperoxidase stains for CD8, TIA-1, and granzyme B. Blood 2002;99(1):268–74.
61. Lundell R, Hartung L, Hill S, et al. T-cell large granular lymphocyte leukemias have multiple phenotypic abnormalities involving pan–T-cell antigens and receptors for MHC molecules. Am J Clin Pathol 2005;124(6):937–46.
62. Chan WC, Wong KF, Jaffe ES, et al. Aggressive NK-cell leukemia. In: Jaffe ES, Harris NL, Stein H, et al, editors. World Health Organisation classification of tumors. Tumors of haematopoietic and lymphoid tissues. Lyon (France): IARC Press; 2001. p. 197–8.
63. Shimoyama M. Diagnostic criteria and clinical subtypes of ATLL. A report from the Lymphoma Study Group (1984–87). Br J Haematol 1991;79(3):428–37.
64. Ohshima K, Suzumiya J, Sato K, et al. Nodal T-cell lymphoma in an HTLV-1 endemic area: proviral HTLV-1 DNA, histological classification and clinical evaluation. Br J Haematol 1998;101(4):703–11.
65. Massone C, Kodama K, Kerl H, et al. Histopathologic features of early (patch) lesions of mycosis fungoides: a morphologic study on 745 biopsy specimens from 427 patients. Am J Surg Pathol 2005;29(4):550–60.
66. Naraghi ZS, Seirafi H, Valikhani M, et al. Assessment of histologic criteria in the diagnosis of mycosis fungoides. Int J Dermatol 2003;42(1):45–52.
67. Wallace ML, Smoller BR. Immunohistochemistry in diagnostic dermatopathology. J Am Acad Dermatol 1996;34(2 Pt 1):163–86.
68. Lu D, Patel KA, Duvic M, et al. Clinical and pathological spectrum of CD8-positive cutaneous T-cell lymphomas. J Cutan Pathol 2002;29(8):465–72.
69. Ralfkiaer E, Jaffe ES. Mycosis fungoides and Sézary syndrome. In: Jaffe ES, Harris NL, Stein H, et al, editors. World Health Organisation classification of tumors. Tumors of haematopoietic and lymphoid tissues. Lyon (France): IARC Press; 2001. p. 216–20.
70. Diwan AH, Prieto VG, Herling M, et al. Primary Sézary syndrome commonly shows low-grade cytologic atypia and an absence of epidermotropism. Am J Clin Pathol 2005;123(4):510–5.
71. Ralfkiaer E, Delsol G, Willemze R, et al. Primary cutaneous CD30-positive T cell lymphoproliferative disorders. In: Jaffe ES, Harris NL, Stein H, et al, editors. World Health Organisation classification of tumors. Tumors of haematopoietic and lymphoid tissues. Lyon (France): IARC Press; 2001. p. 221–4.
72. Macgrogan G, Vergier B, Dubus P, et al. CD30-positive cutaneous large cell lymphomas: a comparative study of clinicopathologic and molecular features of 16 cases. Am J Clin Pathol 1996;105(4):440–50.
73. El Shabrawi-Caelen L, Kerl H, Cerroni L. Lymphomatoid papulosis: reappraisal of clinicopathologic presentation and classification into subtypes A, B, and C. Arch Dermatol. 2004;140(4):441–7.
74. Boulland ML, Wechsler J, Bagot M, et al. Primary CD30-positive cutaneous T-cell lymphomas and lymphomatoid papulosis frequently express cytotoxic proteins. Histopathology 2000;36(2):136–44.

75. Chan JK, Jaffe ES, Ralfkiaer E. Extranodal NK/T cell lymphoma, nasal type. In: Jaffe ES, Harris NL, Stein H, et al, editors. World Health Organisation classification of tumors. Tumors of haematopoietic and lymphoid tissues. Lyon (France): IARC Press; 2001. p. 204–7.

76. Jaffe ES, Chan JK, Su IJ, et al. Report of the workshop on nasal and related extranodal angiocentric T/natural killer cell lymphomas: definitions, differential diagnosis, and epidemiology. Am J Surg Pathol 1996;20(1):103–11.

77. Isaacson P, Wright D, Ralfkiaer E, et al. Enteropathy-type T cell lymphoma. In: Jaffe ES, Harris NL, Stein H, et al, editors. World Health Organisation classification of tumors. Tumors of haematopoietic and lymphoid tissues. Lyon (France): IARC Press; 2001. p. 208–9.

78. Chott A, Haedicke W, Mosberger I, et al. Most CD56+ intestinal lymphomas are CD8+CD5− T-cell lymphomas of monomorphic small to medium size histology. Am J Pathol 1998;153(5):1483–90.

79. deLeeuw R, Zettl A, Klinker E, et al. Whole genome analysis and HLA genotyping of enteropathy-type T-cell lymphoma reveals two distinct lymphoma subtypes. Gastroenterology 2007;132(5):1902–11.

80. Jaffe ES, Ralfkiaer E. Hepatosplenic T-cell lymphoma. In: Jaffe ES, Harris NL, Stein H, et al, editors. World Health Organization classification of tumors. Tumors of haematopoietic and lymphoid tissues. Lyon (France): IARC Press; 2001. p. 210–1.

81. Cooke CB, Krenacs L, Stetler-Stevenson M, et al. Hepatosplenic T-cell lymphoma: a distinct clinicopathologic entity of cytotoxic gamma delta T-cell origin. Blood 1996;88(11):4265–74.

82. Vega F, Medeiros LJ, Gaulard P. Hepatosplenic and other gammadelta T-cell lymphomas. Am J Clin Pathol 2007;127(6):869–80.

83. Gonzalez CL, Medeiros LJ, Braziel RM, et al. T-cell lymphoma involving subcutaneous tissue: a clinicopathologic entity commonly associated with hemophagocytic syndrome. Am J Surg Pathol 1991;15(1):17–27.

84. Jaffe ES, Ralfkiaer E. Subcutaneous panniculitis-like T cell lymphoma. In: Jaffe ES, Harris NL, Stein H, et al, editors. World Health Organisation classification of tumors. Tumors of haematopoietic and lymphoid tissues. Lyon (France): IARC Press; 2001. p. 212–3.

85. Sen F, Rassidakis GZ, Jones D, et al. Apoptosis and proliferation in subcutaneous panniculitis-like T-cell lymphoma. Mod Pathol 2002;15(6):625–31.

86. Salhany KE, Macon WR, Choi JK, et al. Subcutaneous panniculitis-like T-cell lymphoma: clinicopathologic, immunophenotypic, and genotypic analysis of alpha/beta and gamma/delta subtypes. Am J Surg Pathol 1998;22(7):881–93.

87. Willemze R, Jansen PM, Cerroni L, et al. Subcutaneous panniculitis-like T-cell lymphoma: definition, classification, and prognostic factors: an EORTC Cutaneous Lymphoma Group study of 83 cases. Blood 2008;111(2):838–45.

88. Jaffe ES, Ralfkiaer E. Angioimmunoblastic T-cell lymphoma. In: Jaffe ES, Harris NL, Stein H, et al, editors. World Health Organisation classification of tumors. Tumors of haematopoietic and lymphoid tissues. Lyon (France): IARC Press; 2001. p. 225–6.

89. Frizzera G, Moran EM, Rappaport H. Angio-immunoblastic lymphadenopathy: diagnosis and clinical course. Am J Med 1975;59(6):803–18.

90. Anagnostopoulos I, Hummel M, Finn T, et al. Heterogeneous Epstein-Barr virus infection patterns in peripheral T-cell lymphoma of angioimmunoblastic lymphadenopathy type. Blood 1992;80(7):1804–12.

91. Ralfkiaer E, Muller-Hermelink HK, Jaffe ES. Peripheral T-cell lymphoma, unspecified. In: Jaffe ES, Harris NL, Stein H, et al, editors. World Health Organisation classification of tumors. Tumors of haematopoietic and lymphoid tissues. Lyon (France): IARC Press; 2001. p. 227–9.
92. Chott A, Augustin I, Wrba F, et al. Peripheral T-cell lymphomas: a clinicopathologic study of 75 cases. Hum Pathol 1990;21(11):1117–25.
93. Takagi N, Nakamura S, Ueda R, et al. A phenotypic and genotypic study of three node-based, low-grade peripheral T-cell lymphomas: angioimmunoblastic lymphoma, T-zone lymphoma, and lymphoepithelioid lymphoma. Cancer 1992; 69(10):2571–82.
94. Delsol G, Ralfkiaer E, Stein H, et al. Anaplastic large cell lymphoma. In: Jaffe ES, Harris NL, Stein H, et al, editors. World Health Organisation classification of tumors. Tumors of haematopoietic and lymphoid tissues. Lyon (France): IARC Press; 2001. p. 230–5.
95. Stein H, Foss HD, Durkop H, et al. CD30+ anaplastic large cell lymphoma: a review of its histopathologic, genetic, and clinical features. Blood 2000; 96(12):3681–95.
96. Falini B. Anaplastic large cell lymphoma: pathological, molecular and clinical features. Br J Haematol 2001;114(4):741–60.
97. Nelson M, Horsman DE, Weisenburger DD, et al. Cytogenetic abnormalities and clinical correlations in peripheral T cell lymphoma. Br J Haematol 2008;141(4)· 461–9.

Molecular Biology and Genetics of Lymphomas

Elena M. Hartmann, MD[a], German Ott, MD[b], Andreas Rosenwald, MD[a],*

KEYWORDS

- Molecular biology • Genetics
- Diffuse large B cell lymphoma • Burkitt lymphoma
- Follicular lymphoma • Mantle cell lymphoma

The current state-of-the-art diagnosis of malignant lymphomas integrates histopathologic, clinical, and genetic features of the disease. While the morphologic and clinical features of various lymphoma entities are detailed elsewhere in this issue, this article highlights important aspects of the molecular biology and genetics of non-Hodgkin lymphomas. Because of space limitations, the authors focus on four major subtypes of B-cell non-Hodgkin lymphoma (B-NHL), namely diffuse large B-cell lymphoma (DLBCL), Burkitt lymphoma (BL), follicular lymphoma (FL), and mantle cell lymphoma (MCL).

To understand the molecular biology of B-NHL, it is essential to take a glimpse at the key events in normal B-cell development and maturation. These include the genetic recombination of the variable, diversity, and joining segments (VDJ) of the B-cell receptor gene in early B-cell stages in the bone marrow, as well as class-switch recombination and the introduction of somatic mutations into B-cell receptor genes during the germinal center (GC) reaction. The physiologic occurrence of DNA remodeling during B-cell development, including double-strand breaks, carries an intrinsic risk for the accidental introduction of genetic alterations. As a consequence, many lymphoma subtypes are characterized by reciprocal chromosomal translocations involving the immunoglobulin gene (*Ig*) loci, and the detection of these typical alterations can provide important diagnostic information. Interestingly, these translocations appear predominantly in the nonproductively rearranged *Ig* loci, suggesting a dependence of the neoplastic cell on B-cell receptor-derived survival signals. Detailed genetic analysis of the *Ig* genes can hint at the stage of B-cell differentiation at which early transforming events occurred. This includes information on whether *Ig* translocation breakpoints occur in the VDJ region or in the class-switch region and the

---

E.M.H. and A.R. are supported by the Interdisciplinary Center for Clinical Research (IZKF), University of Würzburg, Germany. G.O. is supported by the Robert-Bosch-Stiftung, Stuttgart, Germany.
[a] Institute of Pathology, University of Würzburg, Josef-Schneider-Strasse 2, 97080 Würzburg, Germany
[b] Department of Clinical Pathology, Robert-Bosch-Krankenhaus, Auerbachstrasse 110, 70376 Stuttgart, Germany
* Corresponding author.
E-mail address: rosenwald@mail.uni-wuerzburg.de (A. Rosenwald).

Hematol Oncol Clin N Am 22 (2008) 807–823
doi:10.1016/j.hoc.2008.07.004
0889-8588/08/$ – see front matter © 2008 Elsevier Inc. All rights reserved.

detection of ongoing or completed somatic hypermutation as an indicator of a transit through the germinal center.

Genetic alterations involving the *Ig* loci can be considered early events of lymphomagenesis in many instances. However, it has become clear over the last few decades that lymphomagenesis is a multistep process, involving the stepwise accumulation of molecular alterations as well as macro- and micro-environmental factors. Detailed cytogenetic analysis and, more recently, the application of high throughput technologies, such as gene-expression profiling, have deepened our understanding of the molecular background of lymphomagenesis. Important molecular features of diffuse large B-cell lymphoma, Burkitt lymphoma, follicular lymphoma, and mantle cell lymphoma are detailed below.

DIFFUSE LARGE B-CELL LYMPHOMA

Diffuse large B-cell lymphoma represents the most common type of B-NHL in Western countries.[1] DLBCL is heterogeneous in view of histologic and clinical features, suggesting the existence of biologically distinct subclasses within this entity. This variability is also reflected on the cytogenetic level, as no single hallmark alteration could be identified so far. The most frequently detected genetic alteration in DLBCL involves a rearrangement of the *BCL6* gene in chromosomal band 3q27 with various translocation partners, resulting in promoter substitution and inadequately sustained BCL6 expression, which can be detected in 30% to 40% of the cases.[2] Alternatively, BCL6 expression can be deregulated by mutations in the 5' regulatory sequences of the gene in a considerable proportion of cases. *BCL6* encodes for a transcriptional repressor of the BTB/POZ zinc-finger family that is physiologically expressed in GC B-cells, but subsequently down-regulated upon terminal differentiation into plasma cells. BCL6 targets a variety of genes, including genes involved in the cell cycle control and maintenance of genomic stability, such as *CDKN1B*/p27, *CCND2*/cyclin D2, and *TP53*, allowing B-cells to sustain the physiologic occurrence of DNA breaks during the GC reaction.[3,4] Furthermore, BCL6 represses expression of genes required for terminal differentiation, such as *PRDM1* and its gene product BLIMP1.[4,5] Deregulation of BCL6 expression might therefore contribute to lymphomagenesis by blocking terminal differentiation and providing resistance to apoptotic signals in response to DNA damage.

A translocation of the *BCL2* gene in chromosomal band 18q21 to the *Ig* locus in 14q32, the hallmark translocation of FL, is found in approximately 20% of DLBCL, and the typical BL translocation t(8;14) involving the *MYC* gene locus in 8q24 is present in approximately 6% of DLBCL. Amplification of the *BCL2*, *MYC*, and *REL* gene loci are found in around 20% of DLBCL. Inactivation of *TP53*, a multifunctional transcription factor that plays a major role in the DNA damage response by mediating cell cycle arrest, DNA repair, or apoptosis, can be detected in approximately 20% of DLBCL and is associated with a more aggressive clinical course.[2]

Comparative genomic hybridization (CGH)-based analysis of a large series of DLBCL revealed as common alteration losses of two regions in chromosome 6q (6q21-q22 and 6q16) and gains in 18q, gains and amplifications in 2p, and gains in chromosomes 3q and 6p.[6]

In addition to the occurrence of chromosomal imbalances, there is increasing evidence that epigenetic changes, such as DNA methylation and histone modification, may play an important role in cancerogenesis. Few studies exist in malignant lymphomas and most published reports focus on the transcriptional silencing of putative tumor suppressor genes through CpG island hypermethylation. In DLBCL, inactivation of the *HIC1* gene by deletion and promoter hypermethylation was shown to be associated with an inferior clinical outcome[7] and a very recent study investigated DNA hypermethylation levels of more than 500 CpG islands in DLBCL and uncovered potential target genes that may be transcriptionally regulated by CpG hypermethylation.[8]

Another important mechanism in the transformation process of DLBCL might be the aberrant targeting of a variety of proto-oncogenes by the process of somatic hypermutation, which is not detectable in normal GC B-cells or in other GC-derived lymphomas. Aberrant somatic mutation of the proto-oncogenes *PIM1*, *MYC*, *RHOH/TTF*, and *PAX5* can be detected in approximately 50% of DLBCL, resulting in nucleotide changes preferentially in the 5' sequences of these genes with potentially oncogenic effects.[9]

Gene-expression profiling studies have contributed substantially to the understanding of the heterogeneity among DLBCL cases. Using cDNA microarrays,[10–12] two different subgroups could be identified. The germinal center B-cell like (GCB) DLBCL subgroup shows strong expression of genes that are highly expressed in normal germinal center B-cells, pointing to a GC B-cell as the cell of origin in this subtype. In contrast, the activated B-cell like (ABC) DLBCL type is characterized by a gene-expression signature with features reminiscent of in vitro activated B-cells, suggesting that this subtype may arise from post-GC B-cells. The ABC DLBCL subtype is further characterized by constitutive activation of the nuclear factor (NF)-κB pathway, and it has been demonstrated in cell-line experiments that the inhibition of NF-κB is toxic to ABC-like, but not GCB-like DLBCL cell lines.[13]

These findings are in line with results from analyses of the *Ig* mutational status that also detected two subgroups within the DLBCL: one with intraclonal heterogeneity as a marker of ongoing somatic hypermutations suggesting a derivation of the malignant clone from a GC B-cell, and one without ongoing somatic mutations, suggesting a post-GC B-cell origin.[14] Furthermore, the gene expression-based subgroups showed remarkable differences in clinical outcome in patients treated with cyclophosphamide doxorubicin vincristin prednisone (CHOP)-like therapy, with a more favorable prognosis of the GCB subgroup, a finding that could be confirmed more recently also for patients treated with rituximab-CHOP.[15] In addition to expression signatures that are associated with a GCB-like or ABC-like phenotype, other molecular signatures with prognostic impact have been identified: namely, the proliferation signature, the lymph node signature, and the major histocompatibility (MHC) class II signature. The proliferation signature includes genes that are highly expressed in dividing cells, and high expression of the proliferation signature genes was shown to be associated with an unfavorable clinical course. High expression of genes belonging to the lymph node signature, which reflects mainly the gene expression of the nonmalignant tumor-infiltrating immune cells, was correlated with a favorable prognosis, and this was also demonstrated for the expression of the MHC class II molecules on the gene expression level (MHC class II signature), as well as by immunohistochemistry.[16] Using Affymetrix arrays, Shipp and colleagues[17] described a 13-gene predictor of survival in DLBCL patients that includes genes involved in apoptotic pathways, such as *NOR1*, *PDE4B*, and *PKC-β*, and suggested some of these genes as potential future therapeutic targets. Using a so-called "consensus clustering approach," Monti and colleagues[18] identified three clusters of differentially expressed genes among DLBCL, which they termed "oxidative phosphorylation (OxPhos)," 'B-cell receptor/proliferation (BCR)," and "host response (HR)" clusters. The HR cluster also underlines the potential role of the tumor microenvironment in the biologic behavior of DLBCL.

GCB DLBCL and ABC DLBCL could be associated with distinct genetic alterations, suggesting profound differences between these subgroups on the molecular level. Typical alterations of GCB DLBCL are the translocation t(14;18)(q32;q21) and the amplification of the *REL* locus in 2p.[11] Conventional[6] and array-based CGH analysis[19,20] confirmed the association between the GCB subtype and gains or amplifications in chromosome 2p and, furthermore, revealed more frequent gains of a chromosomal region in 12q as a characteristic feature of the GCB DLBCL. ABC DLBCL carry more frequent gains in chromosomes 3q and 18q, as well as losses in 6q. Interestingly, the deleted region in 6q includes the *PRDM1* gene locus (6q21-q22.1), whose gene product BLIMP1 is a target of BCL6 (vide supra). Indeed, mutational analysis of *PRDM1/BLIMP1* revealed its inactivation by mutations in a considerable proportion of ABC DLBCL, suggesting that *BLIMP1* inactivation may play a pathogenetic role in this subset of DLBCL.[21,22]

New insights into the aberrant activation of oncogenic pathways in DLBCL subtypes may ultimately lead to the development of new therapeutic strategies that are particularly needed for the prognostically unfavorable ABC DLBCL subgroup. Given that ABC DLBCL-derived cell lines strongly depend on signaling through the NF-κB pathway, therapeutic interference with this pathway may be an attractive future option. NF-κB is a transcription factor involved in the regulation of B- and T-cell development, proliferation, and survival, and its deregulation has been implied in the pathogenesis of several lymphoma subtypes (reviewed in[23]). A recent RNA interference screen provided evidence that inhibition of CARD11, a protein that participates in the constitutive NF-κB activation in ABC DLBCL by small hairpin RNAs, was toxic to ABC DLBCL, but not to GCB DLBCL cell lines.[24] Moreover, Lenz and colleagues[25] found activating mutations of *CARD11* in a DLBCL subset that likely contribute to the constitutive activation of the NF-κB pathway in these cases. Therefore, CARD11 might represent a novel, promising molecular target for a subset of DLBCL. A schematic overview of molecular alterations in DLBCL is provided in **Fig. 1**.

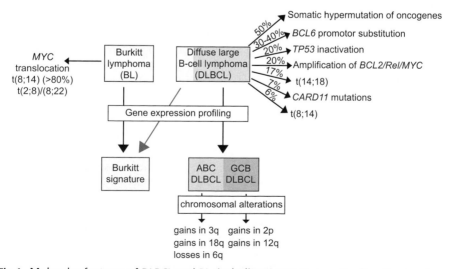

Fig. 1. Molecular features of DLBCL and BL, including common genetic alterations and molecular signatures defined by gene-expression profiling (for details see text).

To translate results from gene-expression profiling studies into clinical practice, two methodologies have been applied: one based on selected immunohistochemical markers and the other on the quantitative measurement of selected genes using polymerase chain reaction (PCR)-based techniques. A large immunohistochemical study employed measurement of CD10, BCL6, and MUM1 protein expression to assign DLBCL cases to the ABC or the GCB DLBCL subgroup.[26] However, the results between this study and various other studies are remarkably inconsistent, which is likely caused by the semiquantitative nature of immunohistochemistry and inter- and intra-observer variations. In a study of 66 DLBCL patients, Lossos and colleagues reported that the quantitative measurement of the expression of six genes, including *LMO2, BCL6, FN1, CCND2, SCYA3,* and *BCL2,* was strongly predictive of clinical outcome.[27] More recently, a monoclonal antibody against LMO2 was developed and in a study of 343 DLBCL specimens, the immunohistochemical detection of LMO2 protein expression provided important prognostic information.[28]

BURKITT LYMPHOMA

Burkitt lymphoma, a highly aggressive B-NHL, comprises three epidemiologic variants, including endemic, sporadic, and immunodeficiency-associated cases. BL is a rapidly proliferating lymphoma, which is displayed by a Ki-67 index of nearly 100%.[1]

The cytogenetic hallmark of all variants of BL is the translocation of the *MYC* gene in chromosome 8q24 to either the immunoglobulin-heavy chain (*IgH*) locus on chromosome 14q32 in more than 80% of cases, or to one of the light chain loci (see **Fig. 1**). This translocation leads to the deregulated expression of the basic helix-loop/helix-leucine zipper-transcription factor *MYC,* which regulates a wide variety of cellular processes including proliferation, differentiation, and apoptosis. Additional transforming events to overcome apoptotic signals as a result of *MYC* over-expression in BL include disturbance of apoptotic signaling via the p14[ARF]-MDM2-p53 axis[29] and the proapoptotic, BH3-only protein BIM, which effectively inhibits BCL2 and other antia-poptotic members of the BCL2 family.[30] Mutations of *TP53* have been detected in at least 30% of BL and, alternatively, over-expression of MDM2 or inactivation of *CDKN2a* have been reported in a fraction of cases.[31] Furthermore, *MYC* mutations are frequently detected in BL and are centered around mutational hotspots; some of these mutations were shown to have increased transforming activity because of failure to induce BIM-mediated apoptosis.[32] Interestingly, the breakpoints affected by the translocation t(8;14) vary between the different variants of BL with respect to their localization to the *MYC* gene as well as within the *IgH* locus. In the endemic cases, the breakpoint on chromosome 8 occurs commonly relatively far 5' from the *MYC* gene (up to >100 kb away; class III breakpoints), and the breakpoint on chromosome 14 usually appears in the VDJ region of the *IgH* locus. In sporadic BL, the breakpoints are either within the first exon or intron of the *MYC* gene (class I breakpoints) or directly 5' to the *MYC* locus (class II breakpoints). Within the *IgH* locus, the breakpoints in the sporadic cases mostly occur in the switch region. The diversity of the breakpoint localization suggests that formation of the translocation takes place at different stages of B-cell development. Specifically, the endemic cases may mostly experience the translocation during VDJ rearrangement in the early B-cell differentiation, whereas in the sporadic cases the recombination occurs more likely during immunoglobulin class-switch events.[33]

BL usually carries relatively few secondary genetic alterations, most frequently gains in 12q, 20q, 22q, Xq, and losses of 13q. Gains or amplifications in 1q and gains in 7q were also described in a substantial subset of cases, and were reported to be associated with a poor clinical outcome.[34] In a small group of patients, the presence of concurrent translocations of MYC and BCL2 (t(14;18)) was reported, and these dual translocations were associated with a particularly poor prognosis.[35]

In 2006, two independent studies employed gene expression profiling to further characterize sporadic BL on the molecular level. Dave and colleagues[36] studied 303 patients with the initial diagnosis of BL, atypical BL, or DLBCL using a custom oligo-nucleotide microarray with 2,524 genes. They constructed a molecular classifier of BL based on the expression of four prominent gene-expression signatures. As expected, because translocations involving the MYC gene are the typical cytogenetic feature of BL, MYC and its target genes were shown to be more highly expressed in BL when compared with DLBCL. Another gene cluster that was found to be expressed at higher levels in BL consisted of a distinct subset of genes expressed in normal germinal center B-cells. Expression of MHC class I genes and NF-κB target genes was reported to be lower in BL compared with DLBCL. Likewise, Hummel and colleagues[37] investigated a large series of mature aggressive B-cell lymphomas that included BL, atypical BL, DLBCL, or unclassifiable mature aggressive non-Hodgkin lymphoma (NHL). These cases were characterized by array CGH and fluorescence in-situ hybridization on the genetic level and by using Affymetrix U133A arrays on the gene-expression level. The investigators developed a core-group extension strategy to define molecular features of BL, an approach that comprised the initial definition of a core group of eight cases that fulfilled all World Health Organization (WHO) criteria for the diagnosis of BL, and the subsequent comparison to the gene-expression profile of the remaining cases. With this strategy, a gene expression signature composed of 58 genes was identified that allowed the classification of the cases into three categories: molecular BL (mBL) (20%), non-mBL (58%), and a relatively large group of intermediate cases (22%) that could not be clearly assigned to one group. In line with the results from Dave and colleagues, target genes of the NF-κB pathway were expressed at lower levels in BL when compared with DLBCL. Furthermore, array CGH analysis revealed that the mBL group was characterized by a low chromosomal complexity: that is, few additional chromosomal alterations apart from the MYC translocation. In contrast, the intermediate and non-mBL group harbored more chromosomal abnormalities (high chromosomal complexity). The presence of a MYC breakpoint in the non-mBL (DLBCL) group was strongly associated with poor clinical outcome in this series of patients.

Importantly, both studies identified a subset of cases diagnosed as DLBCL according to current WHO criteria, but with a typical gene expression profile of BL (see **Fig. 1**). Whether these patients may benefit from intensified treatment approaches will have to be examined in future clinical studies.

GRAY ZONE BETWEEN BURKITT LYMPHOMA AND DIFFUSE LARGE B-CELL LYMPHOMA

Classic BL cases that fulfill all of the diagnostic criteria of the WHO classification can be diagnosed with a high inter- and intra-observer agreement. However, the differential diagnosis between atypical BL and other aggressive lymphomas, especially DLBCL, can be difficult in the diagnostic setting, because morphologic and immunophenotypical features may overlap. Furthermore, on the genetic level, translocations involving the MYC gene, although a typical cytogenetic feature of BL, are not restricted to this entity and can be also found in 5% to 10% of DLBCL.[2] However, the precise discrimination between BL and DLBCL is of significant clinical importance because of the different therapeutic approaches used in the treatment of these patients.

Although gene-expression profiling delineates BL on the molecular level from DLBCL, at the same time it broadens this diagnostic category, because the gene-expression defined BL group includes some cases with morphologic features of DLBCL. Further studies are required to characterize these cases and the group of intermediate cases that could not be clearly assigned to the BL or non-BL (DLBCL) category in the study by Hummel and colleagues. On the cytogenetic level, cases from the intermediate group showed more frequently *MYC* breakpoints when compared with the non-BL group and, occasionally, non-*Ig* partners were involved in this translocation.

FOLLICULAR LYMPHOMA

Follicular lymphoma comprises approximately 30% of adult NHL.[1] Although the clinical course is, in general, relatively indolent with an overall median survival of 8 to 10 years, it displays a wide variability. In some FL patients, the lymphoma progresses slowly over many years, whereas others have a poor prognosis because of progressive disease or transformation to an aggressive lymphoma.[38]

The typical cytogenetic alteration of FL is the translocation t(14;18)(q32;q21), which can be detected in approximately 85% of the cases. This translocation juxtaposes the *BCL2* gene on chromosome 18q21 to the *IgH* enhancer on chromosome 14, leading to constitutive expression of BCL2. BCL2 belongs to a family of pro- and antiapoptotic proteins that share at least one BCL2 homology domain and govern the activation of the intrinsic or mitochondrial apoptotic pathway in response to cytotoxic events, including DNA damage, cell cycle perturbation, and oncogene activation.[39] BCL2 itself potently inhibits apoptosis and, thus, deregulated expression of BCL2 as a consequence of the t(14;18) leads to impaired apoptotic signaling.

Two major lines of evidence indicate that this alteration alone is not sufficient to produce a fully malignant phenotype. First, *BCL2/Ig* transgenic mice indeed showed a B-cell lymphoproliferation, but progression to frank lymphoma appeared only in a small proportion of cases and with long latency.[40,41] Second, it was demonstrated by several groups that B-cells harboring a t(14;18) can be detected in the peripheral blood or hyperplastic lymphatic tissues of healthy individuals.[42,43] These findings indicate that the formation of FL requires additional pathogenetic events, for example the acquisition of secondary molecular alterations, which may be facilitated by the prolonged life span of a B-cell harboring the t(14;18).

This hypothesis is supported by cytogenetic studies that detected at least one secondary chromosomal alteration in addition to the t(14;18) in the majority of FL.[44] The most frequently reported aberrations in FL include gains in chromosomes 1q, 2p, 7, 8q, 12q, 18q and X, as well as losses in 1p, 6q, 10q, 13q and 17p.[45] Among these alterations, losses of chromosome 1p as well as of the long or short arm of chromosome 17, and gains of 1q, 12, and X were identified as late events and negative prognostic markers.[46,47] An interesting pathogenetic model proposes two ways of karyotypic evolution in FL following the primary t(14;18). One route includes the acquisition of a 6q deletion or 1q gain, which is followed by a 1p deletion leading to a poor prognosis. In contrast, gains of chromosome 7, 8, or 18 appear to be associated with a good prognosis.[46,48] Although most FL harbor the t(14;18), approximately 15% of cases lack this translocation. In a subset of these tumors, gains of 18q could be detected that may represent an alternative mechanism of BCL2 over-expression. However, the majority of FL lacking the t(14;18) do not show BCL2 expression and, thus, the underlying pathogenetic mechanisms in this subset are only poorly characterized.[49]

Transformation of FL into a more aggressive lymphoma, most commonly DLBCL, is reported in 10% to 60% of the cases, and this event confers a poor clinical prognosis.

Recurrent cytogenetic abnormalities associated with transformation include gains of chromosomes 7, 12q, and X and losses of 4q, 13q, and 17p. Inactivation of *TP53* in 17p13.1, the *CDKN2a* gene in 9p21.3, and a deregulated expression of *MYC* are most commonly associated with transformation of FL to DLBCL.[50]

Despite their longevity in vivo, FL cells are difficult to maintain in vitro, suggesting their dependence on additional growth stimuli possibly provided from the tumor microenvironment. Gene-expression profiling studies demonstrated that besides intrinsic features of the tumor cells, nonmalignant tumor infiltrating inflammatory cells contribute importantly to the clinical outcome in FL patients. By analyzing gene-expression data from 191 FL patient samples collected at the time of diagnosis, Dave and colleagues[51] identified two highly synergistic gene-expression signatures that allowed the definition of patient subgroups with a widely disparate clinical outcome. Importantly, these gene-expression signatures originated mostly from the nonmalignant bystander cells, and were therefore termed "immune response" (IR) 1 and 2. The IR 1 signature included genes encoding T-cell markers: for example, *CD7, CD8B1, ITK, LEF1*, and *STAT4*, and genes expressed at high levels in macrophages, like *ACTN1* and *TNFSF13B*. High expression of these genes was associated with good prognosis. The IR2 signature contained genes expressed by macrophages and follicular dendritic cells (*TLR5, FCGR1A, SEPT10, LGMN*, and *C3AR1*), and high expression was correlated with an unfavorable clinical course. These findings led to several follow-up studies that aimed at a more detailed characterization of the microenvironment in FL and a definition of prognostically meaningful markers in FL using immunohistochemical markers. Some studies reported that increased infiltration of lymphoma-associated macrophages, detected by immunohistochemistry targeting CD68, is associated with a poor prognosis, and others that increased numbers of tumor-infiltrating lymphocytes expressing CD4 and FOXP3 had a favorable impact on outcome;[52–54] however, these studies varied considerably regarding study design and results. A very recent study[55] investigated the role of the immune response in FL by means of reverse transcription-PCR and immunohistochemistry, and found the number of lymphoma-associated macrophages and CD7+ T-cells as prognostically useful markers, thereby confirming the results of Dave and colleagues[36] and Farinha and colleagues.[52] Furthermore, high expression of the chemokine receptor CCR1, which participates in the recruitment of monocytes during inflammatory processes, was found to be associated with poor prognosis[55] and transformation of FL into DLBCL.[56]

The conflicting results of the immunohistochemical studies may be partially explained by the fact that complex molecular gene-expression signatures may not easily be captured by the application of relatively few immunohistochemical markers. In addition, the study cohorts in many published series were relatively small and treatment was heterogeneous. To what extent immunohistochemical markers can contribute prognostic information in FL specimens at the time of diagnosis will have to be examined in more detail in future studies with defined patient inclusion criteria and homogeneous therapy.

MANTLE CELL LYMPHOMA

Mantle cell lymphoma is an aggressive B-NHL and accounts for approximately 3% to 10% of all NHL.[1] With current therapeutic approaches, MCL has a poor clinical outcome with an overall median survival of approximately 4 years, but the clinical course shows a considerable variability, with survival times ranging from only a few months to more than 10 years.[57]

The typical cytogenetic aberration of MCL is the translocation t(11;14)(q13;q32), which can be detected in almost all cases. This translocation leads to the juxtaposition of the CCND1 gene on chromosome 11q13 to the IgH enhancer on chromosome 14, resulting in over-expression of its gene product cyclin D1, a D-type cyclin that is usually not expressed at high levels in lymphoid cells. D-type cyclins are key regulators of the cell cycle and control the G1/S-phase transition by binding and activating the cyclin-dependent kinases (CDK) 4 and 6 upon mitogenic stimulation, followed by the activation of cyclin E/CDK 2 complexes, which further promote S-phase entry. The active cyclin D1/CDK4/6 complex hyperphosphorylates the retinoblastoma protein (RB), resulting in the release of E2F transcription factors, which mediate cell cycle progression.[58] Over-expression of cyclin D1 may promote G1/S-phase transition independently from mitogenic stimuli via two mechanisms: first, by phosphorylating and thereby overcoming the suppressive effects of RB and, second, by titrating the CDK inhibitor p27 away from cyclin E/CDK 2 complexes, leading to acceleration of the late G1 phase. In line with this hypothesis were findings that in MCL cells, most p27 protein is sequestered by cyclin D1/CDK4 or 6 complexes, which makes it undetectable by immunohistochemical approaches.[59] Furthermore, it was shown that upon mitogenic signals, cyclin E/CDK2 can in turn also phosphorylate p27 and thereby trigger its ubiquitination and degradation.[60] Indeed, increased proteasomal degradation of p27 was reported in MCL.[61]

The CCND1 gene locus includes 5 exons, which can be alternatively spliced resulting in two major mRNA transcript variants of approximately 4.5 kb (isoform a) and 1.7 kb (isoform b) length. The isoform b lacks exon 5, resulting in an altered C-terminus on the protein level, which contains regulatory motifs involved in protein degradation and nuclear export.[62] This isoform seems to have higher transforming properties in vitro,[63] but recent studies indicate that the isoform b does not play a crucial role in MCL pathogenesis.[64,65] However, cyclin D1 mRNA was found in MCL in two main transcripts of 4.5-kb and 1.5-kb length, both containing the whole coding region but differing in the length of their 3' untranslated region (UTR). The shorter transcripts were shown to be more stable because of the lack of destabilizing AUUUA sequences in the 3'UTR, resulting in higher cyclin D1 levels, a higher proliferation, and an inferior clinical outcome.[66] Interestingly, these shorter transcripts were shown to be truncated variants of the cyclin D1 isoform a and not of the alternatively spliced cyclin D1b mRNA.[67]

Although the t(11;14) can be detected in nearly all MCL and is therefore considered essential in the pathogenesis of MCL, there is evidence from transgenic mouse models that cyclin D1 over-expression alone is insufficient for lymphomagenesis, and that additional alterations are required to promote malignant transformation.[68,69] In support of this hypothesis, MCL carry a high number of secondary molecular alterations in addition to the t(11;14). In CGH-based studies, the most frequently detected alterations include gains in 3q, 7p, 8q, 12q, and 18q and losses in 1p, 6q, 8p, 9p, 9q, 11q, 13q, and 17p[70,71] and, at higher resolution, many of these regions could be confirmed and refined by array CGH.[72,73]

Single-gene alterations that were identified to be involved in the pathogenesis of MCL play important roles in either cell cycle regulation or the DNA damage response (Fig. 2) (for detailed review see).[74,75] These include deletions of the CDKN2a locus on 9p21, amplification of BMI1 on 10p11,[76] and amplifications of CDK4 on 12q14.[77] The CDKN2a locus generates two different proteins by alternative splicing, p16^{INK4a} and p14^{ARF}. The protein p16^{INK4a} acts as an inhibitor of CDK4 and 6, and thereby maintains RB in its hypophosphorylated, antiproliferative state. Protein p14^{ARF} stabilizes p53 by preventing its MDM2-mediated degradation. Deletion of the CDKN2a locus thus impairs simultaneously both the cell cycle regulatory and the DNA damage response

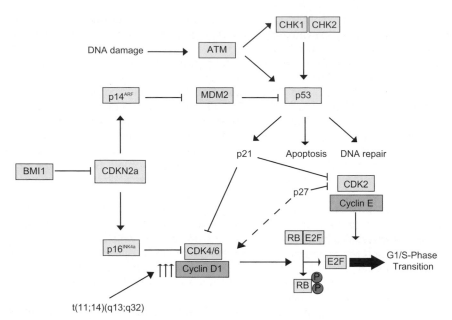

Fig. 2. Overview of perturbed cell cycle regulation and DNA damage response in mantle cell lymphoma. Molecules with increased expression or function in MCL are colored in orange; molecules with decreased expression or function are colored in green. The characteristic translocation t(11;14)(q13;q32) leads to constitutive over-expression of cyclin D1 and, thus, to inappropriate cell cycle progression in the absence of mitogenic stimuli (for details see text).

pathway: loss of functional p16[INK4a] may cooperate with the increased cyclin D1 levels in MCL to further enhance cell cycle progression, and loss of functional p14[ARF] impairs adequate reaction in response to DNA damage. In line with these functions, alterations of the *CDKN2a* locus in MCL were shown to be associated with high proliferation of the tumor cells and an aggressive clinical course.[66,78] Interestingly, in some aggressive MCL with a wild-type status of *CDKN2a*, gene amplification and over-expression of *BMI-1*, which acts as a transcriptional repressor of *CDKN2a*,[76] have been described. Furthermore, amplification and over-expression of *CDK4* has been described in a sub-set of MCL, and patients with concurrent inactivation of *p53* suffer from particularly aggressive disease. Recently, mutations in *RB* resulting in lack of protein expression were detected in a MCL cell line and single, highly proliferating MCL cases.[79] Interestingly, these mutations occurred in cases with concurrent *TP53* inactivation but wild-type *CDKN2a*, supporting the hypothesis that double inactivation of both the cell cycle and DNA-damage response pathways leads to particularly aggressive tumors, but that alterations of more than one member of each pathway may not provide additional biologic advantage for the malignant clone.

The high degree of genetic instability that is characteristic of MCL (including numerous secondary chromosomal alterations and the occurrence of tetraploid karyotypes)[80] suggests that alterations of the DNA damage response pathway may represent another important pathogenetic mechanism in this lymphoma. Alterations affecting the DNA damage response pathway comprise the frequent inactivation of the *ATM* gene localized in 11q22-23 (in about 40%–75% of the cases)[81] and, infrequently, down-regulation of its downstream targets CHK1/2,[82,83] as well as inactivation of *TP53* in 17p13 and over-expression of MDM2, a negative regulator of p53.[77,84] *ATM* encodes for a protein kinase that is activated in response to DNA damage, particularly DNA double-strand breaks, and phosphorylates several proteins involved in cell cycle checkpoint control, DNA repair, and apoptosis, suggesting that its inactivation may contribute to the observed chromosomal instability in MCL. *ATM* inactivation by deletion or mutation was found to be associated with an increased number of chromosomal imbalances;[85] however, this alteration seems to have no influence on tumor cell proliferation or clinical behavior,[66] indicating that it might occur as an early event in lymphomagenesis. Inactivation of *TP53* is found infrequently in MCL cases with classic morphology, but in approximately 30% of cases with blastoid morphology, and was shown to be associated with a poor prognosis.[86,87]

Apart from the commonly detected alterations affecting genes associated with cell cycle or DNA damage-response pathways, amplification of the antiapoptotic *BCL2* gene[88] and homozygous deletion of the proapoptotic *BCL2L11/BIM* gene on 2q13 were reported in MCL cell lines.[89] However, these alterations were only occasionally found in primary MCL tumors.

In gene-expression profiling experiments, a small subset of cyclin D1 negative cases with typical, MCL-like morphology and immunophenotype was identified that did not differ in gene expression from cyclin D1-positive MCL. Therefore, these cases may represent bona fide MCL and, interestingly, some of these cases showed over-expression of cyclin D2 or D3,[66,90] possibly as an alternative molecular mechanism to drive cell cycle progression. In addition, gene-expression profiling defined a powerful predictor of outcome in MCL, termed the "proliferation signature," which encompasses the expression levels of 20 proliferation-associated genes. This survival predictor allows the definition of prognostic subgroups of MCL patients with a widely disparate clinical outcome and appears superior to the predictive power of other molecular markers that have been defined to date.[66]

SUMMARY

In the last decade, we have made significant progress in our understanding of the molecular biology and the definition of underlying genetic alterations in B-NHL which, in part, may explain the clinical heterogeneity that is present even within defined lymphoma entities. Newly available technologies and their application in the analysis of morphologically well-defined B-NHL subtypes have helped to reveal distinct molecular and genetic features of many entities. In DLBCL, gene-expression profiling studies identified at least two distinct biologic subtypes, namely ABC DLBCL and GCB DLBCL, which differ in their underlying molecular features, divergent activation of oncogenic pathways, and clinical course. The detailed analysis of specific pathways, such as the NF-κB pathway, may result in the identification of pivotal molecules that can be targeted therapeutically in the future. One recent example includes the discovery of activating mutations of *CARD11* in a subset in ABC DLBCL that might be responsible for the potent activation of NF-κB in these cases.

Expression profiling also defined a molecular signature of Burkitt lymphoma, and therefore sharpened the molecular border between DLBCL and BL. Some DLBCL, however, that were classified according to current diagnostic criteria provided by the WHO classification, showed a clear gene-expression profile of BL. This discrepancy will have to be resolved in the future and prospective clinical trials will have to answer the question whether these "discrepant DLBCL" cases will benefit from alternative (ie, more aggressive) therapeutic approaches.

Characterization of follicular lymphoma on the molecular level suggests that a complex interaction between the malignant cells and the surrounding immunologic network might be a major determinant of the clinical behavior of this lymphoma. Further studies are needed to determine the influence of the distinct cell populations of the tumor microenvironment (eg, subpopulations of T-cells and macrophages) in more detail.

The molecular analysis of MCL predominantly revealed alterations in the cell cycle and DNA damage-response pathways, resulting in increased tumor cell proliferation as a major pathogenetic and prognostic theme in this entity. A gene expression-based proliferation signature might serve as a quantitative integrator of various molecular alterations and may constitute a powerful predictor of outcome that could guide therapeutic decisions in the future.

REFERENCES

1. Jaffe ES, Stein H, Vardiman JW, editors. World Health Organization classification of tumors. Pathology and genetics of tumours of haematopoetic and lymphoid tissues. Lyon (France): IARC Press; 2001.
2. Lossos IS. Molecular pathogenesis of diffuse large B-cell lymphoma. J Clin Oncol 2005;23(26):6351–7.
3. Phan RT, Dalla-Favera R. The BCL6 proto-oncogene suppresses p53 expression in germinal-centre B cells. Nature 2004;432(7017):635–9.
4. Shaffer AL, Yu X, He Y, et al. BCL-6 represses genes that function in lymphocyte differentiation, inflammation, and cell cycle control. Immunity 2000;13(2): 199–212.
5. Shaffer AL, Lin KI, Kuo TC, et al. Blimp-1 orchestrates plasma cell differentiation by extinguishing the mature B cell gene expression program. Immunity 2002; 17(1):51–62.
6. Bea S, Zettl A, Wright G, et al. Diffuse large B-cell lymphoma subgroups have distinct genetic profiles that influence tumor biology and improve gene-expression-based survival prediction. Blood 2005;106(9):3183–90.
7. Stocklein H, Smardova J, Macak J, et al. Detailed mapping of chromosome 17p deletions reveals HIC1 as a novel tumor suppressor gene candidate telomeric to TP53 in diffuse large B-cell lymphoma. Oncogene 2008;27(18):2613–25.
8. Pike BL, Greiner TC, Wang X, et al. DNA methylation profiles in diffuse large B-cell lymphoma and their relationship to gene expression status. Leukemia 2008;22(5): 1035–43.
9. Pasqualucci L, Neumeister P, Goossens T, et al. Hypermutation of multiple proto-oncogenes in B-cell diffuse large-cell lymphomas. Nature 2001;412(6844):341–6.
10. Wright G, Tan B, Rosenwald A, et al. A gene expression-based method to diagnose clinically distinct subgroups of diffuse large B cell lymphoma. Proc Natl Acad Sci U S A 2003;100(17):9991–6.
11. Rosenwald A, Wright G, Chan WC, et al. The use of molecular profiling to predict survival after chemotherapy for diffuse large-B-cell lymphoma. N Engl J Med 2002;346(25):1937–47.
12. Alizadeh AA, Eisen MB, Davis RE, et al. Distinct types of diffuse large B-cell lymphoma identified by gene expression profiling. Nature 2000;403(6769): 503–11.
13. Davis RE, Brown KD, Siebenlist U, et al. Constitutive nuclear factor kappaB activity is required for survival of activated B cell-like diffuse large B cell lymphoma cells. J Exp Med 2001;194(12):1861–74.

14. Lossos IS, Okada CY, Tibshirani R, et al. Molecular analysis of immunoglobulin genes in diffuse large B-cell lymphomas. Blood 2000;95(5):1797–803.
15. Lenz G, Wright G, Dave S, et al. Gene expression signatures predict overall survival in diffuse large B cell lymphoma treated with rituximab and CHOP-like chemotherapy. ASH Annual Meeting Abstracts 2007;110(11):348.
16. Rimsza LM, Roberts RA, Miller TP, et al. Loss of MHC class II gene and protein expression in diffuse large B-cell lymphoma is related to decreased tumor immunosurveillance and poor patient survival regardless of other prognostic factors: a follow-up study from the Leukemia and Lymphoma Molecular Profiling Project. Blood 2004;103(11):4251–8.
17. Shipp MA, Ross KN, Tamayo P, et al. Diffuse large B-cell lymphoma outcome prediction by gene-expression profiling and supervised machine learning. Nat Med 2002;8(1):68–74.
18. Monti S, Savage KJ, Kutok JL, et al. Molecular profiling of diffuse large B-cell lymphoma identifies robust subtypes including one characterized by host inflammatory response. Blood 2005;105(5):1851–61.
19. Tagawa H, Suguro M, Tsuzuki S, et al. Comparison of genome profiles for identification of distinct subgroups of diffuse large B-cell lymphoma. Blood 2005; 106(5):1770–7.
20. Chen W, Houldsworth J, Olshen AB, et al. Array comparative genomic hybridization reveals genomic copy number changes associated with outcome in diffuse large B-cell lymphomas. Blood 2006;107(6):2477–85.
21. Pasqualucci L, Compagno M, Houldsworth J, et al. Inactivation of the PRDM1/ BLIMP1 gene in diffuse large B cell lymphoma. J Exp Med 2006;203(2):311–7.
22. Tam W, Gomez M, Chadburn A, et al. Mutational analysis of PRDM1 indicates a tumor-suppressor role in diffuse large B-cell lymphomas. Blood 2006;107(10): 4090–100.
23. Jost PJ, Ruland J. Aberrant NF-kappaB signaling in lymphoma: mechanisms, consequences, and therapeutic implications. Blood 2007;109(7):2700–7.
24. Ngo VN, Davis RE, Lamy L, et al. A loss-of-function RNA interference screen for molecular targets in cancer. Nature 2006;441(7089):106–10.
25. Lenz G, Davis RE, Ngo VN, et al. Oncogenic CARD11 mutations in human diffuse large B cell lymphoma. Science 2008;319(5870):1676–9.
26. Hans CP, Weisenburger DD, Greiner TC, et al. Confirmation of the molecular classification of diffuse large B-cell lymphoma by immunohistochemistry using a tissue microarray. Blood 2004;103(1):275–82.
27. Lossos IS, Czerwinski DK, Alizadeh AA, et al. Prediction of survival in diffuse large-B-cell lymphoma based on the expression of six genes. N Engl J Med 2004;350(18):1828–37.
28. Natkunam Y, Farinha P, Hsi ED, et al. LMO2 protein expression predicts survival in patients with diffuse large B-cell lymphoma treated with anthracycline-based chemotherapy with and without rituximab. J Clin Oncol 2008;26(3):447–54.
29. Grandori C, Cowley SM, James LP, et al. The Myc/Max/Mad network and the transcriptional control of cell behavior. Annu Rev Cell Dev Biol 2000;16:653–99.
30. O'Connor L, Strasser A, O'Reilly LA, et al. Bim: a novel member of the Bcl-2 family that promotes apoptosis. Embo J 1998;17(2):384–95.
31. Lindstrom MS, Wiman KG. Role of genetic and epigenetic changes in Burkitt lymphoma. Semin Cancer Biol 2002;12(5):381–7.
32. Hemann MT, Bric A, Teruya-Feldstein J, et al. Evasion of the p53 tumour surveillance network by tumour-derived MYC mutants. Nature 2005;436(7052): 807–11.

33. Boxer LM, Dang CV. Translocations involving c-myc and c-myc function. Oncogene 2001;20(40):5595–610.
34. Garcia JL, Hernandez JM, Gutierrez NC, et al. Abnormalities on 1q and 7q are associated with poor outcome in sporadic Burkitt's lymphoma. A cytogenetic and comparative genomic hybridization study. Leukemia 2003;17(10): 2016–24.
35. Kanungo A, Medeiros LJ, Abruzzo LV, et al. Lymphoid neoplasms associated with concurrent t(14;18) and 8q24/c-MYC translocation generally have a poor prognosis. Mod Pathol 2006;19(1):25–33.
36. Dave SS, Fu K, Wright GW, et al. Molecular diagnosis of Burkitt's lymphoma. N Engl J Med 2006;354(23):2431–42.
37. Hummel M, Bentink S, Berger H, et al. A biologic definition of Burkitt's lymphoma from transcriptional and genomic profiling. N Engl J Med 2006;354(23):2419–30.
38. Horning SJ. Follicular lymphoma: have we made any progress? Ann Oncol 2000; 11(Suppl 1)):23–7.
39. Letai AG. Diagnosing and exploiting cancer's addiction to blocks in apoptosis. Nat Rev Cancer 2008;8(2):121–32.
40. McDonnell TJ, Korsmeyer SJ. Progression from lymphoid hyperplasia to high-grade malignant lymphoma in mice transgenic for the t(14; 18). Nature 1991;349(6306): 254–6.
41. McDonnell TJ, Deane N, Platt FM, et al. BCL-2-immunoglobulin transgenic mice demonstrate extended B cell survival and follicular lymphoproliferation. Cell 1989;57(1):79–88.
42. Liu Y, Hernandez AM, Shibata D, et al. BCL2 translocation frequency rises with age in humans. Proc Natl Acad Sci U S A 1994;91(19):8910–4.
43. Limpens J, de Jong D, van Krieken JH, et al. Bcl-2/JH rearrangements in benign lymphoid tissues with follicular hyperplasia. Oncogene 1991;6(12):2271–6.
44. Horsman DE, Connors JM, Pantzar T, et al. Analysis of secondary chromosomal alterations in 165 cases of follicular lymphoma with t(14;18). Genes Chromosomes Cancer 2001;30(4):375–82.
45. Viardot A, Barth TF, Moller P, et al. Cytogenetic evolution of follicular lymphoma. Semin Cancer Biol 2003;13(3):183–90.
46. Hoglund M, Sehn L, Connors JM, et al. Identification of cytogenetic subgroups and karyotypic pathways of clonal evolution in follicular lymphomas. Genes Chromosomes Cancer 2004;39(3):195–204.
47. Viardot A, Moller P, Hogel J, et al. Clinicopathologic correlations of genomic gains and losses in follicular lymphoma. J Clin Oncol 2002;20(23):4523–30.
48. de Jong D. Molecular pathogenesis of follicular lymphoma: a cross talk of genetic and immunologic factors. J Clin Oncol 2005;23(26):6358–63.
49. Horsman DE, Okamoto I, Ludkovski O, et al. Follicular lymphoma lacking the t(14;18)(q32;q21): identification of two disease subtypes. Br J Haematol 2003; 120(3):424–33.
50. Lossos IS, Levy R. Higher grade transformation of follicular lymphoma: phenotypic tumor progression associated with diverse genetic lesions. Semin Cancer Biol 2003;13(3):191–202.
51. Dave SS, Wright G, Tan B, et al. Prediction of survival in follicular lymphoma based on molecular features of tumor-infiltrating immune cells. N Engl J Med 2004;351(21):2159–69.
52. Farinha P, Masoudi H, Skinnider BF, et al. Analysis of multiple biomarkers shows that lymphoma-associated macrophage (LAM) content is an independent predictor of survival in follicular lymphoma (FL). Blood 2005;106(6):2169–74.

53. Lee AM, Clear AJ, Calaminici M, et al. Number of CD4+ cells and location of forkhead box protein P3-positive cells in diagnostic follicular lymphoma tissue microarrays correlates with outcome. J Clin Oncol 2006;24(31):5052–9.
54. Carreras J, Lopez-Guillermo A, Fox BC, et al. High numbers of tumor-infiltrating FOXP3-positive regulatory T cells are associated with improved overall survival in follicular lymphoma. Blood 2006;108(9):2957–64.
55. Byers RJ, Sakhinia E, Joseph P, et al. Clinical quantitation of immune signature in follicular lymphoma by RT-PCR based gene expression profiling. Blood 2008; 111(9):4764–70.
56. Glas AM, Kersten MJ, Delahaye LJ, et al. Gene expression profiling in follicular lymphoma to assess clinical aggressiveness and to guide the choice of treatment. Blood 2005;105(1):301–7.
57. Campo E, Raffeld M, Jaffe ES. Mantle-cell lymphoma. Semin Hematol 1999;36(2): 115–27.
58. Lundberg AS, Weinberg RA. Control of the cell cycle and apoptosis. Eur J Cancer 1999;35(14):1886–94.
59. Quintanilla-Martinez L, Davies-Hill T, Fend F, et al. Sequestration of p27Kip1 protein by cyclin D1 in typical and blastic variants of mantle cell lymphoma (MCL): implications for pathogenesis. Blood 2003;101(8):3181–7.
60. Sheaff RJ, Groudine M, Gordon M, et al. Cyclin E-CDK2 is a regulator of p27Kip1. Genes Dev 1997;11(11):1464–78.
61. Chiarle R, Budel LM, Skolnik J, et al. Increased proteasome degradation of cyclin-dependent kinase inhibitor p27 is associated with a decreased overall survival in mantle cell lymphoma. Blood 2000;95(2):619–26.
62. Solomon DA, Wang Y, Fox SR, et al. Cyclin D1 splice variants. Differential effects on localization, RB phosphorylation, and cellular transformation. J Biol Chem 2003;278(32):30339–47.
63. Lu F, Gladden AB, Diehl JA. An alternatively spliced cyclin D1 isoform, cyclin D1b, is a nuclear oncogene. Cancer Res 2003;63(21):7056–61.
64. Marzec M, Kasprzycka M, Lai R, et al. Mantle cell lymphoma cells express predominantly cyclin D1a isoform and are highly sensitive to selective inhibition of CDK4 kinase activity. Blood 2006;108(5):1744–50.
65. Krieger S, Gauduchon J, Roussel M, et al. Relevance of cyclin D1b expression and CCND1 polymorphism in the pathogenesis of multiple myeloma and mantle cell lymphoma. BMC Cancer 2006;6:238.
66. Rosenwald A, Wright G, Wiestner A, et al. The proliferation gene expression signature is a quantitative integrator of oncogenic events that predicts survival in mantle cell lymphoma. Cancer Cell 2003;3(2):185–97.
67. Wiestner A, Tehrani M, Chiorazzi M, et al. Point mutations and genomic deletions in CCND1 create stable truncated cyclin D1 mRNAs that are associated with increased proliferation rate and shorter survival. Blood 2007;109(11): 4599–606.
68. Bodrug SE, Warner BJ, Bath ML, et al. Cyclin D1 transgene impedes lymphocyte maturation and collaborates in lymphomagenesis with the myc gene. Embo J 1994;13(9):2124–30.
69. Lovec H, Grzeschiczek A, Kowalski MB, et al. Cyclin D1/bcl-1 cooperates with myc genes in the generation of B-cell lymphoma in transgenic mice. Embo J 1994;13(15):3487–95.
70. Bea S, Ribas M, Hernandez JM, et al. Increased number of chromosomal imbalances and high-level DNA amplifications in mantle cell lymphoma are associated with blastoid variants. Blood 1999;93(12):4365–74.

71. Salaverria I, Zettl A, Bea S, et al. Specific secondary genetic alterations in mantle cell lymphoma provide prognostic information independent of the gene expression-based proliferation signature. J Clin Oncol 2007;25(10):1216–22.

72. Rubio-Moscardo F, Climent J, Siebert R, et al. Mantle-cell lymphoma genotypes identified with CGH to BAC microarrays define a leukemic subgroup of disease and predict patient outcome. Blood 2005;105(11):4445–54.

73. Kohlhammer H, Schwaenen C, Wessendorf S, et al. Genomic DNA-chip hybridization in t(11;14)-positive mantle cell lymphomas shows a high frequency of aberrations and allows a refined characterization of consensus regions. Blood 2004;104(3):795–801.

74. Jares P, Colomer D, Campo E. Genetic and molecular pathogenesis of mantle cell lymphoma: perspectives for new targeted therapeutics. Nat Rev Cancer 2007;7(10):750–62.

75. Fernandez V, Hartmann E, Ott G, et al. Pathogenesis of mantle-cell lymphoma: all oncogenic roads lead to dysregulation of cell cycle and DNA damage response pathways. J Clin Oncol 2005;23(26):6364–9.

76. Bea S, Tort F, Pinyol M, et al. BMI-1 gene amplification and over-expression in hematological malignancies occur mainly in mantle cell lymphomas. Cancer Res 2001;61(6):2409–12.

77. Hernandez L, Bea S, Pinyol M, et al. CDK4 and MDM2 gene alterations mainly occur in highly proliferative and aggressive mantle cell lymphomas with wild-type INK4a/ARF locus. Cancer Res 2005;65(6):2199–206.

78. Pinyol M, Hernandez L, Cazorla M, et al. Deletions and loss of expression of p16INK4a and p21Waf1 genes are associated with aggressive variants of mantle cell lymphomas. Blood 1997;89(1):272–80.

79. Pinyol M, Bea S, Pla L, et al. Inactivation of RB1 in mantle-cell lymphoma detected by nonsense-mediated mRNA decay pathway inhibition and microarray analysis. Blood 2007;109(12):5422–9.

80. Ott G, Kalla J, Ott MM, et al. Blastoid variants of mantle cell lymphoma: frequent bcl-1 rearrangements at the major translocation cluster region and tetraploid chromosome clones. Blood 1997;89(4):1421–9.

81. Schaffner C, Idler I, Stilgenbauer S, et al. Mantle cell lymphoma is characterized by inactivation of the ATM gene. Proc Natl Acad Sci U S A 2000;97(6):2773–8.

82. Tort F, Hernandez S, Bea S, et al. Checkpoint kinase 1 (CHK1) protein and mRNA expression is downregulated in aggressive variants of human lymphoid neoplasms. Leukemia 2005;19(1):112–7.

83. Tort F, Hernandez S, Bea S, et al. CHK2-decreased protein expression and infrequent genetic alterations mainly occur in aggressive types of non-Hodgkin lymphomas. Blood 2002;100(13):4602–8.

84. Hartmann E, Fernandez V, Stoecklein H, et al. Increased MDM2 expression is associated with inferior survival in mantle-cell lymphoma, but not related to the MDM2 SNP309. Haematologica 2007;92(4):574–5.

85. Camacho E, Hernandez L, Hernandez S, et al. ATM gene inactivation in mantle cell lymphoma mainly occurs by truncating mutations and missense mutations involving the phosphatidylinositol-3 kinase domain and is associated with increasing numbers of chromosomal imbalances. Blood 2002;99(1):238–44.

86. Greiner TC, Moynihan MJ, Chan WC, et al. p53 mutations in mantle cell lymphoma are associated with variant cytology and predict a poor prognosis. Blood 1996;87(10):4302–10.

87. Louie DC, Offit K, Jaslow R, et al. p53 overexpression as a marker of poor prognosis in mantle cell lymphomas with t(11;14)(q13;q32). Blood 1995;86(8):2892–9.

88. de Leeuw RJ, Davies JJ, Rosenwald A, et al. Comprehensive whole genome array CGH profiling of mantle cell lymphoma model genomes. Hum Mol Genet 2004;13(17):1827–37.
89. Tagawa H, Karnan S, Suzuki R, et al. Genome-wide array-based CGH for mantle cell lymphoma: identification of homozygous deletions of the proapoptotic gene BIM. Oncogene 2005;24(8):1348–58.
90. Fu K, Weisenburger DD, Greiner TC, et al. Cyclin D1-negative mantle cell lymphoma: a clinicopathologic study based on gene expression profiling. Blood 2005;106(13):4315–21.

Staging and Evaluation of the Patient with Lymphoma

Bruce D. Cheson, MD

KEYWORDS

- Response criteria • Non-Hodgkin's lymphoma
- Hodgkin lymphoma • PET Scan

PRETREATMENT EVALUATION

Patients with non-Hodgkin's lymphoma (NHL) or Hodgkin's lymphoma (HL) most often present for medical attention because of signs or symptoms referable to enlarged lymph nodes or other disease-related symptoms, such as fevers, night sweats, or fatigue. They less often present with secondary effects of lymphoma on critical organs, such as bone marrow, lung, liver, spleen, or kidneys. Because of the nonspecific nature of these findings, months may elapse before the diagnosis of lymphoma is considered. Less often, enlarged lymph nodes or splenomegaly may be incidental findings during evaluation for other medical issues.

Once the diagnosis of lymphoma has been established by an experienced pathologist, a comprehensive history and physical examination provide the basis for subsequent assessment and appropriate management. The presence or absence of constitutional symptoms should be noted: fevers less than 38°C, night sweats, or unintentional weight loss of greater than 10% of body weight during the 6 months before the time of diagnosis. Other lymphoma-related complaints, including fatigue, pruritus and, in HL, alcohol-induced pain in an involved node-bearing area, should be similarly noted.[1] The history should also include questions regarding possible etiologies for the lymphoma, risk factors for HIV, or other infection-associated lymphomas. The patient should also be queried for performance status as a baseline for treatment-induced improvement or because eligibility for clinical trials may require a certain level of function. A family history may identify other members with lymphomas, chronic lymphocytic leukemia (CLL), or autoimmune disorders.

At the time of the physical examination, notation of the location and size of all lesions should be recorded by accurate two-dimensional measurements as a baseline against which to compare subsequent determinations. The extent of the liver and spleen below their respective mid-costal margins should also be noted.

Georgetown University Hospital, Lombardi Comprehensive Cancer Center, 3800 Reservoir Road, NW, Washington, DC 20007, USA
E-mail address: bdc4@georgetown.edu

Hematol Oncol Clin N Am 22 (2008) 825–837
doi:10.1016/j.hoc.2008.07.015
0889-8588/08/$ – see front matter © 2008 Elsevier Inc. All rights reserved.

hemonc.theclinics.com

Baseline laboratory studies should include a complete blood count, with careful examination of the peripheral blood smear to evaluate for the presence of circulating lymphoma cells, liver chemistries, a lactate dehydrogenase (LDH) as an indicator of tumor mass, and a serum uric acid, potassium, calcium, and phosphorus, which may identify a patient at increased risk for tumor lysis syndrome with therapy. A unilateral bone marrow aspirate with a biopsy, with a goal of at least 2 cm in length, are necessary.[2,3] The marrow should be classified as being involved with lymphoma or not and, if positive, the histologic subtype of lymphoma should be noted because of the possibility of a discordant histology. The percent cellularity should be recorded, especially in patients who are being considered for radioimmunotherapy where a hypocellular specimen precludes the use of such agents. Immunohistochemical assessment may help distinguish benign from lymphomatous infiltrates, and flow cytometry may also be of use in identifying small amounts of involvement. A serum protein electrophoresis may identify a paraprotein, especially in patients with lymphoplasmacytic lymphoma, CLL/ small lymphocytic lymphoma, or marginal zone lymphoma where it suggests bone marrow involvement. Nevertheless, this information rarely impacts on patient management.

Newer technologies, including molecular and cytogenetic studies, such as bcl-2 or bcl-6 on blood or bone marrow, or DNA microarray analysis may improve diagnostic accuracy and identify prognostically distinct subsets of histologies; these tests are currently investigational, but in the future may help direct therapy.

RESPONSE ASSESSMENT

In the absence of effective therapies, assessment of response is almost irrelevant. However, as an increasing number of effective treatments become available, standardized measures of evaluation become critical.

Prior to 1999, the lack of standardized measures led to variability among clinical trials groups and cancer centers in how response to therapy was evaluated and, thus, impeded comparisons of study results. Response was sometimes assessed prospectively, other times retrospectively, with disparity as to the size of a "normal" lymph node. The importance of standardization was emphasized by an analysis of the rituximab pivotal trial, in which minor differences in the definition of a normal-size lymph node resulted in major differences in the percentage of patients considered to have attained a complete remission.[4]

To address these issues, an International Working Group (IWG) composed of clinicians, radiologists, and pathologists with expertise in the evaluation and management of patients with lymphoma, developed guidelines that standardized how responses were assessed and defined response categories and endpoint definitions.[2] These recommendations were widely adopted by clinical trial groups and regulatory agencies. However, over time, that the need for revisions became apparent. For example, the IWG criteria relied on physical examination, with its marked inter- and intra-observer variability, CT scans, and single photon emission computerized tomography gallium scans, the latter no longer being widely used.

A major problem with the original IWG criteria was the misinterpretation of the term "complete remission/unconfirmed" (CRu). CRu was originally proposed to designate two types of responses: the first were in patients with curable histologies, such as Hodgkin's lymphoma or diffuse large B-cell lymphoma, with a large mass before therapy and for whom treatment resulted in a disappearance of all detectable tumor except for persistence of that mass, but which had decreased by at least 75% on CT scan. In as many as 90% of cases, these lesions are scar tissue or fibrosis rather than active tumor.[5,6] Instead, CRu was often applied to situations in which the sum of the product of the diameters (SPD) of multiple nodes decreased by at least 75%, even in patients with incurable histologies, which would more appropriately be considered partial responses. One consequence has been an artificial inflation of CR rates. The second type of CRu included patients with bone marrow involvement before treatment who fulfilled all of the conditions for a CR following therapy, except that the bone marrow was considered by the pathologist to be morphologically indeterminate. Instead, the term was also assigned to patients who did not undergo a repeat biopsy to confirm a complete response.

The increasing availability of 18-fluorodeoxyglucose positron emission tomography (FDG-PET) has resulted in a major change in lymphoma patient management. PET has been proposed for diagnosis (where it is not useful because of a lack of specificity), staging, prognosis, directing therapy, restaging, and after-treatment surveillance.[3,7–29]

Pretreatment staging determines the extent of disease and helps direct therapy. For decades, the Ann Arbor system has been used to determine the stage or extent of disease based on physical examination and bone marrow evaluation, with CT scans subsequently incorporated. The original rationale was to distinguish patients who might be candidates for radiation therapy from those with more extensive disease, who might require systemic treatment.[30]

Whether PET should be incorporated into the Ann Arbor staging system is controversial (**Table 1**). PET is highly sensitive in detecting nodal and extranodal involvement by most histologic subtypes of lymphoma and may provide complementary information to conventional staging methods, such as CT and bone marrow biopsy.[7,11,13,14,19,24,31–41]

Most common lymphoma histologies (eg, diffuse large B-cell NHL, follicular NHL, mantle cell NHL, HL) are routinely FDG-avid with a sensitivity that exceeds 80% and a specificity of about 90%, which is superior to CT.[31,32,35] PET and CT are 80% to 90% concordant in staging of patients with diffuse large B-cell lymphoma, follicular lymphoma, and mantle cell lymphoma.[13,35] In those patients with discordant results, PET typically results in upstaging because of the additional presumed sites of nodal,

Table 1 Recommended timing of PET (PET/CT) scans in lymphoma clinical trials				
Histology	Pretreatment	Mid-Treatment	Response Assessment	Posttreatment Surveillance
Routinely FDG avid				
DLBCL	Yes[a]	Clinical trial	Yes	No
HL	Yes[a]	Clinical trial	Yes	No
Follicular NHL	No[b]	Clinical trial	No[b]	No
MCL	No[b]	Clinical trial	No[b]	No
Variably FDG avid				
Other aggressive NHLs	No[b]	Clinical trial	No[c]	No
Other indolent NHLs	No[b]	Clinical trial	No[c]	No

Abbreviations: CR, complete remission; DLBCL, diffuse large B-cell lymphoma; MCL, mantle-cell lymphoma; ORR, overall response rate.
[a] Recommended but not required pretreatment.
[b] Recommended only if OPR/CR is a primary study and point.
[c] Recommended only if PET is positive pretreatment.
Data from Cheson BD, Pfistner B, Juweid ME, et al. Revised response criteria for malignant lymphoma. J Clin Oncol. 2007;25:580.

hepatic, or splenic disease. Concordance of PET and CT in determining clinical stage occurs in only about 60% to 80% of patients with Hodgkin's lymphoma.[7,11,19,24,37–39] Although PET identifies more lesions than CT, PET alone cannot replace CT for pre-treatment staging.[7,11,19,38]

In a meta-analysis of FDG-PET in staging of patients with lymphoma,[41] the pooled sensitivity for 14 studies with patient-based data was 90.9% (95% confidence interval or CI, 88.0–93.4) with a false-positive rate of 10.3% (95% CI, 7.4–13.8). The maximum joint sensitivity and specificity was 87.8% (95% CI, 85.0–90.7), with an apparently higher sensitivity and false-positive rate in patients with HL compared with NHL. The pooled sensitivity for seven studies with lesion-based data was 95.6% (95% CI, 93.9–97.0) with a false-positive rate of only 1.0% (95% CI, 0.6–1.3). The maximum sensitivity and specificity was 95.6% (95% CI, 93.1–98.1). Thus, PET detects more occult lymphomatous sites than contrast enhanced CT and bone marrow biopsy.[13,19,24,34,35,40,42]

PET can detect bone or bone marrow involvement in lymphoma patients with a negative iliac crest bone marrow biopsy, confirmed by histopathology or MRI.[42–44] However, PET alone is unreliable in detecting limited bone marrow involvement.[44] In patients with extensive bone and bone marrow involvement by PET, the bone marrow biopsy is typically positive. Diffusely increased bone marrow uptake on PET may also be because of reactive myeloid hyperplasia, such as with the use of myeloid growth factors.[43] PET-positive bone and bone marrow findings should be confirmed by biopsy or MRI if a change in treatment will be based on these findings. Thus, PET cannot substitute for bone marrow biopsy in lymphoma staging.

Despite the superior sensitivity and specificity of PET compared with CT, PET is currently not part of standard lymphoma staging primarily because of its expense and the generally small percentage of patients (approximately 15%–20%) in whom PET detects additional disease sites that modify clinical stage, and even fewer patients (approximately 10%–15%) for whom this modification alters management or outcome.[14,35,45]

PET/CT is more sensitive and specific than contrast-enhanced full dose CT for evaluation of nodal and extranodal lymphomatous involvement.[40,46] Schaefer and colleagues[40] reported that the sensitivity of PET/CT and contrast-enhanced CT for lymph node involvement in patients with HL or high grade NHL was 94% and 88%, while the specificity was 100% and 86%, respectively. For organ involvement, the sensitivity of PET/CT and contrast-enhanced CT was 88% and 50%, while the specificity was 100% and 90%, respectively. Tatsumi and colleagues[46] evaluated 1,537 anatomic sites in 20 patients with HL and 33 patients with NHL on an unenhanced low-dose PET/CT scanner. There were 1,489 sites concordant between PET and CT, and among the 48 discordant sites, PET correctly identified 40 sites as true positives or true negatives by biopsy or clinical follow-up.

The CT portion of the PET/CT examination for initial staging using intravenous contrast may permit a more accurate assessment of the liver and spleen compared with unenhanced CT.[28] PET/CT may represent a reasonable choice as a single-imaging modality for staging routinely FDG-avid lymphomas. The increased radiation associated with PET would be, in part, offset by the reduced radiation dose associated with the low- compared with full-dose CT.

PET/CT may be of particular value before therapy for patients who appear to have stage I or II disease and for whom involved field radiation therapy is being considered (**Fig. 1**), as additional sites of involvement would require systemic treatment. Thus, while PET may identify additional lesions during staging, prospective trials are needed to document an impact on patient outcome.

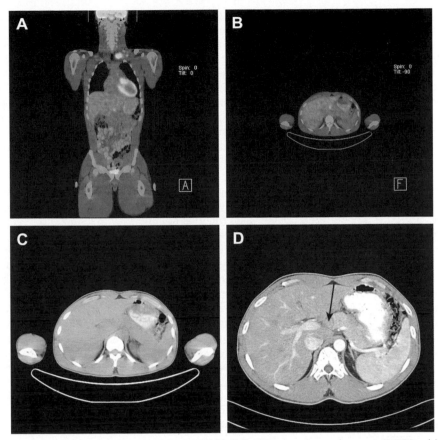

Fig. 1. Patient with nodular sclerosing Hodgkin's lymphoma who underwent CT/PET, which demonstrated supradiaphragmatic disease, with a suggestion of an intraabdominal lymph node (*A*, *B*). This node was not visible on the CT portion of the PET/CT scan (*C*). Contrast-nhanced CT was required to confirm that the patient had stage III disease (*D*).

In a recent systematic review, Kwee and colleagues[47] evaluated the role of CT and FDG-PET in staging of lymphomas. Of the 19 studies that were eligible for analysis, 3 investigated CT and 17 investigated PET. Nine of the latter included patients with Hodgkin's lymphoma, but only one of these was as part of initial staging with sensitivity and specificity of 87.5% and 100%, respectively. In the single staging study including patients with non-Hodgkin's lymphoma, the sensitivity was 83.3% with 100% lesion-based specificity. Four studies evaluated PET/CT fusion scans, but only one for initial staging.[48] The investigators concluded that CT remains the standard for staging, with FDG-PET being superior for restaging. While PET/CT was found to be superior to either modality alone, they felt that further study was needed to determine the most accurate and cost-effective method for lymphoma staging.

RECOMMENDATIONS FOR THE USE OF PET IN CLINICAL TRIALS

The clinical use of FDG-PET has far exceeded the validation of this technology in clinical trials. Juweid and colleagues[22] were the first to integrate PET into the IWG criteria in NHL. PET not only increased the number of complete remissions in patients with diffuse large B-cell NHL, but it eliminated CRus, and provided a better separation of the progression-free survival curves between CR and partial remission (PR) patients. This information, along with the increasing availability of FDG-PET, stimulated interest in revising the IWG response criteria. The German Competence Network Malignant Lymphoma facilitated this process by convening the International Harmonisation Project (IHP), including an international committee of lymphoma clinical investigators, pathologists, and nuclear medicine physicians to review the IWG and other proposed response criteria (eg, RECIST), and to determine how best to clarify and improve them to ensure transparency among clinical trials groups.[49]

The major outcomes of the IHP were a standardization of performance and interpretation of PET in lymphoma clinical trials,[28] recommended indications for the use of FDG-PET in clinical trials (see **Table 1**), and new response criteria incorporating PET, as well as bone marrow immunohistochemistry (**Table 2**).[3] Visual assessment is currently considered adequate for determining whether a PET scan is positive, and using the standardized uptake value (SUV) is not currently the standard.[28] What proportion of a reduction in SUV correlates with response is being evaluated. A positive scan was defined as focal or diffuse FDG uptake above background in a location incompatible with normal anatomy or physiology. Exceptions include mild and diffusely increased FDG uptake at the site of moderate or large-sized masses with an intensity that is lower than or equal to the mediastinal blood pool, hepatic or splenic nodules 1.5 cm with FDG uptake lower than the surrounding liver/spleen uptake, and diffusely increased bone marrow uptake within weeks following treatment.[28] Areas of necrosis may be FDG-avid within an otherwise negative residual mass, and a follow-up scan in a few months may confirm this clinical impression. Residual masses greater than or equal to 2 cm in greatest transverse diameter with FDG activity visually exceeding that of mediastinal blood pool structures are considered PET-positive, whereas residual masses 1.1 cm to 1.9 cm are considered PET-positive only if their activity exceeds surrounding background activity. However, the numerous causes of false-positive scans must be ruled out, including sarcoidosis, infection, or inflammation.[50]

Another major outcome of the IHP was a revision of the IWG response criteria.[3] The new recommendations for PET scans in clinical trials took into consideration the variability in FDG-avidity among the various lymphoma histologic subtypes, and the relevant endpoints of clinical trials (see **Table 1**). For example, PET was recommended as standard for the initial evaluation of patients with routinely FDG-avid, potentially curable lymphomas (eg, DLBCL, HL) to define the extent of disease and to provide a baseline against which to compare after-treatment studies. It is also useful in confirming whether a patient has limited-stage disease and, thus, who might be a candidate for local radiation only. For the FDG-avid but incurable histologies (eg, follicular lymphoma and low-grade and mantle cell lymphoma) PET is warranted only if complete response is a primary endpoint of the trial because time-dependent endpoints (eg, progression-free survival) are generally of greater importance.

Numerous studies have demonstrated that interim PET scans predict progression-free and overall survival.[8–10,23,24,26,27,51–53] Gallamini and colleagues[54] demonstrated that PET after two cycles of chemotherapy was a more potent predictor of outcome in Hodgkin's lymphoma than the standard International Prognostic Score. Several investigators have demonstrated that PET after one or two cycles has even stronger predictive value than a scan performed later during or after therapy.[24,27,52,54] Unfortunately, no available data demonstrate that altering treatment on the basis of PET results improves patient outcome. This critically important issue is currently being addressed in a number of clinical trials.

Table 2
Revised response criteria for assessing response in clinical trials

Response	Definition	Nodal Masses	Spleen, Liver	Bone Marrow
Complete remission	Disappearance of all evidence of disease	a) FDG-avid or PET+ before therapy mass of any size if PET−, regress to normal size on CT scan b) Variably FDG-avid or PET−,	Not palpable, lesions disappeared	Infiltrate cleared, if indeterminate by morphology, must be negative by immunohistochemistry
Partial remission	Regression of measurable disease and no new sites	≥ 50% decrease in SPD of up to 6 largest dominant masses. No increase in size of other nodes. a) FDG-avid or PET+ at previously involved site b) Variably FDG-avid or PET−: regression on CT.	≥ 50% decrease in SPD of nodules or greatest transverse diameter of single nodule, no increase in size of liver or spleen	
Stable disease	Failure to attain CR, PR, or PD	a) FDG-avid or PET+ before therapy, PET+ only at previously + sites of disease, no new lesions on PET or CT. b) Variably FDG-avid or PET−: no change in previous lesions on CT.		
Relapsed or progressive disease (PD)	New lesion or increase by ≥ 50% from nadir of previously involved sites	New lesion > 1.5 cm in any axis; ≥ 50% increase in longest diameter of previously identified node > 1 cm in short axis or in the SPD of more than 1 node. Lesions PET+ if FDG-avid lymphoma or PET+ before therapy, otherwise use CT.	≥ 50% increase from nadir in SPD of previous lesions	New or recurrent involvement

Data from Cheson BD, Pfistner B, Juweid ME, et al. Revised response criteria for malignant lymphoma. J Clin Oncol 2007;25:582.

In a study by Moskowitz and colleagues[54], 87 patients who had DLBCL were treated with an intensive R-cyclophosphamide-hydroxydaunorubicin-oncovin-prednisone regimen for four cycles delivered every 14 days followed by a PET scan. Patients who had a negative scan received three cycles of ifosfamide, carboplatin and etoposide (ICE) and observation. Patients who had a positive interim PET scan underwent a biopsy. Those patients who had a negative biopsy received three cycles of ICE, whereas those who had a positive biopsy received ICE for two cycles, rituximab plus ICE for one cycle, and were followed by an autologous stem cell transplant. The negative predictive value of the PET scan was 89%. However, the positive predictive value was only 26% with only four positive biopsies, but 27 that were negative, giving an 87% false positive rate. There was no difference in event-free survival between patients who had a positive or negative PET scan. The intensity of the rituximab-containing regimen, the timing of the scan, and the definition of a positive scan may have contributed to these findings.

PET is essential for restaging the potentially curable lymphoma histologies following completion of therapy. However, when indicated, PET scans should not be performed until at least 6 to 8 weeks following completion of therapy to reduce the likelihood of a false-positive result.[28] In these patients, where a complete remission is required for cure, therapeutic intervention is generally indicated if residual disease is present. However, PET is not recommended in the after-treatment assessment of the remaining histologies unless the PET scan was positive before treatment and if complete response rate is a primary endpoint of a clinical study.

FOLLOW-UP EVALUATION

The most important components of monitoring patients following treatment are a careful history and physical examination along with complete blood count and serum chemistries, including LDH and other relevant blood tests. Recently, the National Comprehensive Cancer Network published recommendations for follow-up of patients with Hodgkin's and non-Hodgkin's lymphoma:[55,56] for patients with Hodgkin's lymphoma in an initial complete remission, follow-up should include an interim history and physical examination every 2 to 4 months for 1 to 2 years, then every 3 to 6 months for the next 3 to 5 years, with annual monitoring for late effects after 5 years. For follicular or other indolent histology lymphoma patients in a complete remission, the recommendation for follow-up was every 3 months for a year then every 3 to 6 months. For diffuse large B-cell NHL, the guidelines proposed every 3 months for 2 years, then every 6 months for 3 years. Imaging studies should be performed when clinically indicated.

Although widely used in clinical practice, there is no evidence to support regular surveillance CT or PET scans. A number of studies in the pre-PET era demonstrated that it is the patient or physician who identifies the relapse more than 80% of the time.[57–60]

Jerusalem[61] reported a series of 36 patients who underwent PET following therapy and every 4 to 6 months thereafter. There were five events detected by PET, one in a patient with known residual disease. Two of the four patients whose relapse 5 to 24 months following treatment was identified by PET already had developed disease-related symptoms, In addition, there were six false-positive studies. Zinzani and colleagues[62] conducted a prospective evaluation of 160 patients with HL and 261 patients with indolent or aggressive NHL who underwent PET at 6, 12, 18, and 24 months after therapy. For the Hodgkin's patients, the likelihood of relapse was negligible after 12 months, and after 18 months for the aggressive NHLs. There was a continuous risk of relapse for the indolent non-Hodgkin's lymphomas. Patients with suspected relapse were biopsied and more than 40% of those with a positive PET but negative CT had a negative biopsy. The investigators concluded that there was no benefit from continued surveillance studies after 18 months.

ISSUES WITH PET(/CT)

A number of important limitations of PET remained to be resolved. Differences in equipment, technique, and variability in interpretation among readers impairs comparisons among studies. Newer technology, such as PET/CT, makes comparisons with older data difficult. Histologic subtypes also differ in FDG-avidity.[13,63–66] Moreover, there are many common causes of false-positive and false-negative PET scans.[22,28,51,67] In addition, the usefulness of PET in clinical trials requires additional prospective validation as is being conducted by the Cancer and Leukemia Group B Lymphoma Committee in multicenter studies.

Consequences of the increase in PET-directed clinical trials and the IHP revised response criteria (see **Table 2**) should include more effective therapies improving the outcome for patients with lymphoma.

REFERENCES

1. Cheson BD. Hodgkin's disease, alcohol and vena caval obstruction. JAMA 1978; 239:23–4.
2. Cheson BD, Horning SJ, Coiffier B, et al. Report of an International Workshop to standardize response criteria for non-Hodgkin's lymphomas. J Clin Oncol 1999; 17:1244–53.
3. Cheson BD, Pfistner B, Juweid ME, et al. Revised response criteria for malignant lymphoma. J Clin Oncol 2007;25:579–86.
4. Grillo-López AJ, Cheson BD, Horning SJ, et al. Response criteria for NHL: importance of "normal" lymph node size and correlations with response rates. Ann Oncol 2000;11:399–408.
5. Surbone A, Longo DL, DeVita VT Jr, et al. Residual abdominal masses in aggressive non-Hodgkin's lymphoma after combination chemotherapy: significance and management. J Clin Oncol 1988;6:1832–7.
6. Radford JA, Cowan RA, Flanagan M, et al. The significance of residual mediastinal abnormality on the chest radiograph following treatment for Hodgkin's disease. J Clin Oncol 1988;6:940–6.
7. Bangerter M, Moog F, Buchmann I, et al. Whole-body 2-[18F]-fluoro-2-deoxy-D-glucose positron emission tomography (FDG-PET) for accurate staging of Hodgkin's disease. Ann Oncol 1998;9:1117–22.
8. Spaepen K, Stroobants S, Dupont P, et al. Prognostic value of positron emission tomography (PET) with fluorine-18 fluorodeoxyglucose ([18F]FDG) after first-line chemotherapy in non-Hodgkin's lymphoma: is [18F]FDG-PET a valid alternative to conventional diagnostic methods? J Clin Oncol 2001;19:414–9.
9. Spaepen K, Stroobants S, Dupont P, et al. Prognostic value of pretransplantation positron emission tomography using fluorine 18-fluorodeoxyglucose in patients with aggressive lymphoma treated with high-dose chemotherapy and stem cell transplantation. Blood 2003;102:53–9.
10. Spaepen K, Stroobants S, Dupont P, et al. Early restaging positron emission tomography with 18F-fluorodeoxyglucose predicts outcome in patients with aggressive non-Hodgkin's lymphoma. Ann Oncol 2002;13:1356–63.

11. Jerusalem G, Beguin Y, Fassotte MF, et al. Whole-body positron emission tomography using 18F-fluorodeoxyglucose compared to standard procedures for staging patients with Hodgkin's disease. Haematologica 2001;86:266–73.

12. Jerusalem G, Beguin Y, Fassotte MF, et al. Whole-body positron emission tomography using 18F-fluorodeoxyglucose for posttreatment evaluation in Hodgkin's disease and non-Hodgkin's lymphoma has higher diagnostic and prognostic value than classical computed tomography scan imaging. Blood 1999;94:429–33.

13. Jerusalem G, Beguin Y, Najjar F, et al. Positron emission tomography (PET) with 18F-fluorodeoxyglucose (18F-FDG) for the staging of low-grade non-Hodgkin's lymphoma (NHL). Ann Oncol 2001;12:825–30.

14. Jerusalem G, Warland V, Najjar F, et al. Whole-body 18F-FDG PET for the evaluation of patients with Hodgkin's disease and non-Hodgkin's lymphoma. Nucl Med Commun 1999;20:13–20.

15. Zinzani PL, Magagnoli M, Chierichetti F, et al. The role of positron emission tomography (PET) in the management of lymphoma patients. Ann Oncol 1999; 10:1141–3.

16. Weihrauch MR, Re D, Scheidhauer K, et al. Thoracic positron emission tomography using ^{18}F-fluorodeoxyglucose for the evaluation of residual mediastinal Hodgkin disease. Blood 2001;98:2930–4.

17. Naumann R, Vaic A, Beuthien-Baumann B, et al. Prognostic value of popsitron emission tomography in the evalaution of post-treatment residual mass in patients with Hodgkin's disease and non-Hodgkin's lymphoma. Br J Haematol 2001;115: 793–800.

18. Kostakoglu L, Leonard JP, Kuji I, et al. Comparison of fluorine-18 fluorodeoxyglucose positron emission tomography and Ga-67 scintigraphy in evaluation of lymphoma. Cancer 2002;94:879–88.

19. Naumann R, Beuthien-Baumann B, Reiss A, et al. Substantial impact of FDG PET imaging on the therapy decision in patients with early-stage Hodgkin's lymphoma. Br J Cancer 2004;90:620–5.

20. Munker R, Glass J, Griffeth LK, et al. Contribution of PET imaging to the initial staging and prognosis of patients with Hodgkin's disease. Ann Oncol 2004;15: 1699–704.

21. Mikhaeel NG, Hutchings M, Fields PA, et al. FDG-PET after two to three cycles of chemotherapy predicts progression-free and overall survival in high-grade non-Hodgkin lymphoma. Ann Oncol 2005;16:1514–23.

22. Juweid M, Wiseman GA, Vose JM, et al. Response assessment of aggressive non-Hodgkin's lymphoma by integrated International Workshop criteria (IWC) and 18F-fluorodeoxyglucose positron emission tomography (PET). J Clin Oncol 2005;23:4652–61.

23. Haioun C, Itti E, Rahmouni A, et al. [18F]fluoro-2-deoxy-D-glucose positron emission tomography (FDG-PET) in aggressive lymphoma: an early prognostic tool for predicting patient outcome. Blood 2005;106:1376–81.

24. Hutchings M, Loft A, Hansen M, et al. Positron emission tomography with or without computed tomography in the primary staging of Hodgkin's lymphoma. Haematologica 2006;91:482–9.

25. Querellou S, Valette F, Bodet-Milin C, et al. FDG-PET/CT predicts outcome in patients with aggressive non-Hodgkin's lymphoma and Hodgkin's disease. Ann Hematol 2006;85:759–67.

26. Gallamini A, Rigacci L, Merli F, et al. Predictive value of positron emission tomography performed after two courses of standard therapy on treatment outcome in advanced stage Hodgkin's disease. Haematologica 2006;91:475–81.

27. Hutchings M, Loft A, Hansen M, et al. FDG-PET after two cycles of chemotherapy predicts treatment failure and progression-free survival in Hodgkin lymphoma. Blood 2006;107:52–9.

28. Juweid ME, Stroobants S, Hoekstra OS, et al. Use of positron emission tomography for response assessment of lymphoma: consensus recommendations of the Imaging Subcommittee of the International Harmonization Project in Lymphoma. J Clin Oncol 2007;25:571–8.

29. Seam P, Juweid ME, Cheson BD. The role of FDG-PET scans in patients with lymphoma. Blood 2007;110:3507–16.

30. Carbone PP, Kaplan HS, Musshoff K, et al. Report of the Committee on Hodgkin's Disease Staging Classification. Cancer Res 1971;31:1860–1.

31. Newman JS, Francis JR, Kaminski MS, et al. Imaging of lymphoma with PET with 2-[F-18]-fluoro-2-deoxy-D-glucose: correlation with CT. Radiology 1994;190: 111–6.

32. Thill R, Neuerburg J, Fabry U, et al. Comparison of findings with 18-FDG PET and CT in pretherapeutic staging of malignant lymphoma. Nuklearmedizin 1997;36:234–9.

33. Moog F, Bangerter M, Diederichs CG, et al. Lymphoma: role of whole-body 2-deoxy-2-[F-18]-D-glucpse (FDG) PET in nodal staging. Radiology 1997;203: 795–800.

34. Moog F, Bangerter M, Diederichs CG, et al. Extranodal malignant lymphoma: detection with FDG PET versus CT. Radiology 1998;206:475–81.

35. Buchmann I, Reinhardt M, Elsner K, et al. 2-(fluorine-18)fluoro-2-deoxy-D-glucose positron emission tomography in the detection and staging of malignant lymphoma. A bicenter trial. Cancer 2001;91:889–99.

36. Blum RH, Seymour JF, Wirth A, et al. Frequent impact of [18F] Fluorodeoxyglucose positron emission tomography on the staging and management of patients with indolent non-Hodgkin's lymphoma. Clin Lymphoma 2004;4:43–9.

37. Partridge S, Timothy A, O'Doherty MJ, et al. 2-Fluorine-18-fluoro-2-deoxy-D glucose positron emission tomography in the pretreatment staging of Hodgkin's disease: influence on patient management in a single institution. Ann Oncol 2000;11: 1273–9.

38. Weihrauch MR, Re D, Bischoff S, et al. Whole-body positron emission tomography using 18F-fluorodeoxyglucose for initial staging of patients with Hodgkin's disease. Ann Hematol 2002;81:20–5.

39. Menzel C, Dobert N, Mitrou P, et al. Positron emission tomography for the staging of Hodgkin's lymphoma—increasing the body of evidence in favor of the method. Ann Oncol 2002;41:430–6.

40. Schaefer NG, Hany TF, Taverna C, et al. Non-Hodgkin lymphoma and Hodgkin disease: coregistered FDG PET and CT at staging and restaging—do we need contrast-enhanced CT? Radiology 2004;232:823–9.

41. Isasi CR, Lu P, Blaufox MD. A metaanalysis of ^{18}F-2-deoxy-2-fluoro-D-glucose positron emission tomography in the staging and restaging of patients with lymphoma. Cancer 2005;104:1066–74.

42. Moog F, Bangerter M, Kotzerke J, et al. 18-F-fluorodeoxyglucose-positron emission tomography as a new approach to detect lymphomatous bone marrow. Blood 1998;16:603–9.

43. Carr R, Barrington SF, Madan B, et al. Detection of lymphoma in bone marrow by whole-body positron emission tomography. Blood 1998;91:3340–6.

44. Pakos EE, Fotopoulos AD, Ioannidis JP. 18F-FDG PET for evaluation of bone marrow infiltration in staging of lymphoma: a meta-analysis. J Nucl Med 2005;46: 958–63.

45. Rodriguez-Vigil B, Gomez-Leon N, Pinilla I, et al. PET/CT in lymphoma: prospective study of enhanced full-dose PET/CT versus unenhanced low-dose PET/CT. J Nucl Med 2006;47:1643–8.
46. Tatsumi M, Cohade C, Nakamoto Y, et al. Direct comparison of FDG PET and CT findings in patients with lymphoma: initial experience. Radiology 2005;237: 1038–45.
47. Kwee TC, Kwee RM, Nievelstein RA. Imaging in staging of malignant lymphoma: a systematic review. Blood 2008;111:504–16.
48. La Fougere C, Hundt W, Brockel N, et al. Value of PET/CT versus PET and CT performed as separate investigations in patients with Hodgkin's disease and non-Hodgkin's lymphoma. Eur J Nuclear Med Mol Imaging 2006;33:1417–25.
49. Pfistner B, Diehl V, Cheson B. International harmonization of trial parameters in malignant lymphoma. Eur J Haematol Suppl 2005, July;(66):53–4.
50. Castellucci P, Nanni C, Farsad M, et al. Potential pitfalls of ^{18}F-FDG PET in a large series of patients treated for malignant lymphoma: prevalence and scan interpretation. Nuclear Medicine Communications 2005;26:689–94.
51. Zinzani PL, Tani M, Fanti S, et al. Early positron emission tomography (PET) restaging: a predictive final response in Hodgkin's disease patients. Ann Oncol 2006;17:1296–300.
52. Kostakoglu L, Goldsmith SJ, Leonard JP, et al. FDG-PET after 1 cycle of therapy predicts outcome in diffuse large cell lymphoma and classic Hodgkin disease. Cancer 2006;107:2678–87.
53. Gallamini A, Hutchings M, Rigacci L, et al. Early interim 2-[18F]fluoro-2-D-glucose positron emission tomography is prognostically superior to international prognostic score in advanced stage Hodgkin's lymphoma: a report from a joint Italian-Danish study. J Clin Oncol 2007;25:3746–52.
54. Moskowitz C, Hamlin PA, Horwitz SM, et al. Phase II trial of dose-dense R-CHOP followed by risk-adapted consolidation with either ICE or ICE and ASCT, based upon the results of biopsy confirmed abnormal interim restaging PET scan, improves outcome in patients with advanced stage DLBCL. Blood 2006;108: 16:[abstract 532].
55. Hoppe RT, Advani RH, Bierman PJ, et al. Hodgkin disease/lymphoma. Clinical Practice Guidelines in Oncology. Journal of the National Comprehensive Cancer Network 2006;4(3):210–30.
56. Zelenetz AD, Advani RH, Buadi F, et al. Non-Hodgkin's lymphoma: Clinical Practice Guidelines in Oncology. Journal of the National Comprehensive Cancer Network 2006;4(3):258–310.
57. Weeks JC, Yeap BY, Canellos GP, et al. Value of follow-up procedures in patients with large-cell lymphoma who achieve a complete remission. J Clin Oncol 1991;9: 1196–203.
58. Oh YK, Ha CS, Samuels BI, et al. Stages I-III follicular lymphoma: role of CT of the abdomen and pelvis in follow-up studies. Radiology 1999;210:483–6.
59. Foltz LM, Song KW, Connors JM. Who actually detects relapse in Hodgkin lymphoma: patient or physician. Blood 2004;104(part 1):853–4 a [abstract 3124].
60. Liedtke M, Hamlin PA, Moskowitz CH, et al. Surveillance imaging during remission identifies a group of patients with more favorable aggressive NHL at time of relapse: a retrospective analysis of a uniformly-treated patient population. Ann Oncol 2006;17:909–13.
61. Jerusalem G, Beguin Y, Fassotte MF, et al. Early detection of relapse by whole-body positron emission tomography in the follow-up of patients with Hodgkin's disease. Ann Oncol 2003;14:123–30.

62. Zinzani PL, Stefoni V, Ambrosini V, et al. FDG-PET in the serial assessment of patients with lymphoma in complete remission. Blood 2007;110(part 1):71 a [abstract 216].
63. Hoffmann M, Kletter K, Diemling M, et al. Positron emission tomography with fluorine-18-2-fluoro-2-deoxy-D-glucose (F18-FDG) does not visualize extranodal B-cell lymphoma of the mucosa-associated lymphoid tissue (MALT)-type. Ann Oncol 1999;10:1185–9.
64. Elstrom R, Guan L, Baker G, et al. Utility of FDG-PET scanning in lymphoma by WHO classification. Blood 2003;101:3875–6.
65. Karam M, Novak L, Cyriac J, et al. Role of fluorine-18 fluoro-deoxyglucose positron emission tomography scan in the evaluation and follow-up of patients with low-grade lymphomas. Cancer 2006;107:175–83.
66. Hoffmann M, Wöhrer S, Becherer A, et al. 18F-fluoro-deoxy-glucose positron emission tomography in lymphoma of mucosa-associated lymphoid tissue: histology makes the difference. Ann Oncol 2006;17:1761–5.
67. Lewis PJ, Salama A. Uptake of fluorine-18-flouorodeoxyglucose in sarcoidosis. J Nucl Med 1994;35:1647–9.

Prognostic Systems for Lymphomas

Anna Johnston, MBBS[a], Gilles Salles, MD, PhD[b],*

KEYWORDS

- Lymphoma • Prognosis • Biomarkers • Micro-arrays

The survival of patients who have newly diagnosed non-Hodgkin's lymphoma (NHL) has improved markedly since the 1990s, with recent estimates of the 5-year survival rate in the United States increasing from 50.4% for patients diagnosed between 1990 and 1992 to 66.8% for patients diagnosed between 2002 and 2004.[1] This improvement can be attributed in part to the introduction of new treatments, such as the addition of rituximab to chemotherapy for patients who have diffuse large B-cell lymphoma (DLBCL).[2] Even with current treatment approaches, however, a substantial minority of patients are not cured of their disease. It is imperative to identify these patients at diagnosis so that novel treatment approaches can be applied while sparing patients who have good prognoses from increased toxicity resulting from unnecessary treatments. Although significant progress has been made in identifying these patients, in particular with the development of robust clinical indices such as the International Prognostic Index,[3] the biologic and clinical heterogeneity of NHL remains a substantial therapeutic challenge.

Well-validated prognostic systems are essential for the management of NHL. They enable accurate assessment of an individual patient's outcome for the purposes of prognostication and treatment selection, and they are a critical foundation for clinical trials of new therapies and new treatment strategies, enabling valid comparisons between trials and the development of strategies tailored to patient risk. Biologic prognostic factors also may enable the identification of patient subgroups that are most likely to benefit from new, targeted therapies.

CLINICAL INDICES FOR NON-HODGKIN'S LYMPHOMA
International Prognostic Index

The landmark International Non-Hodgkin's Lymphoma Prognostic Factors Project[3] was a collaborative effort of 16 institutions and cooperative groups in the United States, Europe, and Canada. The analysis of pretreatment characteristics of 2031

[a] Service d'Hématologie, Hospices Civils de Lyon, 69495 Pierre Benite, Lyon, France
[b] Service d'Hématologie, Hospices Civils de Lyon, Université Lyon-1, 69495 Pierre Benite, Lyon, France
* Corresponding author.
E-mail address: gilles.salles@chu-lyon.fr (G. Salles).

Hematol Oncol Clin N Am 22 (2008) 839–861
doi:10.1016/j.hoc.2008.07.012   hemonc.theclinics.com
0889-8588/08/$ – see front matter © 2008 Elsevier Inc. All rights reserved.

patients who had aggressive lymphoma treated with anthracycline-containing chemotherapy between 1982 and 1987 led to the development of the International Prognostic Index (IPI) based on five routinely obtained pretreatment clinical factors: age (≤ 60 vs. >60 years), tumor stage (stage I or II [localized] disease versus stage III or IV [advanced] disease), the number of extranodal sites of disease (≤ 1 vs. >1), Eastern Cooperative Oncology Group performance status (0 or 1 vs. ≥ 2), and serum lactate dehydrogenase (LDH) level (≤ 1 times normal vs. >1 times normal). Based on the number of presenting risk factors, patients can be assigned into one of four risk groups with overall survival at 5 years ranging from 26% to 73% (**Fig. 1**). A similarly valid age-adjusted index was developed for patients less than 60 years of age incorporating three risk factors: stage, performance status, and serum LDH. It should be noted that the IPI was developed before the widespread availability of positron emission tomography (PET) for lymphoma staging, and the impact of different methods of staging on the predictive value of the IPI has not been evaluated. Also, the assessment of performance status in the clinic is somewhat subjective.

Since its development the IPI has been validated in a wide variety of histologies and clinical scenarios including indolent NHL,[4,5] follicular lymphoma,[5–7] DLBCL,[8] peripheral T-cell lymphoma (PTCL) including systemic anaplastic large-cell lymphoma,[9–14] AIDS-related lymphomas,[15] transformed NHL,[16] and relapsed aggressive NHL.[17]

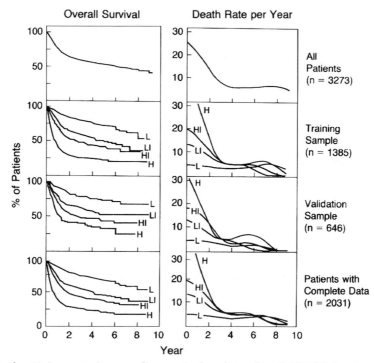

Fig. 1. Kaplan-Meier survival curves of aggressive lymphoma (mostly DLBCL) showing different IPI subgroups. The left panels show Kaplan-Meier survival curves for the four risk groups. H, high risk; HI, high-intermediate risk; L, low risk; LI, low-intermediate risk. The right panels show death rates during the study period. (*From* The International Non-Hodgkin's Lymphoma Prognostic Factors Project. A predictive model for aggressive non-Hodgkin's lymphoma. N Engl J Med 1993;329(14):990; with permission. Copyright © 1993, Massachusetts Medical Society.)

There are, however, a number of situations in which the IPI does not perform well. Although the IPI is prognostic for survival in follicular lymphoma, it has limited discriminating power, because most patients are classified in the favorable and intermediate-risk groups, with only approximately 13% of patients falling into the high-risk group.[18] In mantle cell lymphoma (MCL), the IPI has been demonstrated to be poorly discriminative in numerous smaller retrospective studies[19–22] and in a recent analysis of a large number of patients included in three clinical trials.[23] The IPI also is of limited value in localized natural killer (NK)/T cell lymphoma, nasal type.[24] In some subtypes of PTCL with an extremely unfavorable prognosis, such as enteropathy-type and hepatosplenic T-cell lymphoma, the outcome is poor even in patients who have low IPI scores. Disease-specific clinical indices have been developed to reflect better the biology of some of these entities.

Follicular Lymphoma International Prognostic Index

The Follicular Lymphoma International Prognostic Index (FLIPI) was the result of another large international cooperative effort[25] and also is based on five simple independent risk factors (hemoglobin < 12 g/dL, serum LDH levels above the upper limit of normal, Ann Arbor stage III–IV, more than four nodal sites, age > 60 years). A score based on these risk factors enables separation of patients into three approximately equal groups with survival at 10 years ranging from 36% in the high-risk group to 71% in the low-risk group (**Table 1**).

The FLIPI has become a useful, and indeed mandatory, tool for comparing patients across different clinical studies and for assessing the value of new biologic prognostic factors. It is slightly more cumbersome than the IPI for assessment in clinical practice, particularly in assessing the number of nodal areas. Although the FLIPI identifies more high-risk patients than the IPI, the 5-year survival rate of this group is still greater than 50%, and only 17% to 20% of patients under the age of 60 years fall into this group.[7,25] In applying the FLIPI in clinical practice, it is important to recognize that the FLIPI score in an individual patient may not necessarily correlate with urgency of treatment.

Mantle Cell Lymphoma International Prognostic Index

The FLIPI has been reported to be a useful prognostic index in MCL in a small series of patients,[26] but it performed poorly in an analysis of 455 patients who had advanced-stage MCL treated within three clinical trials.[23] An analysis of prognostic factors from this study led to the development of the MCL International Prognostic Index (MIPI), based on four clinical factors (age, performance status, LDH level, and leukocyte

Table 1
Prediction of follicular lymphoma patients' outcomes based on the FLIPI index

Number of Risk Factors[a]	FLIPI Score	Proportion of Patients (%)	Overall Survival (%)	
			At 5 Years	At 10 Years
0 or 1	Low	36	91	71
2	Intermediate	37	78	51
3 to 5	High	27	53	36

[a] Factors adversely affecting survival in the FLIPI include age greater than 60 years; Ann Arbor stage III–IV; more than four nodal sites; serum LDH level greater than the upper limit of normal; and hemoglobin level < 12 g/dL.

From Solal-Celigny P, Roy P, Colombat P, et al. Follicular lymphoma international prognostic index. Blood 2004;104(5):1261; with permission. Copyright © 2004 American Society of Hematology.

count), which separated patients into three equilibrated groups with significantly different prognoses. This study did not include patients who had stage I and II disease, and these findings await validation in an independent patient population. Although the authors of this study also developed a simplified algorithm, the MIPI is more complex to calculate than the IPI and thus may not be applied so readily in the clinic, but it may prove to be particularly useful in the comparison of clinical trials and validation of biologic prognostic markers.

Other Disease-Specific Clinical Indices

Peripheral T-cell lymphoma
A prognostic index for PTCL, not otherwise specified (NOS) (PIT), has been described from a retrospective study that also validated the prognostic validity of the IPI.[10] The PIT was reported to have slightly better accuracy than the IPI, but its clinical impact is questionable.

Extranodal natural killer/T-cell lymphoma
In a large series of Korean patients who had extranodal NK/T-cell lymphoma, Lee and colleagues[27] found that regional lymph node involvement, B symptoms, stage, and LDH level were the four prognostic factors retained in multivariate analyses. They used these four factors to devise a new prognostic model which was superior to the IPI in identifying patients in the higher-risk groups.

Clinical Prognostic Indices in the Era of Targeted Therapies

The value of individual prognostic factors and prognostic models may change with the introduction of new therapies that have different mechanisms of action. The IPI and the FLIPI were developed before the introduction of immunochemotherapy, and thus their predictive ability requires revalidation with new standard therapies that include rituximab. Sehn and colleagues[28] performed a retrospective analysis of 365 patients treated with cyclophosphamide, hydroxydaunorubicin, vincristine, and prednisone (CHOP) or with cyclophosphamide, hydroxydaunorubicin, vincristine, and prednisone plus rituximab (R-CHOP) in the province of British Columbia to confirm the validity of the IPI in this setting and to investigate whether a different grouping of prognostic factor scores could enhance the prognostic capacity of the IPI. They found that the IPI remains predictive in patients treated with R-CHOP but that it did not distinguish between patients at low and low-intermediate risk or between patients at intermediate-high and high risk, instead dividing patients into two risk groups. They proposed a regrouping of the IPI risk factors (the "revised" IPI or R-IPI) that allowed identification of three risk groups—very good, good, and poor—with 4-year overall survival rates of 94%, 79%, and 55%, respectively. Importantly in this study, with R-CHOP neither the IPI nor the R-IPI identified a group with a survival rate of less than 50%, suggesting a very real need for biologic prognostic markers to identify high-risk patients accurately.

In the larger, prospective RICOVER-60 trial of the German High-Grade Non-Hodgkin Lymphoma Study Group,[23] which included 1222 patients over the age of 60 years, the IPI separated both the CHOP- and the R-CHOP–treated patients into four significantly different risk groups. A recently completed analysis of the Groupe d'Etude des Lymphomes de l'Adulte (GELA) LNH98-5 trial (Gilles Salles, MD, PhD, unpublished data) also confirmed the prognostic significance of the original IPI groupings, suggesting that a revision of the IPI may not be necessary in rituximab-treated patients.

The German Low-Grade Lymphoma Study Group[29] examined the predictive value of the FLIPI in a prospective trial of patients who had advanced-stage FL that compared first-line R-CHOP with CHOP. In the 338 patients treated with R-CHOP who were evaluated for the FLIPI, the distribution of patients into the three risk groups was similar to that of the CHOP-treated patients (14% low risk, 41% intermediate risk, and 45% high risk). The major efficacy end point of this trial was time to treatment failure, and the FLIPI was able to separate high-risk patients from intermediate- and low-risk patients. It was not able to discriminate between intermediate- and low-risk patients treated with either R-CHOP or CHOP, however, possibly because of the small number of patients included in this trial. The investigators also found a regrouping of prognostic factors may have superior discriminative power. In the GELA–Groupe Ouest Est d'Etude des Leucémies et Autres Maladies du Sang (GOELAMS) FL2000 study, the FLIPI also was found to predict outcome after 5 years of follow-up in rituximab-treated patients (**Fig. 2**).

In the cohort of 455 patients from which the MIPI was developed,[23] 31% had received rituximab in initial therapy, and exploratory analyses found that the inclusion of primary rituximab treatment as a covariate did not change the final prognostic model. Thus the MIPI is valid in patients treated with chemotherapy with or without rituximab.

Further data from ongoing prospective trials will assist in the assessment of the prognostic capacity of the IPI and the FLIPI in rituximab-treated patients, although both these indices seem to retain their validity in this setting. It remains to be confirmed whether a redistribution of the IPI factors is necessary. It is imperative that prospective trials of new therapies include assessment of established clinical and biologic prognostic factors so the ongoing relevance of these prognostic factors can be determined.

BIOLOGIC PROGNOSTIC SYSTEMS

Because a PubMed search using the terms "prognosis" and "non-Hodgkin's lymphoma" yields more than 10,000 citations, it is clear that the confines of this article do not allow a discussion of all the parameters that have been shown to influence the prognosis of patients who have non-Hodgkin's lymphoma. This article therefore addresses the parameters that are encountered most frequently in routine clinical practice (morphology, cytogenetics, some individual prognostic biomarkers, PET) as well as those systems that are highly likely to be of importance in the future (gene-expression profiling and its applications), with a focus on the most frequent histologic subtypes.

MORPHOLOGY
Diffuse Large B-Cell Lymphoma

Apart from the distinct subtypes of mediastinal large-B cell lymphoma and intravascular large B-cell lymphoma, the 2001 World Health Organization (WHO) classification recognizes four variants of DLBCL (centroblastic, immunoblastic, T-cell/histiocyte-rich, anaplastic), but with poor intraobserver and interobserver reproducibility.[30] Although morphology is important in identifying distinct disease entities (in particular mediastinal large B-cell lymphoma), data are insufficient to support the use of morphologic features as prognostic factors in this disease.[31]

Follicular Lymphoma

Classic morphologic parameters identified on biopsy specimens, such as grading or the presence of diffuse areas, have not been reproducibly found to be of prognostic significance in different series and have not been adopted worldwide as standard prognostic criteria. Some reports indicate that grade 3 follicular lymphoma (3a or 3b) may have a distinct outcome,[32,33] but this finding seems to be restricted to patient

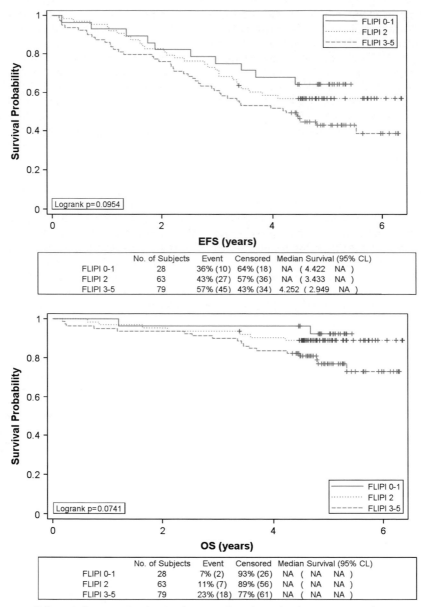

Fig. 2. Validity of the FLIPI in rituximab-treated patients in the FL2000 study. Top panel: event-free survival (EFS). Bottom panel: overall survival (OS). (Gilles Salles, MD, PhD, unpublished data, 2008.)

cohorts treated without anthracyclines. Many investigators consider grade 3b as a distinct entity and manage these patients like patients who have DLBCL.[34]

Peripheral T-Cell Lymphoma

Several morphologic variants have been recognized among the group of PTCL, NOS, but their prognostic significance is not established.[35]

CYTOGENETICS

Conventional cytogenetic studies are not part of the routine management of patients who have lymphoma in many centers. Recurring cytogenetic changes have been found in most subtypes in NHL. The molecular basis of many of these changes is understood, and a few are discussed in the subsequent sections. Some abnormalities have diagnostic rather than prognostic significance (eg, t(14;18)(q32;q21) in follicular lymphoma and t(11;14)(q13;q32) in MCL), and the prognostic impact of some of the recurrent abnormalities is uncertain because of disparate results in different studies. The frequency of detection of cytogenetic abnormalities depends on the method of detection used, including fluorescent in situ hybridization (FISH) and polymerase chain reaction (PCR) techniques that show much higher sensitivity than conventional cytogenetics. The use of different methodologies may explain some of the inconsistencies in the results from different studies.

In follicular lymphoma, some recurrent cytogenetic findings have been found to be associated with an adverse outcome including del(17p), +12 and abnormalities of 6q.[36,37] In DLBCL, t(14;18) (which is found in 13%–20% of cases using FISH) has been recognized recently to be a marker of germinal center (GC)-derived DLBCL (see the later section on gene-expression profiling).[38,39] This finding eventually may account for the favorable prognosis of cases with t(14;18) found in some series. In some studies translocations affecting the *MYC* oncogene have been found to be associated with poor prognosis in DLBCL. In one of the two recent studies that defined a molecular signature for Burkitt's lymphoma, 220 mature aggressive B-cell lymphomas were studied using gene-expression profiling, interphase FISH, and array-based comparative genomic hybridization (CGH). Of the 155 cases of DLBCL included in this study, 21% had a chromosomal breakpoint at the myc locus in association with complex chromosomal changes, and these patients had a significantly worse survival, independent of stage and age.[40]

The dismal outcomes of the so-called "double-hit" lymphomas, which harbor a 8q24/*C-MYC* rearrangement in association with a 18q21/*BCL*-2 or 3q27/*BCL*-6 rearrangement, have been recognized for some time. Although this combination is associated with transformed follicular NHL, it also may be seen in de novo DLBCL (often with Burkitt-like morphology) and, rarely, in other B-cell lymphomas.[2,40–42]

Among the T-cell lymphomas, detection of t(2;5)(p23;q35) in anaplastic large-cell lymphoma is a very important prognostic marker associated with the nucleophosmin-anaplastic lymphoma kinase (*NPM-ALK*) fusion protein and with a substantially better prognosis than seen in cases that lack the translocation and expression of the ALK protein.[43]

As discussed in the section on gene-expression profiling, new techniques such as CGH and array-based CGH enable a more comprehensive analysis of genomic aberrations associated with different lymphoma subtypes that have demonstrated prognostic value in some cases.

INDIVIDUAL PROGNOSTIC BIOMARKERS

A discussion of all of the individual biomarkers that have been assessed for prognosis in NHL is beyond the scope of this article. This discussion is restricted to a few of the better-characterized markers and their relationship to prognosis. Considerable controversy remains about the significance of some of these biomarkers. There are insufficient data to determine how their detection should modify the therapeutic strategy in an individual patient. As with clinical indices, new treatments such as rituximab have been shown to modify the prognostic value of biomarkers in some instances.

Apoptotic Proteins

BCL-2
BCL-2 is an anti-apoptotic protein located on the inner mitochondrial membrane.[44] Overexpression of BCL-2 can result from the t(14;18)(q32;q21), which brings the *BCL-2* gene under the control of the immunoglobulin heavy-chain promoter, but over-expression also can result from amplification of the *BCL-2* gene.[45] BCL-2 is expressed in most cases of follicular lymphoma, but its prognostic value seems to be in DLBCL where it is expressed in 47% to 58% cases.[45] Although translocations involving *BCL-2* have not been shown to correlate with outcome, most studies show inferior survival of patients who have DLBCL whose tumors have high BCL-2 protein expression.[46,47] It seems, however, that rituximab can mitigate the negative prognostic effect of BCL-2 expression in DLBCL.[48]

Cell-Cycle Regulatory Molecules

TP53
p53 is a transcription factor that induces the expression of genes involved in cell-cycle arrest or apoptosis in response to various toxic and oncogenic stimuli.[49] *TP53* muta-tions and stabilization of the p53 protein are associated with more aggressive clinical behavior and treatment resistance in follicular lymphoma; marginal zone lymphoma, and MCL.[49] Mutations in *TP53* have been associated with shorter survival in DLBCL in some studies, but not in others.[45] Available evidence suggests that *TP53* mutations and p53 overexpression are markers of poor prognosis in aggressive T-cell lymphomas.[50,51]

Ki-67
Ki-67 is a nuclear antigen associated with cell proliferation that is not found in resting cells and is detected using immunohistochemistry (IHC) (**Fig. 3**).[52] The prognostic sig-nificance of Ki67 in DLBCL is controversial. Although some studies have shown that high expression of Ki67 (>60% or 80%, depending on the study) is an adverse prog-nostic factor,[52,53] this finding has not been confirmed in other studies, including a study from the Nordic Lymphoma Group.[54] Different cutoffs for positivity may be one reason for the discrepancies. It also is possible that the relationship between Ki67 expression and prognosis may not be linear, and that tumors with low levels of expression may be resistant to chemotherapy.[54] Ki67 is an independent quantitative prognostic marker in MCL, and a recent study suggested that it retains its predictive

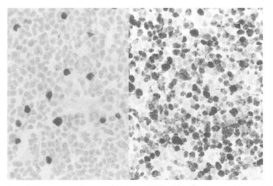

Fig. 3. Ki67 staining, low (*left panel*) and high (*right panel*), in mantle cell lymphoma. (*Cour-tesy of* Françoise Berger, Lyon, France.)

capacity in patients treated with immunochemotherapy.[55] In a tissue microarray (TMA) study of PTCL, Ki67 greater than or equal to 80% was found to be an adverse prognostic factor for PTCL, unspecified type.[56] Ki67 expression also was found to correlate with the proliferation signature in gene-expression profiling studies of nodal PTCL discussed in the next section (although not with survival in this small study).[57]

GENE-EXPRESSION PROFILING AND ITS APPLICATIONS FOR PROGNOSTIC EVALUATION

Clinical prognostic indices such as the IPI have been very helpful in defining different prognostic subgroups in NHL, but there is a substantial minority of patients whose clinical course is not well reflected by such indices in both aggressive and indolent NHL. For example, for young patients in the IPI low-risk group (0–1 risk factors) treated with six cycles of rituximab and CHOP-like combination chemotherapy, the 3-year EFS rate is 79%; thus 21% of patients will suffer progressive disease under therapy and require additional treatment.[58] Conversely, a significant proportion of patients in the high-risk groups of the FLIPI and IPI will be long-term survivors of follicular lymphoma and DLBCL, respectively.

Gene-expression profiling is a powerful technique that enables the simultaneous analysis of thousands of known genes or expressed sequence tags in tumor specimens. Microarrays constructed using cDNA or oligonucleotides are used to analyze mRNA extracted from tumor specimens. Various detection methods, coupled to computers equipped with special software, are used to measure levels of gene expression, generating a gene-expression profile for that sample.

Different methods of analysis can be applied to data sets containing gene-expression profiles of multiple tumor samples in attempts to define unique molecular signatures. Supervised analytic approaches depend on prior knowledge about the tumor samples, whereas unsupervised approaches disregard prior knowledge and can be used to look for hitherto unrecognized subgroups.[59] Unsupervised approaches have resulted in the cell-of-origin classification of DLBCL, which has prognostic significance independent of the IPI.[60]

In addition to elucidating the biology of different subtypes of NHL and identifying potential therapeutic targets, gene-expression profiling is the basis of a number of molecular classifications of NHL and has been used to generate molecular and immunohistochemical prognostic tools.

Gene-expression profiling is expensive, requiring the extraction of RNA from fresh or frozen tissue and technology and expertise that are not available in routine diagnostic hematology laboratories. Thus numerous investigators have looked at the feasibility of translating the findings into more widely applicable techniques such those based on PCR and IHC. IHC can be performed on whole-tissue sections or TMAs, a technique that allows high-throughput analysis of multiple tumor specimens. As a recent international collaborative study of TMAs in DLBCL demonstrated,[61] however, highly variable results may be obtained from different laboratories because of different techniques and interpretation. This finding highlights the need for harmonization of techniques and interpretation before these techniques can be used outside clinical trials. Although it is hoped that the data derived from gene expression-profiling studies will lead to robust algorithms that may predict the clinical course of patients who have NHL at diagnosis, at the present time these data are investigational and cannot be used to modify treatment strategies. A Cancer and Leukemia Group B trial currently underway comparing R-CHOP versus etoposide, prednisone, vincristine, cyclophosphamide, and adriamycin plus rituximab in patients who had DLBCL is the first to incorporate prospective molecular profiling.

Studies of Prognosis in Different Non-Hodgkin's Lymphoma Subtypes Using Gene-Expression Profiling

Diffuse large B-cell lymphoma

DLBCL is recognized as a very heterogeneous disease, and morphologic subclassification fails to account for the variability in outcome.[31] Alizadeh and colleagues[60] used a cDNA microarray to characterize gene expression in DLBCL and identified two distinct groups of DLBCL, GC B-like and activated B-like, with very different prognoses. The 5-year survival rate for patients who had GC B-like DLBCL was 76%, compared with 16% for patients who had activated B-like DLBCL. This cell-of-origin classification was able to distinguish patients who had distinct prognoses despite having the same IPI score and has been confirmed with models using 100 genes[62] and 27 genes[63] instead of the original 375 genes. These subsequent two reports also have identified a third category, but with poor concordance.[64]

In addition to confirming the prognostic significance of the cell-of-origin model, the study by Rosenwald and colleagues[62] identified particular genes that correlated with outcome and then combined these genes in a multivariate model that was able to categorize patients who had the same IPI score into good and poor prognostic groups (**Fig. 4**).

Shipp and colleagues[65] used a supervised approach to define prognostic subgroups using oligonucleotide arrays, by comparing molecular signatures in "cured" patients with those from patients who had "fatal/refractory" disease. The resulting algorithm classified 58 patients who had de novo DLBCL into two groups with very different 5-year overall survival rates (70% vs. 12%) and was able to subdivide the different IPI groups further.

Gene-expression profiling also has established primary mediastinal DLBCL as a distinct subgroup of DLBCL with similarities to classic Hodgkin's lymphoma[66,67] and a more favorable clinical outcome.

Lossos and colleagues[68] used qualitative real-time PCR (RT-PCR) to measure the expression of 36 genes that had been reported to be predictive of survival in 66 patients who had DLBCL. They then selected the six most predictive genes to construct a prognostic model that was able to identify patients at a higher risk of death in each IPI risk group. This model was found to be valid using previously reported microarray data.[62,65] Thus they confirmed that the powerful predictive capacity of microarrays may be distilled down to smaller numbers of genes that can be measured with more widely available techniques.

One of the genes included in this six-gene model, *BCL6-6*, is a proto-oncogene that is necessary for GC formation and is considered to be a hallmark of NHL derived from GC cells. Although *BCL-6* gene rearrangements have not been found to have prognostic significance in DLBCL, the expression of BCL-6 (mRNA or protein) is strongly correlated with superior survival, independent of the IPI.[45,69] As with BCL-2, however, it seems that the prognostic significance of BCL-6 protein expression may be eliminated by the addition of rituximab to chemotherapy. In a recent United States Intergroup study that compared CHOP with R-CHOP, BCL-6 positivity predicted a superior outcome only in CHOP-treated patients; BCL-6 status did not influence the outcome of patients treated with R-CHOP.[70]

Applying the technique of CGH to cases that had been characterized by gene-expression profiling, Bea and colleagues[71] found that the DLBCL subgroups (GC B-like, activated B-like, and primary mediastinal B-cell lymphoma) differed in the frequency of particular chromosomal changes and identified a chromosome region (3p11-p12) that was associated with a poor outcome in DLBCL and that added prognostic information to the survival model based on gene expression.

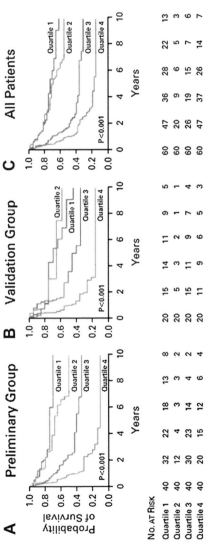

Fig. 4. Gene-expression profiling can predict outcome in DLBCL. Kaplan–Meier estimates of overall survival in patients who have DLBCL in (*A*) the preliminary group, (*B*) the validation group, and (*C*) all patients. (*From* Rosenwald A, et al. The use of molecular profiling to predict survival after chemotherapy for diffuse large-B-cell lymphoma. N Engl J Med 2002;346(25):1943; with permission. Copyright © 2002, Massachusetts Medical Society.)

Finally, two studies using gene-expression profiling have been able to define a molecular signature that distinguishes Burkitt's lymphoma from DLBCL.[40,72] Given the different prognoses and treatment of these two entities, this distinction is a critical one, and molecular diagnosis of Burkitt's lymphoma should be incorporated in prospective clinical trials.

Translation of gene-expression profiling findings in diffuse large B-cell lymphoma using immunohistochemical approaches Hans and colleagues[73] developed a TMA to classify cases of de novo DLBCL into GC B-like or activated B-like lymphoma using the expression of three antigens (CD10, bcl-6, and MUM-1). Using a cDNA microarray as the reference standard, the TMA model demonstrated reasonable sensitivity in designating cases of DLBCL as GC B-like or non–GC-B-like. In fact, when the predictive accuracy of the TMA was compared with that of the cDNA microarray, the TMA was more accurate in predicting overall survival. As the investigators pointed out, that superiority may be result from contamination of the cDNA microarray by nontumor mRNA or from discordance between mRNA and protein expression. The predictive impact of the cell-of-origin classification has been confirmed using the same or a similar algorithm in 68 patients who had de novo DLBCL treated with chemotherapy[74] and in a group of 66 patients who had high-risk DLBCL and received autologous transplantation as first-line treatment.[75] In another study of 128 cases of de novo DLBCL that used standard IHC on tissue sections rather than a TMA, however, the GC versus non-GC distinction had not effect on survival,[76] and Moskowitz and colleagues[77] found that cell of origin (as defined by the Hans algorithm) did not predict survival in a group of patients who had relapsed and refractory DLBCL undergoing salvage treatment and ASCT.

More recently, the prognostic impact of the cell of origin as defined by IHC was examined in a group of patients treated with R-CHOP and compared with a control group of chemotherapy-treated patients. Although in the chemotherapy-treated group the survival of the patients who had a GC phenotype was superior to that of the patients who had a non-GC phenotype, the immunohistochemically defined GC phenotype did not predict outcome in the patients treated with R-CHOP.[78] Preliminary data from the GELA and other groups, however, indicate that the cell of origin as defined by gene-expression profiling retains its prognostic significance in patients treated with R-CHOP.[79,80]

Follicular Lymphoma

Gene-expression profiling studies reveal that follicular lymphoma is a more biologically homogeneous disease than DLBCL at diagnosis.[81] These studies also have demonstrated the critical role of the host immune response in determining the clinical course of patients who have follicular lymphoma. Investigators from the Leukemia Lymphoma Molecular Profiling Project (LLMPP) examined the gene-expression profiles of 286 follicular lymphoma specimens and identified two gene signatures that together were strongly associated with patient survival.[82] Intriguingly, these two signatures, termed "immune response-1" (IR-1) and "immune response-2" (IR-2), were found to originate from the nonmalignant infiltrating immune cells. IR-1, associated with a good response, included genes encoding T-cell markers and macrophages, whereas IR-2 was associated with an adverse outcome and included genes preferentially expressed in macrophages and dendritic cells.

Using these two "survival signatures," investigators were able to segregate the patient population into four groups with distinct outcomes and, importantly, identified a subgroup comprising a quarter of patients that had a very poor outcome and a median survival of 3.9 years.

Since these initial findings substantial effort has gone into delineating the role of the various cells involved in the immune response to follicular lymphoma and their relationship to patient outcome. It is clear that much work remains to be done in this area, with conflicting results from a number of studies possibly relating to different methodologies and patient selection. Farinha and colleagues,[83] using TMAs to study a group of 99 homogenously treated patients, found that the group with increased numbers of CD68-positive macrophages (>15/high power field) had a poorer prognosis. This finding has been corroborated in 194 patients included in the FL2000 study by the GELA, although, interestingly, in this trial the unfavorable impact of high macrophage content was observed predominantly in patients who did not receive rituximab.[84] Another study, however, found that a higher infiltration of CD68+ macrophages was identified more frequently in patients who had low-risk features.[85] T-cell numbers and subsets also have been studied for their association with prognosis using techniques including flow cytometry and IHC.[85–88] In one study that used flow cytometry, higher numbers of CD8+ cells in lymph node biopsies at diagnosis were associated with a superior outcome.[88] Two studies have identified T-regulatory cells, defined by positivity for FOXP3, as being associated with a better outcome.[86,87] A recent study of 60 frozen lymph nodes from patients who had follicular lymphoma used RT-PCR to measure the levels of 35 genes associated with the immune response to follicular lymphoma in parallel with IHC studies. They found that CCR1, a marker of monocyte activation, was associated with a shorter survival interval and confirmed that a high number of CD68+ macrophages was an adverse prognostic marker (Blood, Byers epub 3 Jan).

Mantle Cell Lymphoma

The important prognostic role of markers of proliferation in MCL has been recognized for some time and was confirmed recently using IHC (see the earlier discussion of Ki67 in the section on individual prognostic biomarkers). A study of gene-expression profiling by the LLMPP consortium led to the development of a gene-expression–based "proliferation signature" of 20 different genes that is able to predict the survival of patients who have MCL in a linear fashion. When represented in quartiles, it could distinguish four groups with median survival ranging from 6.7 years to 0.83 years.[89] This proliferation signature also could be represented by as few as four genes, suggesting the feasibility of reproducing this system using RT-PCR.

T-Cell Lymphoma

Fewer data are available on gene-expression profiling in T-cell lymphoma. Molecular profiling can distinguish between different types of T-cell lymphoma, including PTCL, T lymphoblastic lymphoma (T-LBL),[90] and well-defined entities in the WHO classification such as angioimmunoblastic lymphoma and anaplastic large-cell lymphoma.[91] As would be suspected from their clinical heterogeneity, cases belonging to PTCL, NOS did not share a single molecular profile in one study but could be separated into three groups; this categorization did not have prognostic significance, however.[91] Robust molecular signatures associated with survival have been more elusive. A recent study of 35 nodal PTCLs (excluding anaplastic large-cell lymphoma), using a cDNA microarray and confirmed using an oligonucleotide array, identified a proliferation signature that was significantly associated with survival.[57] A study of gene-expression profiling of CTCL skin lesions also identified three groups with significant differences in event-free survival.[92]

Table 2
Summary of major clinical and biologic prognostic factors in diffuse large B-cell lymphoma, follicular lymphoma, peripheral T-cell lymphoma, and mantle cell lymphoma

Disease Entity	Prognostic Factors	Clinical	Imaging	Morphology	Cytogenetic	Molecular: Gene-Expression Profiling	Molecular: Single Marker
Diffuse large B-cell lymphoma	Established	IPI[3]	Early PET[94-97]	Subtype: primary mediastinal DLBCL[67]	t(14;18) plus 8q24/c-myc[2,41,42]	GC B-cell versus ABC[60,62,63] "cured" versus "fatal/refractory"[65]	BCL-6 expression[68-70] BCL-2 expression[46,47]
	Possible	Bulky disease >7.5 cm[58]			t(14;18) alone[38,39] gains involving 3p11-p12[71]		Ki67[52-54] TP53[45]
	Not generally useful/unproven			Variants: centroblastic, immunoblastic, T-cell/histiocyte-rich, anaplastic[31]			
Follicular lymphoma	Established	IPI,[5-7] FLIPI[25]			del(17p) trisomy 12 6q anomalies[36,37]	Immune response (IR-1 versus IR-2)[82]	
	Possible			Grade 3b[34] CD68+ macrophage content[83,84] CD8+ T cells content[88] Increased T-regulatory cells[86,87]			Host immune gene polymorphisms[93]
	Not generally useful/unproven			Grading (apart from recognition of type 3b)			

Lymphoma	Validity					
Mantle cell lymphoma	Established			High mitotic rate[30]		Ki-67[55]
	Possible	MIPI[23]		Blastic or pleomorphic variant[30]	Proliferation signature[89]	
	Not useful	IPI FLIPI[23]				
Peripheral T-cell lymphoma	Established	IPI[9-14]	Early PET[94,95,97]	t(2;5)[43]		ALK[43]
	Possible	PIT[10]			Proliferation signature[57]	Ki67[56] TP53[50,51]
	Not generally useful/unproven			Morphologic variants within PTCL, NOS[35]		

PROGNOSTIC EVALUATION IN NON-HODGKIN'S LYMPHOMA BY EXAMINATION OF THE HOST GENOME

Results from gene-expression profiling studies in follicular lymphoma and DLBCL have highlighted the importance of the host immune response in determining the outcome of patients who have NHL. Differences in host metabolism also may be of importance in chemotherapy-treated patients. Studies of the host genome, using techniques such as single-nucleotide polymorphism (SNP) genotyping, show great promise as a method of identifying clinically useful prognostic biomarkers.

Single-Nucleotide Polymorphism Genotyping

SNP genotyping of host immune and cytokine genes has been used to find biologic markers of lymphoma risk. An elegant study recently used this technique to investigate the prognostic impact of host immune gene polymorphisms on survival in follicular lymphoma.[93] The investigators hypothesized that germ-line variations in immune genes could account for the variability of survival in follicular lymphoma. Using complex statistical approaches, they were able to identify four SNPs (respectively located in the *IL8*, *IL2*, *IL12B*, and *IL1RN* genes), enabling them to build a strong outcome predictor, with estimates of 5-year survival rates ranging from 96% to 58%.

THE ROLE OF POSITRON EMISSION TOMOGRAPHY IN PROGNOSIS

It has been demonstrated convincingly that 18F-fluorodeoxyglucose (FDG)-PET performed after one to four cycles of induction chemotherapy ('early FDG-PET') is a strong independent predictor of outcome in patients who have aggressive NHL.[94–97] Spaepen and colleagues[95] in their study of 70 patients who had aggressive NHL (67% of whom had DLBCL) found that the result of early FDG-PET scanning was in fact a stronger prognostic factor than the pretreatment IPI. In the study by Haioun and colleagues,[94] which included 90 patients who had newly diagnosed aggressive lymphoma (94% of whom had DLBCL), a negative FDG-PET after two cycles of chemotherapy predicted a 2-year event-free survival rate of 82% compared with 43% (*P*<.001) for patients who were FDG-PET positive. Importantly the prognostic value of PET scanning was independent of IPI risk group and of the type of treatment given (intensification with high-dose therapy and autologous transplantation, or not, and treatment with rituximab, or not). Studies currently are underway in France, Germany, and Canada examining whether a change in treatment strategy according to the results of an early FDG-PET scan can improve the currently poor outcome of patients who have DLBCL and a positive mid-treatment FDG-PET scan.

A PERSPECTIVE ON FUTURE DIRECTIONS

A number of technologic advances are likely to facilitate the development of useful and accessible biologic prognostic tools. One of the major limitations of the application of powerful gene-expression profiling techniques for prognostic evaluation has been the need to use fresh or frozen tissues. Two recently presented abstracts suggest that in the future these techniques may be able to be applied to formalin-fixed paraffin-embedded tissues.[98,99]

The recognition of the prognostic importance of the host immune response, particularly in follicular lymphoma, has resulted in a large number of studies attempting to elucidate the complex interplay of host and tumoral factors. In this regard studies of the host genome using SNP genotyping seem particularly appealing, given the widespread accessibility of these techniques. Preliminary reports suggest the interest of these techniques in other histologies and in the elucidation of host metabolic pathways that may determine response to treatment.[100]

Although array-based CGH is a useful technique for identifying genetic aberrations that play a role in the development and progression of lymphomas, it is not widely applicable. A recent paper described a multiplex PCR-based assay that may be used to detect gains and losses of genes of possible prognostic importance in DLBCL. Using this approach, the authors of the study developed a single assay, based on the copy number of four genes, that had prognostic value independent of the IPI.[101]

The great challenges that remain are the development of robust biologic prognostic markers that can be used in routine clinical practice and the prospective validation of such prognostic markers. International and multicenter collaboration will be necessary to meet these challenges, and in this regard consortiums, such as the Lunenburg Lymphoma Biomarker Consortium should prove invaluable.

SUMMARY

At present the most robust prognostic tools remain clinical indices, although, as discussed, they have clear limitations. Clinicians should use these well-validated indices to assess the prognosis of patients who have NHL and to select an optimal therapeutic strategy. Substantial progress has been made in identifying molecular prognostic markers that in the future should enable adaptation of treatment strategies according to the patient's biologic risk profile (**Table 2**). New prognostic systems require prospective validation in well-designed studies. As a number of studies have demonstrated, the introduction of new therapies may change the predictive value of established prognostic markers, and thus there is an ongoing need for revalidation. Biologic prognostic systems need to be integrated with clinical and imaging findings, particularly in view of the growing role of FDG-PET as a prognostic tool. An ongoing challenge will be the development of prognostic systems based on the expanding molecular understanding of NHL that can be applied in routine diagnostic hematology laboratories.

REFERENCES

1. Pulte D, Gondos A, Brenner H. Ongoing improvement in outcomes for patients diagnosed as having non-hodgkin lymphoma from the 1990s to the early 21st century. Arch Intern Med 2008;168:469–76.
2. Sehn LH, Donaldson J, Chhanabhai M, et al. Introduction of combined CHOP plus rituximab therapy dramatically improved outcome of diffuse large B-cell lymphoma in British Columbia. J Clin Oncol 2005;23:5027–33.
3. The international non-hodgkin's lymphoma prognostic factors project. A predictive model for aggressive non-hodgkin's lymphoma. N Engl J Med 1993;329: 987–94.
4. Hermans J, Krol AD, van Groningen K, et al. International Prognostic Index for aggressive non-Hodgkin's lymphoma is valid for all malignancy grades. Blood 1995;86:1460–3.
5. Lopez-Guillermo A, Montserrat E, Bosch F, et al. Applicability of the International Index for aggressive lymphomas to patients with low-grade lymphoma. J Clin Oncol 1994;12:1343–8.
6. Decaudin D, Lepage E, Brousse N, et al. Low-grade stage III-IV follicular lymphoma: multivariate analysis of prognostic factors in 484 patients–a study of

the Groupe d'Etude des Lymphomes de l'Adulte. J Clin Oncol 1999;17: 2499–505.

7. Perea G, Altes A, Montoto S, et al. Prognostic indexes in follicular lymphoma: a comparison of different prognostic systems. Ann Oncol 2005;16:1508–13.

8. Armitage JO, Weisenburger DD. New approach to classifying non-Hodgkin's lymphomas: clinical features of the major histologic subtypes. Non-Hodgkin's Lymphoma Classification Project. J Clin Oncol 1998;16:2780–95.

9. Gisselbrecht C, Gaulard P, Lepage E, et al. Prognostic significance of T-cell phenotype in aggressive non-hodgkin's lymphomas. Blood 1998;92:76–82.

10. Gallamini A, Stelitano C, Calvi R, et al. Peripheral T-cell lymphoma unspecified (PTCL-U): a new prognostic model from a retrospective multicentric clinical study. Blood 2004;103:2474–9.

11. Savage KJ, Chhanabhai M, Gascoyne RD, et al. Characterization of peripheral T-cell lymphomas in a single North American institution by the WHO classification. Ann Oncol 2004;15:1467–75.

12. Sonnen R, Schmidt W-P, Muller-Hermelink HK, et al. The International Prognostic Index determines the outcome of patients with nodal mature T-cell lymphomas. British Journal of Haematology 2005;129:366–72.

13. Escalón M, Liu N, Yang Y, et al. Prognostic factors and treatment of patients with T-cell non-Hodgkin lymphoma. Cancer 2005;103:2091–8.

14. Ansell SM, Habermann TM, Kurtin PJ, et al. Predictive capacity of the International Prognostic Factor Index in patients with peripheral T-cell lymphoma. J Clin Oncol 1997;15:2296–301.

15. Mounier N, Spina M, Gabarre J, et al. AIDS-related non-Hodgkin lymphoma: final analysis of 485 patients treated with risk-adapted intensive chemotherapy. Blood 2006;107:3832–40.

16. Micallef INM, Remstein ED, Ansell SM, et al. The International Prognostic Index predicts outcome after histological transformation of low-grade non-Hodgkin lymphoma. Leukemia and Lymphoma 2006;47:1794–9.

17. Blay JY, Gomez F, Sebban C, et al. The International Prognostic Index correlates to survival in patients with aggressive lymphoma in relapse: analysis of the PARMA Trial. Blood 1998;92:3562–8.

18. Bastion Y, Coiffier B. Is the International Prognostic Index for aggressive lymphoma patients useful for follicular lymphoma patients? J Clin Oncol 1994;12: 1340–2.

19. Velders GA, Kluin-Nelemans JC, De Boer CJ, et al. Mantle-cell lymphoma: a population-based clinical study. J Clin Oncol 1996;14:1269–74.

20. Samaha H, Dumontet C, Ketterer N, et al. Mantle cell lymphoma: a retrospective study of 121 cases. Leukemia 1998;12:1281–7.

21. Oinonen R, Franssila K, Teerenhovi L, et al. Mantle cell lymphoma: clinical features, treatment and prognosis of 94 patients. European Journal of Cancer 1998;34:329–36.

22. Tiemann M, Schrader C, Klapper W, et al. Histopathology, cell proliferation indices and clinical outcome in 304 patients with mantle cell lymphoma (MCL): a clinicopathological study from the European MCL Network. British Journal of Haematology 2005;131:29–38.

23. Hoster E, Dreyling M, Klapper W, et al. A new prognostic index (MIPI) for patients with advanced-stage mantle cell lymphoma. Blood 2008;111:558–65.

24. Kim TM, Park YH, Lee S-Y, et al. Local tumor invasiveness is more predictive of survival than International Prognostic Index in stage IE/IIE extranodal NK/T-cell lymphoma, nasal type. Blood 2005;106:3785–90.

25. Solal-Celigny P, Roy P, Colombat P, et al. Follicular Lymphoma International Prognostic Index. Blood 2004;104:1258–65.
26. Moller MB, Pedersen NT, Christensen BE. Mantle cell lymphoma: prognostic capacity of the Follicular Lymphoma International Prognostic Index. British Journal of Haematology 2006;133:43–9.
27. Lee J, Suh C, Park YH, et al. Extranodal natural killer T-cell lymphoma, nasal-type: a prognostic model from a retrospective multicenter study. J Clin Oncol 2006;24:612–8.
28. Sehn LH. Optimal use of prognostic factors in non-hodgkin lymphoma. Hematology Am Soc Hematol Educ Program 2006;295–302.
29. Buske C, Hoster E, Dreyling M, et al. The Follicular Lymphoma International Prognostic Index (FLIPI) separates high-risk from intermediate- or low-risk patients with advanced-stage follicular lymphoma treated front-line with rituximab and the combination of cyclophosphamide, doxorubicin, vincristine, and prednisone (R-CHOP) with respect to treatment outcome. Blood 2006;108:1504–8.
30. Jaffe ES, Harris NL, Stein H, et al. Pathology and genetics of tumours of Haematopoietic and Lymphoid tissues. Lyon: IARC Press; 2001.
31. Salar A, Fernandez de Sevilla A, Romagosa V, et al. Diffuse large B-cell lymphoma: Is morphologic subdivision useful in clinical management? Eur J Haematol 1998;60:202–8.
32. Hans CP, Weisenburger DD, Vose JM, et al. A significant diffuse component predicts for inferior survival in grade 3 follicular lymphoma, but cytologic subtypes do not predict survival. Blood 2003;101:2363–7.
33. Ganti AK, Weisenburger DD, Smith LM, et al. Patients with grade 3 follicular lymphoma have prolonged relapse-free survival following anthracycline-based chemotherapy: the Nebraska Lymphoma Study Group Experience. Ann Oncol 2006;17:920–7.
34. Ott G, Katzenberger T, Lohr A, et al. Cytomorphologic, immunohistochemical, and cytogenetic profiles of follicular lymphoma: 2 types of follicular lymphoma grade 3. Blood 2002;99:3806–12.
35. Savage KJ. Aggressive Peripheral T-Cell Lymphomas (Specified and Unspecified Types). Hematology Am Soc Hematol Educ Program 2005;2005:267–77.
36. Tilly H, Rossi A, Stamatoullas A, et al. Prognostic value of chromosomal abnormalities in follicular lymphoma. Blood 1994;84:1043–9.
37. Hoglund M, Sehn L, Connors JM, et al. Identification of cytogenetic subgroups and karyotypic pathways of clonal evolution in follicular lymphomas. Genes Chromosomes Cancer 2004;39:195–204.
38. Huang JZ, Sanger WG, Greiner TC, et al. The t(14;18) defines a unique subset of diffuse large B-cell lymphoma with a germinal center B-cell gene expression profile. Blood 2002;99:2285–90.
39. Barrans SL, Evans PAS, O'Connor SJM, et al. The t(14;18) is associated with germinal center-derived diffuse large B-cell lymphoma and is a strong predictor of outcome. Clin Cancer Res 2003;9:2133–9.
40. Hummel M, Bentink S, Berger H, et al. A biologic definition of burkitt's lymphoma from transcriptional and genomic profiling. N Engl J Med 2006;354:2419–30.
41. Le Gouill S, Talmant P, Touzeau C, et al. The clinical presentation and prognosis of diffuse large B-cell lymphoma with t(14;18) and 8q24/c-MYC rearrangement. Haematologica 2007;92:1335–42.
42. Kanungo A, Medeiros LJ, Abruzzo LV, et al. Lymphoid neoplasms associated with concurrent t(14;18) and 8q24//c-MYC translocation generally have a poor prognosis. Mod Pathol 2005;19:25–33.

43. Gascoyne RD, Aoun P, Wu D, et al. Prognostic significance of anaplastic lymphoma kinase (ALK) protein expression in adults with anaplastic large cell lymphoma. Blood 1999;93:3913–21.
44. Hockenbery D, Nunez G, Milliman C, et al. Bcl-2 is an inner mitochondrial membrane protein that blocks programmed cell death. Nature 1990;348:334–6.
45. Lossos IS, Morgensztern D. Prognostic biomarkers in diffuse large B-cell lymphoma. J Clin Oncol 2006;24:995–1007.
46. Hermine O, Haioun C, Lepage E, et al. Prognostic significance of bcl-2 protein expression in aggressive non-Hodgkin's lymphoma. Groupe d'Etude des Lymphomes de l'Adulte (GELA). Blood 1996;87:265–72.
47. Gascoyne RD, Adomat SA, Krajewski S, et al. Prognostic significance of Bcl-2 protein expression and Bcl-2 gene rearrangement in diffuse aggressive non-hodgkin's lymphoma. Blood 1997;90:244–51.
48. Mounier N, Briere J, Gisselbrecht C, et al. Rituximab plus CHOP (R-CHOP) overcomes bcl-2–associated resistance to chemotherapy in elderly patients with diffuse large B-cell lymphoma (DLBCL). Blood 2003;101:4279–84.
49. Sanchez-Beato M, Sanchez-Aguilera A, Piris MA. Cell cycle deregulation in B-cell lymphomas. Blood 2003;101:1220–35.
50. Pescarmona E, Pignoloni P, Puopolo M, et al. p53 over-expression identifies a subset of nodal peripheral T-cell lymphomas with a distinctive biological profile and poor clinical outcome. Journal of Pathology 2001;195:361–6.
51. Moller MB, Gerdes A-M, Skjodt K, et al. Disrupted p53 function as predictor of treatment failure and poor prognosis in B- and T-cell Non-hodgkin's lymphoma. Clin Cancer Res 1999;5:1085–91.
52. Grogan TM, Lippman SM, Spier CM, et al. Independent prognostic significance of a nuclear proliferation antigen in diffuse large cell lymphomas as determined by the monoclonal antibody Ki-67. Blood 1988;71:1157–60.
53. Miller TP, Grogan TM, Dahlberg S, et al. Prognostic significance of the Ki-67-associated proliferative antigen in aggressive non-Hodgkin's lymphomas: a prospective Southwest Oncology Group trial. Blood 1994;83:1460–6.
54. Jerkeman M, Anderson H, Dictor M, et al. Assessment of biological prognostic factors provides clinically relevant information in patients with diffuse large B-cell lymphoma—a Nordic Lymphoma Group study. Annals of Hematology 2004;83:414–9.
55. Determann O, Hoster E, Ott G, et al. Ki-67 predicts outcome in advanced-stage mantle cell lymphoma patients treated with anti-CD20 immunochemotherapy: results from randomized trials of the European MCL Network and the German Low Grade Lymphoma Study Group. Blood 2008;111:2385–7.
56. Went P, Agostinelli C, Gallamini A, et al. Marker expression in peripheral T-cell lymphoma: a proposed clinical-pathologic prognostic Score. J Clin Oncol 2006;24:2472–9.
57. Cuadros M, Dave SS, Jaffe ES, et al. Identification of a proliferation signature related to survival in nodal peripheral T-cell lymphomas. J Clin Oncol 2007;25:3321–9.
58. Pfreundschuh M, Trümper L, Österborg A, et al. CHOP-like chemotherapy plus rituximab versus CHOP-like chemotherapy alone in young patients with good-prognosis diffuse large-B-cell lymphoma: a randomised controlled trial by the MabThera International Trial (MInT) Group. The Lancet Oncology 2006;7:379–91.
59. Quackenbush J. Microarray analysis and tumor classification. N Engl J Med 2006;354:2463–72.

60. Alizadeh AA, Eisen MB, Davis RE, et al. Distinct types of diffuse large B-cell lymphoma identified by gene expression profiling. Nature 2000;403:503–11.
61. de Jong D, Rosenwald A, Chhanabhai M, et al. Immunohistochemical prognostic markers in diffuse large B-cell lymphoma: validation of tissue microarray as a prerequisite for broad clinical applications–a study from the lunenburg lymphoma biomarker consortium. J Clin Oncol 2007;25:805–12.
62. Rosenwald A, Wright G, Chan WC, et al. The Use of Molecular Profiling to Predict Survival after Chemotherapy for Diffuse Large-B-Cell Lymphoma. N Engl J Med 2002;346:1937–47.
63. Wright G, Tan B, Rosenwald A, et al. A gene expression-based method to diagnose clinically distinct subgroups of diffuse large B cell lymphoma. Proceedings of the National Academy of Sciences 2003;100:9991–6.
64. Abramson JS, Shipp MA. Advances in the biology and therapy of diffuse large B-cell lymphoma: moving toward a molecularly targeted approach. Blood 2005; 106:1164–74.
65. Shipp MA, Ross KN, Tamayo P, et al. Diffuse large B-cell lymphoma outcome prediction by gene-expression profiling and supervised machine learning. Nat Med 2002;8:68–74.
66. Savage KJ, Monti S, Kutok JL, et al. The molecular signature of mediastinal large B-cell lymphoma differs from that of other diffuse large B-cell lymphomas and shares features with classical Hodgkin lymphoma. Blood 2003;102:3871–9.
67. Rosenwald A, Wright G, Leroy K, et al. Molecular diagnosis of primary mediastinal B cell lymphoma identifies a clinically favorable subgroup of diffuse large B cell lymphoma related to hodgkin lymphoma. J. Exp. Med 2003;198:851–62.
68. Lossos IS, Czerwinski DK, Alizadeh AA, et al. Prediction of survival in diffuse large-B-cell lymphoma based on the expression of six genes. N Engl J Med 2004;350:1828–37.
69. Lossos IS, Jones CD, Warnke R, et al. Expression of a single gene, BCL-6, strongly predicts survival in patients with diffuse large B-cell lymphoma. Blood 2001;98:945–51.
70. Winter JN, Weller EA, Horning SJ, et al. Prognostic significance of Bcl-6 protein expression in DLBCL treated with CHOP or R-CHOP: a prospective correlative study. Blood 2006;107:4207–13.
71. Bea S, Zettl A, Wright G, et al. Diffuse large B-cell lymphoma subgroups have distinct genetic profiles that influence tumor biology and improve gene-expression-based survival prediction. Blood 2005;106:3183–90.
72. Dave SS, Fu K, Wright GW, et al. Molecular diagnosis of burkitt's lymphoma. N Engl J Med 2006;354:2431–42.
73. Hans CP, Weisenburger DD, Greiner TC, et al. Confirmation of the molecular classification of diffuse large B-cell lymphoma by immunohistochemistry using a tissue microarray. Blood 2004;103:275–82.
74. Zinzani PL, Dirnhofer S, Sabattini E, et al. Identification of outcome predictors in diffuse large B-cell lymphoma. Immunohistochemical profiling of homogeneously treated de novo tumors with nodal presentation on tissue micro-arrays. Haematologica 2005;90:341–7.
75. van Imhoff GW, Boerma E-JG, van der Holt B, et al. Prognostic impact of germinal center-associated proteins and chromosomal breakpoints in poor-risk diffuse large B-cell lymphoma. J Clin Oncol 2006;24:4135–42.
76. Colomo L, Lopez-Guillermo A, Perales M, et al. Clinical impact of the differentiation profile assessed by immunophenotyping in patients with diffuse large B-cell lymphoma. Blood 2003;101:78–84.

77. Moskowitz CH, Zelenetz AD, Kewalramani T, et al. Cell of origin, germinal center versus nongerminal center, determined by immunohistochemistry on tissue microarray, does not correlate with outcome in patients with relapsed and refractory DLBCL. Blood 2005;106:3383–5.

78. Nyman H, Adde M, Karjalainen-Lindsberg M-L, et al. Prognostic impact of immunohistochemically defined germinal center phenotype in diffuse large B-cell lymphoma patients treated with immunochemotherapy. Blood 2007;109:4930–5.

79. Lenz G, Wright G, Dave S, et al. Gene expression signatures predict overall survial in diffuse large B cell lymphoma treated with rituximab and chop-like chemotherapy. Blood (ASH Annual Meeting Abstracts) Nov 2007;110:348.

80. Jais J-P, Haioun C, Molina T, et al. The expression of 16 genes related to the cell of origine and immune response predicts survival in elderly patients with Diffuse large B-cell lymphoma treated with CHOP and Rituximab. Leukemia 2008 Jul 10. [Epub ahead of print].

81. Glas AM, Knoops L, Delahaye L, et al. Gene-expression and immunohistochemical study of specific T-cell subsets and accessory cell types in the transformation and prognosis of follicular lymphoma. J Clin Oncol 2007;25:390–8.

82. Dave SS, Wright G, Tan B, et al. Prediction of Survival in Follicular Lymphoma Based on Molecular Features of Tumor-Infiltrating Immune Cells. N Engl J Med 2004;351:2159–69.

83. Farinha P, Masoudi H, Skinnider BF, et al. Analysis of multiple biomarkers shows that lymphoma-associated macrophage (LAM) content is an independent predictor of survival in follicular lymphoma (FL). Blood 2005;106:2169–74.

84. Canioni D, Salles G, Mounier N, et al. High numbers of tumor-associated macrophages have an adverse prognostic value that can be circumvented by rituximab in patients with follicular lymphoma enrolled onto the GELA-GOELAMS FL-2000 trial. J Clin Oncol 2008;26:440–6.

85. Alvaro T, Lejeune M, Salvado M-T, et al. Immunohistochemical patterns of reactive microenvironment are associated with clinicobiologic behavior in follicular lymphoma patients. J Clin Oncol 2006;24:5350–7.

86. Carreras J, Lopez-Guillermo A, Fox BC, et al. High numbers of tumor-infiltrating FOXP3-positive regulatory T cells are associated with improved overall survival in follicular lymphoma. Blood 2006;108:2957–64.

87. Lee AM, Clear AJ, Calaminici M, et al. Number of CD4+ cells and location of forkhead box protein P3-positive cells in diagnostic follicular lymphoma tissue microarrays correlates with outcome. J Clin Oncol 2006;24:5052–9.

88. Wahlin BE, Sander B, Christensson B, et al. CD8+ T-cell content in diagnostic lymph nodes measured by glow cytometry is a predictor of survival in follicular lymphoma. Clin Cancer Res 2007;13:388–97.

89. Rosenwald A, Wright G, Wiestner A, et al. The proliferation gene expression signature is a quantitative integrator of oncogenic events that predicts survival in mantle cell lymphoma. Cancer Cell 2003;3:185–97.

90. Martinez-Delgado B, Melendez B, Cuadros M, et al. Expression profiling of T-cell lymphomas differentiates peripheral and lymphoblastic lymphomas and defines survival related genes. Clin Cancer Res 2004;10:4971–82.

91. Ballester B, Ramuz O, Gisselbrecht C, et al. Gene expression profiling identifies molecular subgroups among nodal peripheral T-cell lymphomas. Oncogene 2005;25:1560–70.

92. Shin J, Monti S, Aires DJ, et al. Lesional gene expression profiling in cutaneous T-cell lymphoma reveals natural clusters associated with disease outcome. Blood 2007;110:3015–27.

93. Cerhan JR, Wang S, Maurer MJ, et al. Prognostic significance of host immune gene polymorphisms in follicular lymphoma survival. Blood 2007;109:5439–46.
94. Haioun C, Itti E, Rahmouni A, et al. [18F]fluoro-2-deoxy-D-glucose positron emission tomography (FDG-PET) in aggressive lymphoma: an early prognostic tool for predicting patient outcome. Blood 2005;106:1376–81.
95. Spaepen K, Stroobants S, Dupont P, et al. Early restaging positron emission tomography with 18F-fluorodeoxyglucose predicts outcome in patients with aggressive non-Hodgkin's lymphoma. Ann Oncol 2002;13:1356–63.
96. Kostakoglu L, Goldsmith SJ, Leonard JP, et al. FDG-PET after 1 cycle of therapy predicts outcome in diffuse large cell lymphoma and classic Hodgkin disease. Cancer 2006;107:2678–87.
97. Mikhaeel NG, Hutchings M, Fields PA, et al. FDG-PET after two to three cycles of chemotherapy predicts progression-free and overall survival in high-grade non-Hodgkin lymphoma. Ann Oncol 2005;16:1514–23.
98. Rimsza LM, LeBlanc ML, Roberts RA, et al. Major Histocompatibility class II (MHCII) and germinal center associated gene expression correlate with overall survival in ritiximab and CHOP-like treated diffuse large B cell lymphoma (DLBCL) patients using formalin fixed paraffin embedded (FFPE) tissues. Blood (ASH Annual Meeting Abstracts) Nov 2007;110:50.
99. Malumbres R, Johnson NA, Sehn LH, et al. Paraffin-based 6-gene model predicts outcome of diffuse large B-cell lymphoma patients treated with R-CHOP. Blood (ASH Annual Meeting Abstracts) Nov 2007;110:49.
100. Cerhan JR, Maurer MJ, Hartge P, et al. Polymorphisms in one-carbon metabolism genes and overall survival in diffuse large B-cell lymphoma (DLBCL). ASH Blood (ASH Annual Meeting Abstracts) Nov 2007;110:49.
101. Jardin F, Ruminy P, Kerckaert J-P, et al. Detection of somatic quantitative genetic alterations by multiplex polymerase chain reaction for the prediction of outcome in diffuse large B-cell lymphomas. Haematologica 2008;93:543–50.

Follicular Lymphoma: Clinical Features and Treatment

Daryl Tan, MBBS, MRCP[a],*, Sandra J. Horning, MD[b]

KEYWORDS

- Follicular • Non-Hodgkin's Lymphoma • Indolent
- Treatment

Follicular lymphoma (FL) is the second most common subtype of non-Hodgkin's lymphoma (NHL) in the Western world, constituting up to 22% of the total cases of NHL.[1] There is geographic variation, with the incidence of FL reported to be lower in Asia. In the West, up to 85% of FL cases have a detectable rearrangement of the B-cell lymphoma 2 (*Bcl-2*) gene, a genetic hallmark of the disease. FL is characterized by an indolent clinical course, with recurrent remissions and relapses. Ultimately FL is the primary or contributing cause of mortality in most patients who have FL. In many cases, the terminal phase of the disease is associated with transformation to an aggressive lymphoma, an event reported to have an incidence ranging from 16% to 60%.[2–5] Recent data indicate that median survivals in FL have increased to 10 or more years, as the result, at least in part, of progress in treatment as detailed in this article.

CLINICAL CHARACTERISTICS

Most patients who have FL present with the disease in the sixth to seventh decade of life, and no gender imbalance is observed. Clinically, patients most often manifest painless peripheral lymphadenopathy involving the cervical, axillary, inguinal, or femoral regions. They may provide a history of waxing and waning lymph node size before diagnosis. Upon complete diagnostic staging, widespread disease usually is observed. Despite advanced disease, constitutional B symptoms of fever, sweats, or weight loss occur in only a small minority of patients. Abdominal and pelvic lymphadenopathy is seen regularly on CT imaging. Intrathoracic adenopathy may be appreciated radiographically but rarely is bulky. Compression of normal structures within the abdominal cavity, marked splenomegaly, pleural effusion, and ascites may be observed but are uncommon. Extranodal disease other than in bone marrow is

[a] Department of Hematology, Singapore General Hospital, Outram Road, Singapore 169608
[b] Department of Medicine/Oncology, Stanford Cancer Center, 875 Blake Wilbur Drive, Suite 2338, Stanford, CA 94305-5821, USA
* Corresponding author.
E-mail address: daryl.tan@sgh.com.sg (D. Tan).

Hematol Oncol Clin N Am 22 (2008) 863–882
doi:10.1016/j.hoc.2008.07.013
0889-8588/08/$ – see front matter © 2008 Elsevier Inc. All rights reserved.

hemonc.theclinics.com

uncommon, although microscopic involvement of the liver as well as the spleen was appreciated when surgical staging was used several decades ago. Unusual and distinct forms of FL beyond the scope of this article occur in pediatric patients and are limited to the gastrointestinal tract and the skin.[6,7] Bone marrow involvement, assessed by percutaneous biopsy, occurs in 60% to 70% of cases. Laboratory abnormalities may include anemia, elevation of lactate dehydrogenase, cytopenias caused by extensive splenic and/or marrow involvement, and, very rarely, circulating tumor cells. Most patients, however, have normal laboratory values at diagnosis. Thus, when the Ann Arbor staging system is used, about 80% of patients are found to have stage III or IV disease, and most of these patients are clinically well.

Clinical heterogeneity within advanced disease at diagnosis is well known to clinicians but has been difficult to categorize. Variability in tumor burden has been captured by summing the products of the diameters of measurable disease, describing the number of nodal sites involved, assessing tumor bulk, and by using other parameters as discussed in the following sections.

PROGNOSTIC INDICATORS

The International Prognostic Index developed for aggressive NHL is only moderately discriminating for FL.[8] The Follicular Lymphoma International Prognostic Index (FLIPI), developed by an international consortium, separates patients into three distinct risk categories for overall survival and provides a balanced distribution of patients.[9] Five factors (age > 60 years, more than four nodal sites, hemoglobin < 12 G/dL, advanced stage, and elevated lactate dehydrogenase level) are combined to create a score that can range from 0 to 5 and to categorize patients as being at low (0–1), intermediate (2), or high (3–5) risk. As shown in **Table 1**, less than 20% of younger patients have high-risk disease. The FLIPI has been validated in multiple reports and has been shown to predict progression-free (PFS) and overall (OS) survival. Notably, the FLIPI continues to be prognostic in the current era of anti-CD20 monoclonal antibody therapy.[10] The FLIPI is a useful tool for communicating clinical trial results and comparing populations across studies. It also can be useful in stratifying patients for clinical studies. Clearly, however, it is not appropriate to use the FLIPI as an exclusive guide to initial therapy. For instance, among multiple recent clinical trials limiting eligibility to patients "requiring treatment" according to protocol specification, fewer than half the patients enrolled had high-risk FLIPI scores.[11,12] Notably, an international registration study suggests that, with modern antibody therapy, improvements in early survival are observed across intermediate- and high-risk groups, reducing the differences between

Table 1 Follicular Lymphoma International Prognostic Index (FLIPI): effect of age			
FLIPI Risk	**% Patients**	**5-Year Survival (%)**	**10-Year Survival (%)**
<60 years			
Low	43	94	77
Intermediate	40	82	57
High	17	63	50
≥60 years			
Low	20	87	65
Intermediate	32	72	47
High	48	47	30

these patients and those at lower risk.[13] Finally, it has been suggested that the number of factors in the high-risk category be adjusted within the context of treatment with rituximab-chemotherapy combinations.[10] Together, these observations indicate that the FLIPI detects differences in the prognosis of patients who have FL that inform clinical investigation but should be used in context for individual patient management.

The Groupe d'Etude Lymphome Folliculaires (GELF) introduced an alternate prognostic system related to tumor burden, which it has used in several clinical trials.[14] Patients who had a high tumor burden had one or more of a series of adverse factors, including marked splenomegaly, a single tumor site larger than 7 cm, three or more nodal sites 3 cm or larger, cytopenias, leukemia, compressive symptoms, or effusions. Modifications of this system have been made over time and also with the inclusion of β2 microglobulin as a laboratory marker of tumor burden. The GELF system of tumor burden, which captures more information about tumor volume and its impact, does not completely overlap with the FLIPI but instead may be viewed as a complementary system.[15]

Prognostic schemas represent the clinical manifestations of the underlying biology of the lymphoma and host. The World Health Organization subclassifies FL into three grades based on the Berard system, in which the number of centroblasts in 10 neoplastic follicles per high power field is counted.[16] These distinctions have limited clinical significance, however, and are poorly reproducible. A study by Hans and colleagues[17] demonstrated that newly diagnosed patients who have stage IIIA and IIIB disease have no significant differences in clinical characteristics, OS, or event-free survival (EFS) when treated with anthracycline-containing chemotherapy regimens. Instead, the presence of a significant diffuse component predicted worse survival.[17] In the forthcoming revision of the World Health Organization classification, grade 3 FL with diffuse areas will be classified as diffuse large B-cell lymphoma, a modification that should lead to greater clarity for both pathologists and clinicians. Meanwhile, clinical pathologists and molecular and cellular biologists have made strides in elucidating FL biology that promise future clinical application.

In addition to morphologic features, cytogenetic features of FL have been associated with prognosis, and with the advent of gene-expression profiling genetic features associated with a rapidly progressive course were described.[18] In a landmark publication, investigators from the National Cancer Institute identified discrete FL gene expression profiles, termed "immune-response 1" and "immune response 2," as powerful predictors of OS.[19] Unexpectedly, the prognostic information was associated with the nonmalignant infiltrating immune component, T cells, and macrophages. This important work spawned multiple investigations of the FL microenvironment with immunohistochemical investigations describing the numbers and location of immune cells and microvasculature.[17,20–22] The somewhat contradictory results in this active area of investigation may be explained, in part, by the context of the findings and the impact of treatment. Another potentially important aspect of FL biology indicating clinical course may be host polymorphisms that predict susceptibility and recently have been reported to correlate with OS.[23] Although considerable work remains in sorting though the complexity host and treatment impact in FL, there is optimism that the clinical prognostic factors in FL soon will be augmented by biologic factors.

CLINICAL COURSE

The clinical course of FL is highly variable, with some patients dying within 5 years of diagnosis and others alive and well more than 30 years later.[24] In general, the disease is sensitive to a variety of therapies at diagnosis but follows a remitting and relapsing course over time. When asymptomatic patients who have a low tumor burden are observed without initial treatment, a management strategy referred to as "watchful waiting," the rate of tumor progression frequently is slow, and spontaneous regressions of disease have been reported.[2] Similarly, disease in patients observed upon relapse after treatment typically follows a indolent course with periods of waxing and waning lymphadenopathy. Alternately, a relatively abrupt increase in tumor size, onset of constitutional or tumor-related symptoms, or new signs and symptoms may herald the transformation of FL to an aggressive NHL. Over time, the development of refractory FL, transformation, or complications of the treatment and immune suppression significantly shorten life expectancy for patients who have FL.[25]

Survival in FL remained unchanged for many years but has improved during the past 2 decades.[25] The data used to define the FLIPI recorded a median survival of 10 years.[9] Data from successive clinical trials conducted by the Southwest Oncology Group (SWOG) indicated that patients who had FL were living longer.[26] Likewise, data from the United States Surveillance, Epidemiology, and End Results program demonstrated survival gains in the FL population.[27] Institutional data from the M.D. Anderson Cancer Center and Stanford University show longer OS in patients who have FL.[28,29] In fact, the Stanford data indicate that median survival in patients diagnosed after 1986 is in excess of 18 years. Although rituximab has greatly affected the management of FL, as described later, it is not solely responsible for these gains, because improved survivals antedated the use of immunotherapy in some series.[29] Although the causes of the longer survivals are not completely explained, they may be related to improved diagnostics, better management including supportive care, increased awareness of and improved outcome for transformed lymphoma, and the expansion of the therapeutic armamentarium with rituximab and various other treatments described later in this article.

TRANSFORMATION

The frequency of histologic transformation to an aggressive lymphoma has been variably estimated from 20% to 60% or even higher in autopsy series.[3,4,30,31] In most clinical series, the risk is about 3% per year. Series differ, however, in the policy of biopsy with each FL recurrence, clinical suspicion for transformation, adequacy of the biopsy sample, and, in some instances, whether a clinical definition of transformation has been met. In general, histologic transformation is associated with very limited survival, less than 12 months in many case series. Investigators at Stanford University reported that individuals who had a limited extent of transformation and who were treatment naïve had better OS, with a median of 1.8 years.[30] In fact, transformed lymphomas prove either to be a fatal evolution of FL or are eradicated successfully with treatment. Recent reports from the British Columbia Cancer Agency and Stanford University indicate that treatment for transformed lymphoma has improved in the last several years, largely through the incorporation of rituximab, which has significantly improved the prognosis of de novo aggressive lymphoma.[32,33]

Researchers from St. Bartholomew's Hospital in England have studied transformed lymphoma carefully in the setting of an institutional policy of biopsying patients who have FL at each relapse.[31] Their data indicate a higher rate of relapse among patients who had high FLIPI scores at diagnosis and advanced-stage disease. Of note, these investigators found a higher risk of transformation with expectant management. An earlier series from the GELF associated the risk of transformation with higher tumor burden.[14] Whether biologic features at diagnosis and/or initial treatment influence the risk of transformation is an area of intense, ongoing investigation.[22] In some series the risk of transformation was seen to plateau by 20 years, but others have observed an ongoing risk.[31]

PRIMARY MANAGEMENT

Several principles have long guided the initial management of FL. First, treatment is not curative for most patients who have advanced disease. For these patients the goal of treatment is to ameliorate signs and symptoms of disease and to maintain treatment for the longest time possible, emphasizing quality of life. With a median age of about 60 years, many patients who have FL are older and may have significant comorbidities that influence treatment decisions. Furthermore, because many patients are asymptomatic and have a limited amount of slow-growing disease, and because conventional treatment is associated with morbidity, close observation has been considered appropriate for selected patients.[2,34] Changes in the last several years have called these principles into question. Specifically, rituximab is a well-tolerated therapy with proven efficacy, alone and in combination. Many new agents on the horizon have novel mechanisms and, in some cases, more targeted effects. Transplantation data have matured. Finally, advances in understanding the biologic underpinnings of FL behavior hold the promise for more tailored management for individual patients. With these points in mind, a review of primary FL treatments follows.

Observation

Stanford investigators popularized the concept of no initial treatment for selected FL patients and reported on the natural history of the disease with this approach.[2,34] The median time to starting treatment in their series was more than 4 years after diagnosis, and median survival rates were comparable with or superior to those of patients treated immediately. In several series, 15% to 20% of patients had received no treatment 10 years or more after diagnosis.[14,35] The rate of histologic transformation was similar in the Stanford series comparing patients enrolled in clinical trials and treated immediately and those who received no initial therapy.[2] Clinical indications for treatment include symptoms arising from progressive local disease, a change in the tempo of the disease, systemic or constitutional symptoms, threatened end-organ function, significant cytopenia caused by marrow infiltration, and transformation to an aggressive histology. Guidelines established by the British National Lymphoma Investigation and GELF groups have been used to determine the appropriateness of initiating treatment or for trial stratification.[14,35] Each of three randomized trials demonstrated no significant difference in OS between the expectant approach of observation and immediate treatment in advanced FL.[14,35,36] The treatment arms in these studies varied from relatively mild single-agent chlorambucil in the United Kingdom study to either interferon-α or prednimustine in the French study or an aggressive regimen of prednisone, cyclophosphamide, doxorubicin, etoposide, procarbazine, methotrexate, vincristine (ProMACE-MOPP) chemotherapy and low-dose total lymphoid irradiation in the United States study. None demonstrated any discernible advantage to immediate treatment in asymptomatic patients who had low-tumor-burden FL. These data supported the approach of watchful waiting in the pre-rituximab era. As discussed in later sections, the tolerability and single-agent activity of rituximab have led to a reconsideration of advisability of deferring treatment and presents an option for patients who are uncomfortable with waiting. To address this issue, an international study is in progress comparing observation and rituximab monotherapy in patients who have advanced-stage, low-tumor-burden FL.

Chemotherapy

Over the years, many studies compared combination and single-agent chemotherapy approaches in FL without determining a significant prolongation in time to progression (TTP) or OS. Historically, response rates of 70% to 80% were achieved with chemotherapy based on the alkylating agents chlorambucil or cyclophosphamide, vincristine, and prednisone (CVP), and the TTP was approximately 2 years.[37,38] Despite enthusiasm for the incorporation of doxorubicin and higher response rates observed, the regimen of cyclophosphamide, doxorubicin, vincristine, prednisone (CHOP) did not significantly prolong TTP compared with oral chlorambucil.[39] A United States study comparing CHOP-bleomycin chemotherapy with oral cyclophosphamide found no significant differences in disease progression or OS.[40] The purine analogue fludarabine represented a novel chemotherapeutic with an impressive response rate (65%) as a single agent.[41] Combination therapies followed with mitoxantrone in the fludarabine (FN), mitoxantrone (FM), and fludarabine, mitoxantrone, and dexamethasone (FMD) regimens and with mitoxantrone and cyclophosphamide (FCM) combination.[42–44] FN was not further pursued in the United States after a phase II study.[43] An international study comparing fludarabine and low-dose CVP found a significantly higher complete response rate for fludarabine.[45] Unfortunately, consistent with prior history, this improved complete response rate did not translate into superior TTP or OS. Together, these data indicated the lack of progress with conventional chemotherapy in FL and increased the interest in alternate approaches such as immunotherapy. Ironically, the success with rituximab has again raised the question of the preferred regimen for combined chemotherapy.

Rituximab

The major therapeutic advance in the treatment of FL during the past several decades is the chimeric, anti-CD20 monoclonal antibody, rituximab. Responses were observed even after single infusions in early-phase studies and at all doses studied.[46] In the pivotal trial in patients who had relapsed disease, the response rate in FL was 60%.[47] The next step was to investigate rituximab monotherapy in untreated patients. More than 70% of patients who have FL with a low tumor burden or other favorable factors responded to rituximab with a TTP of about 2 years.[48,49] Complete responses occurred in a little more than a third of cases. Although the familiar pattern of continued relapses in FL was observed, a subset of 15% of patients was alive and disease-free at 7 years, and 91% of the patients were alive at that time.[50] Based on the brevity of the 4-week course of rituximab, the favorable safety profile of this agent, and the ability to re-treat patients successfully, extended or maintenance courses of rituximab were administered both to treatment-naïve and to chemotherapy-treated patients.[48,51] Extended courses of treatment resulted in longer remissions with an excellent safety profile. For instance, the Swiss Group for Clinical Cancer Research (SAKK) reported that a prolonged rituximab treatment of four additional infusions every 2 months improved TTP from 12 to 23 months ($P = .02$) after a standard rituximab induction.[51] These experiences led to the next question: the optimal schedule and duration of maintenance rituximab.

In a European study conducted by the SAKK, a short maintenance schedule of four treatments every 2 months was compared with a prolonged maintenance, in which rituximab was administered every 2 months until the disease became refractory to rituximab. Similarly, the Eastern Cooperative Oncology Group (ECOG) 4402 trial entails initiating four weekly doses of rituximab for all patients who have low-tumor-burden, advanced-stage FL and randomly assigning responders to rituximab maintenance (a single dose of rituximab administered every 3 months until progression) or to re-treatment with rituximab only on progression.[52] This trial builds upon a randomized phase II study in previously treated patients in which median PFS was 31.3 months in the maintenance arm (four weekly doses of rituximab administered every 6 months for a maximum of four courses or until progression) versus 7.4 months in the re-treatment group, but neither arm was clearly superior with regard to the duration of rituximab benefit.[48] As noted earlier, an ongoing international trial led by investigators in the United Kingdom features a quality-of-life instrument in the context of an extended course of rituximab monotherapy versus watchful waiting.

Rituximab in Combination with Chemotherapy

The efficacy of rituximab, together with its unique mechanism of action and lack of he-matologic toxicity, suggested that combined chemotherapy and rituximab would be safe and effective. The remarkable data in **Table 2** describe the results of several ran-domized, controlled trials in which the quality of response, TTP, and, in some cases, OS were improved when conventional chemotherapy was combined with rituxi-mab.[11,12,15,53] Eligibility for each of four studies was limited to patients who met crite-ria for requiring treatment. The rituximab plus CHOP (R-CHOP) study of the German Low-Grade Study Group (GLSG) had a second randomization to autologous trans-plantation or interferon for young patients and two different schedules of interferon for older patients.[12] Interferon also was integrated into the treatment program in the studies of melphalan, cyclophosphamide, and prednisone with or without rituximab (MCP ± R) and of cyclophosphamide, hydroxydaunomycin, teniposide, prednisone with or without rituximab (CHVP ± R).[15,53]

Table 2
Randomized trials of chemotherapy plus CD20-based therapies versus chemotherapy in patients who had previously untreated FL

Study (Reference)	N Patients	Therapy Required	3-Year PFS (%)	P-Value
Marcus[11,54]				
CVP	321	Yes	35	<.0001
R-CVP			65	
Hiddemann[12]				
CHOP +[a]	428	Yes	63	.0004
R-CHOP +[a]			84	
Herold[53]				
MCP + IFN	196	Yes	52	<.0001
R-MCP + IFN			80	
Salles[15]				
CHVP-IFN	359	Yes	62	.003
R-CHVP-IFN			78	
Hochster[55]				
CVP	287	No	36	<.0001
CVP + R			62	
Hagenbeek[66]				
CT[b]	414	No	28	.001
CT + RIT[b]			46	

Abbreviation: INF, interferon.
 [a] Interferon versus autotransplantation for young patients and high-versus low-dose interferon for older patients.
 [b] Chemotherapy of choice; RIT = 90-Y ibritumomab tiuxetan.

Despite differences in the chemotherapy regimen, study design, and ancillary therapies, the impact of rituximab on the TTP in the experimental arms was notably similar. Although the results are dramatic, each of these studies illustrates a continued relapse pattern. In three of the four rituximab-chemotherapy trials, the OS was significantly longer in rituximab-treated patients, and these trials were the first randomized, controlled trials to demonstrate a significant advance in the treatment of stage III–IV FL.[12,53,54] It will be of great interest to determine the impact and use of rituximab as second-line treatment within the context of this international experience.

The ECOG 1496 study studied rituximab in combination with chemotherapy for consolidation/maintenance following CVP chemotherapy in advanced indolent lymphoma.[55] As detailed in **Table 2**, PFS in patients who had FL was significantly prolonged in the rituximab arm versus the observation arm (4.3 vs. 1.5 years).[55] The E1496 study included patients who had low and high tumor burden. The survival difference in this study did not meet statistical significance, although a strong trend ($P = .06$) was observed in patients who had high tumor burden. These results, and those with R-CVP and the other combinations, raise the question as to whether maintenance rituximab would further lengthen PFS and, possibly, OS. Among rituximab-naïve patients who had recurrent FL, maintenance rituximab prolonged PFS after chemotherapy alone or after chemotherapy combined with rituximab.[56] The objective of the recently completed international Primary Rituximab and Maintenance trial in patients who have untreated FL is to determine if maintenance rituximab results in superior outcomes after rituximab-chemotherapy induction.

Radioimmunotherapy

Radioimmunotherapy (RIT) allows the delivery of radiation with a unique radiobiology to lymphoma cells while minimizing the exposure of nonmalignant cells. Two radioimmunoconjugates that target the CD20 antigen, ^{131}I-tositumomab (Bexxar) and ^{90}Y-ibritutomab tiuxetan (Zevalin), have been approved for the treatment of recurrent FL.[57,58] These radioimmunoconjugates resulted in high response rates relative to alternate or historical therapies in the relapsed/refractory setting. A subset of patients had prolonged remissions, and activity was demonstrated after failure of rituximab.[59-62] Kaminski and colleagues[63] used ^{131}I-tositumomab in untreated patients who had advanced-stage FL, achieving a complete response rate of 75%. After a median follow-up of 5.1 years, the 5-year PFS rate was 59%, with a median PFS of 6.1 years. Thereafter, the SWOG administered six cycles of CHOP chemotherapy followed 4 to 8 weeks later by ^{131}I-tositumomab to an unselected group of patients who had advanced FL, achieving a complete response rate of 69%.[64] The 5-year PFS rate was 67%. A phase III Intergroup trial led by the SWOG comparing R-CHOP with CHOP plus ^{131}I-tositumomab has been completed recently, and results are eagerly awaited. Smaller phase II studies have used RIT after chemotherapy.[65] Recently, results from the European First-Line Indolent (FIT) study were reported.[66] In this design, patients who responded to a choice of induction chemotherapies were assigned randomly to ^{90}Y-ibritutomab tiuxetan consolidation or to observation. The median PFS of 37 months in the RIT arm was significantly longer than the 13.5 months in the control arm. Of note, although results were limited to chemotherapy responders, PFS on the RIT arm in this trial was shorter than the phase II published data with ^{131}I-tositumomab alone or following chemotherapy. The FIT trial data are presented in **Table 2** for comparison with the phase III rituximab and combination chemotherapy results.

Autologous Hematopoietic Cell Transplantation

After demonstrating efficacy and safety for recurrent FL, high-dose chemoradiotherapy and autologous hematopoietic cell transplantation (AHCT) were used following chemotherapy induction by Freedman and colleagues[67] Clinical remission was long relative to chemotherapy alone, and molecular remissions were achieved in a subset of patients. A number of further phase II institutional experiences also demonstrated promising results with AHCT, yielding prolonged PFS compared with historical controls.[68–70] AHCT has been investigated in three prospective, randomized cooperative group trials (see **Table 3**). In the study of Sebban and colleagues,[71] EFS was not significantly different in the study arms, possibly because of the differences in the duration of treatment, but a survival benefit was observed for AHCT. The study by Deconinck and colleagues[72] showed a significant advantage for AHCT in EFS, but a statistically significant difference in OS was not achieved. The GLSG study reported significantly longer EFS after AHCT but no survival difference to date.[73] Because these studies were performed in the pre-rituximab era, they are difficult to interpret in light of modern treatment. Results of the CHOP versus R-CHOP study with a second randomization to AHCT or interferon in young patients (see **Table 2**) should provide valuable information.[12] Because AHCT studies are complicated by an increased risk of secondary leukemia and do not demonstrate consistent OS benefits, this therapeutic maneuver in first remission should be considered investigative, particularly in the setting of marked improvement with the new standard treatment of rituximab and combination chemotherapy.

Adoptive Immunotherapy

Patient-specific vaccine designed to provoke a humoral and/or cellular immune response against the clonal surface immunoglobulin (idiotype) unique to each patient who has FL is an attractive and novel therapeutic strategy.[74] The optimal setting for vaccination is the minimal residual disease state after adequate recovery of the immune system from chemotherapy. Three phase III trials have studied idiotype vaccinations versus sham vaccination in patients responding to chemotherapy cytoreduction (**Table 4**). Results from two of these studies have been released recently and are disappointing, in that no benefit was seen in vaccinated patients.[75,76] The third trial uses a more aggressive induction chemotherapy and limits the vaccine randomization

Table 3
Randomized trials of high-dose therapy followed by autologous hematopoietic cell transplantation in first remission of FL

Study (Reference)	Experimental Arm	Control Arm	Event-Free Survival (%)	Time (Years)	Overall Survival (%)
Sebban/GELA[71]	CHOP + TBI/Cy	CHVP + IFN	45 versus 36 ($P = .5$)	7	86 versus 74 ($P = .05$)
Deconinick/ GOELAMS[72]	CHVP + TBI/Cy	CHVP + IFN	60 versus 48 ($P<.05$)	5	NS
Lenz/GLSG[73]	CHOP + TBI/Cy	CHOP + IFN	65 versus 33 ($P<.0001$)	5	NA[a]

Abbreviations: Cy, cyclophosphamide; GELA, Groupe d'Etude des Lymphomes de l'Adulte; GOELAMS, Groupe Ouest Est d'Etude des Leucémies et Autres Maladies du Sang; IFN, interferon; NA, not available; NS, not significant; TBI, total-body irradiation.
[a] Not available.

Table 4
Phase III trials of consolidative idiotype vaccination for FL

Study (Reference)	Induction Treatment	Manufacturing	Accrual	Result
Genitope/(MyVax)[75]	CVP	Recombinant	Completed	NSD
Favrille/(FavId)[76]	Rituximab	Recombinant	Completed	NSD
NCI/Biovest/(Biovaxld)	PACE	Hybridoma	Ongoing	Pending

Abbreviations: NCI, National Cancer Institute; NSD, no significant difference; PACE, prednisone, adriamycin, cyclophosphamide, and etoposide.

to complete responders. This study continues in progress. In a study involving 40 patients who had FL treated with a series of tumor-specific idiotype vaccinations after cytoreduction with chemotherapy at Stanford University, the generation of specific immune response was associated with prolonged TTP (7.9 years) compared with historical controls.[77] Similarly, patients who mounted an immune response to the idiotype target had significantly longer PFS in the study conducted by Genitope, Inc.[75] These results suggest that differences in the FL host and tumor are prognostically significant. Although the experience with lymphoma vaccines has not met expectations, immunotherapy enthusiasts are encouraged by new approaches to enhancing antigen presentation such as the use of dendritic cells and other means of enhancing the immunogenicity of tumor or stimulating the immune response.

Stage I–II Disease

About 15% to 25% of patients who have FL present with limited-stage disease.[78] As summarized in **Table 5** % of patients who have stage I–II FL have prolonged PFS after radiotherapy alone; therefore regional or involved-field radiotherapy is the standard of care.[79–83] There are limited data to determine whether chemotherapy confers further benefit.[84] In some series, larger tumor size was associated with treatment failure.[80,82] Because accurate staging is critical in the potential cure of stage I–II disease with radiotherapy, there has been interest in improved diagnostics. Wirth and colleagues[85] reported that in positron emission tomography, fluorodeoxyglucose avidity was demonstrated in 97% of patients in whom disease was evident on conventional assessment; 31% of patients were upstaged, and the radiotherapy portal was enlarged in another 14%. These data suggest the potential for functional imaging to improve radiotherapy cure rates by excluding cases with more advanced disease. To date, therapeutics targeted against CD20 have not been studied adequately in limited FL.

Table 5
Results of radiotherapy in early-stage FL

Study (Reference)	N Patients	Time (Years)	Relapse-Free Survival (%)	Overall Survival (%)
Mac Manus[79]	177	15	40	44
Wilder et al[80]	80	15	66 (stage I)	49
			26 (stage II)	40
Guadagnolo et al[82]	106	15	39	62
Pendlebury et al[81]	58	10	43	79
Peterson et al[83]	460	10	41	62

THERAPY OF RECURRENT FOLLICULAR LYMPHOMA
CD20-Based Therapies

Rituximab was approved for the treatment of relapsed or recurrent FL in 1997. In the pivotal trial conducted by McLaughlin and colleagues,[47] a 48% response rate, a 6% complete response rate and a median duration of response of 13 months were seen after 4 weekly injections of rituximab (375 mg/m^2) in indolent lymphomas. These data were corroborated in further studies in patients who had relapsed disease. Because more patients now are exposed to rituximab as primary therapy, data for re-treatment with rituximab are relevant. Davis and colleagues[86] described a response rate of 40% and complete response rate of 11% upon rituximab re-treatment as well as the surprising finding that the median TTP was 18 months, longer than the median initial TTP after rituximab monotherapy. An international study evaluated the role of rituximab in both induction and maintenance in patients who had relapsed or refractory FL who had no prior exposure to anthracycline or rituximab.[56] Median PFS was significantly longer after R-CHOP than after CHOP (33 months vs. 20 months), and maintenance rituximab after the second randomization also significantly improved PFS from the time of the second randomization, regardless of induction. In another study in recurrent FL, rituximab in combination with FCM yielded better outcomes than chemotherapy alone.[44]

As noted previously, RIT is approved for patients who have recurrent FL. Relatively high overall response rates of 60% to 80% were observed in the pivotal studies, although PFS generally was less than 1 year.[57,58,61,87] In recurrent FL, RIT yields higher response rates than rituximab monotherapy.[58] Furthermore, RIT is active in patients who have FL recurrent after rituximab exposure.[61,87] The major toxicity of RIT is myelosuppression; the use of RIT is limited to patients who have less than 25% marrow involvement and adequate marrow reserve. Secondary leukemia and minimal residual disease have been observed after RIT, although all prior exposures contribute to this complication, so ascribing causality is a challenge.[88] Secondary leukemia has been reported in patients who have had an initial course of chemotherapy plus RIT only.[89] Current interest is focused on the assessment of RIT earlier in the disease course and to incorporate RIT as consolidation after induction chemotherapy.

Transplantation

Several phase II studies have investigated a variety of conditioning regimens plus AHCT in relapsed FL. PFS in these studies is significantly longer than reported in historical controls managed with conventional chemotherapy.[90,91] For instance, Freedman and colleagues[92] described 42% rate of DFS at 8 years. Patients in molecular remission, as determined by a bone marrow negative for a Bcl2/IgH rearrangement, had markedly higher DFS at 8 years than patients who had molecular evidence of disease (83% vs. 19%, $P = .0001$).[92] A single phase III trial compared conventional versus high-dose therapy and AHCT in patients who had chemosensitive FL.[93] Although the study was underpowered, it demonstrated a significant benefit in both PFS and OS for the patients who underwent transplantation. More recently, long-term follow-up from the St. Bartholomew's group indicates that 48% of patients who have FL enjoy durable remissions for 12 years after AHCT.[94] This outcome has renewed interest in the role and timing of transplantation in FL in combination with anti-CD20–based therapies. Concerns about the use of AHCT are related to secondary leukemia, a complication that seems to be lower when total body irradiation is not included in the preparatory regimen.[91] Furthermore, this therapeutic option generally is limited to patients in complete response or who have minimal disease, requiring continued disease sensitive to chemotherapy.

Allogeneic hematopoietic cell transplantation (allotransplantation) generally has been assessed in patients who have unfavorable, multiply recurrent FL. Although durable remissions have been reported with this approach, enthusiasm for the efficacy of results has been offset by treatment-related mortality. The International Bone Marrow Transplant Registry reported on myeloablative allotransplants from HLA-identical donors in 176 patients who had FL.[91] The recurrence rate was low, at 19%, but the non-relapse treatment-related mortality was 30%, primarily because of infections and graft-versus-host disease. The European Blood and Marrow Transplant Registry Group (EBMT) and others have reported similar findings.[95,96]

A graft-versus-lymphoma effect has been observed in patients who have recurrent FL after allotransplantation, based on the ability to achieve remission subsequent to donor lymphocyte infusions.[97,98] This observation and the desire to reduce treatment-related mortality were the impetus for exploring reduced-intensity conditioning as a means of achieving immunosuppression before allotransplantation. Applying this approach with a nonmyeloablative conditioning regimen of fludarabine and cyclophosphamide, Khouri and colleagues[99,100] reported a 2-year DFS rate of 84% and a 10% treatment-related mortality. In a recent update at a median follow-up time of 56 months, the estimated OS and PFS rates at 6 years were 85% and 83%, respectively.[101] The incidence of chronic graft-versus-host disease was 51%. The EBMT reported retrospective registry data for 52 patients who underwent nonmyeloablative allotransplantation. The 100-day treatment-related mortality was 11.5%, but the 2-year treatment-related mortality was a high 30%, highlighting the potentially high risk of chronic graft-versus-host disease. In this study, the 2-year PFS and OS rates were 54% and 65%, respectively.[101] A phase II trial with the objective of validating the data of Khouri and colleagues is in process by the United States Clinical Trials Network. At this time allotransplantation represents an important area of ongoing investigation.

New Agents

Multiple agents in FL are in various levels of active development. A novel chemotherapeutic agent with the properties of an alkylating agent and a purine analogue, bendamustine, resulted in a 75% response rate and a 25% complete response rate in relapsed FL.[102] Preliminary data from a phase III trial comparing the combination of bendamustine and rituximab versus R-CHOP demonstrate encouraging efficacy and safety in untreated FL.[103] The proteosome inhibitor bortezomib, approved for multiple myeloma and mantle cell lymphoma, has been used as a single agent in FL.[104] Several trials exploring bortezomib in combination with other agents, including rituximab, in relapsed FL now are underway.

New monoclonal antibodies being studied in FL include galiximab, a primatized IgG1 anti-CD80 with modest single-agent activity (11%).[105] A phase I/II study evaluating galiximab in combination with rituximab demonstrated an overall response rate of 66% (33% complete response/unconfirmed complete response; 33% partial response) with a favorable toxicity profile at the recommended dose.[106] Epratuzumab is directed against the CD22 antigen, which is strongly expressed by follicular B cells. Single-agent activity included a 24% response rate; in combination with rituximab, a response rate of 67% was reported.[107,108] Other monoclonal antibodies being investigated in early-phase clinical trials include anti-CD40 antibody (SGN40) and a new generation of anti-CD20 antibodies that are humanized or fully human and, in one case, nonfucosylated. These new anti-CD20 antibodies have been engineered to have greater cytotoxicity though antibody-dependent cellular cytotoxicity, complement-dependent toxicity, or both. Other new approaches include lenalidomide, an immunomodulatory drug with multiple properties. In a phase II study as monotherapy in relapsed/refractory FL, lenalidomide demonstrated an overall response rate of 32% (7/22).[109] As noted earlier, immunotherapists continue to try to harness adaptive immunity through novel approaches, including new vaccine approaches.

SUMMARY

During the last 2 decades, overall survival in FL has improved. The explanation for this advance is not clear, but the expanding number of therapeutic alternatives, particularly rituximab, must play a leading role. When combined with chemotherapy, rituximab has profoundly affected the duration of remission in patients who have advanced disease, and it is the first treatment to demonstrate a survival benefit in multiple studies. Rituximab plus chemotherapy is established as the new standard for patients who have FL requiring treatment. Rituximab monotherapy is well tolerated and effective, potentially offering an alternative to asymptomatic patients who have a low tumor burden, who historically have been managed with initial observation. Key clinical trials in progress will inform the therapeutic choice in this setting. Although patients who have FL enjoy longer remissions and OS with current treatments, recurrence of disease continues to provide a challenge and an opportunity for alternative treatments. RIT is a highly active treatment that is being studied in important clinical trials. Maintenance therapy with rituximab extends remission after chemotherapy in untreated patients and after rituximab-chemotherapy in patients who have relapsed disease. Results are awaited with this approach in untreated patients who have advanced disease. The role of transplantation and the use of this option within the sequence of treatment alternatives in FL is the subject of ongoing inquiry. Newer treatments with promise include antibodies directed against other surface antigens, anti-CD20 antibodies engineered for greater efficacy, bendamustine, bortezomib, and lenalidomide. With these developments and more agents on the horizon, there is optimism that patient outcomes can be improved further. Participation in clinical trials is essential to realize this promise.

The management of FL remains an art based on clues at diagnosis and throughout the clinical course, where risk of transformation influences decisions for re-sampling lymphoma tissues. Looking forward, unmasking the biologic basis for clinical heterogeneity, particularly to the extent that the clinical course becomes more predictable, should refine treatment approaches to maximize quality of life and longevity. Advances in biomarker discovery and diagnostics development will require annotated biospecimens, which are particularly valuable in the context of clinical trials.

REFERENCES

1. A clinical evaluation of the International Lymphoma Study Group classification of non-Hodgkin's lymphoma. The non-Hodgkin's lymphoma classification project. Blood 1997;89:3909–18.
2. Horning SJ, Rosenberg SA. The natural history of initially untreated low-grade non-Hodgkin's lymphomas. N Engl J Med 1984;311:1471–5.
3. Acker B, Hoppe RT, Colby TV, et al. Histologic conversion in the non-Hodgkin's lymphomas. J Clin Oncol 1983;1:11–6.
4. Garvin AJ, Simon RM, Osborne CK, et al. An autopsy study of histologic progression in non-Hodgkin's lymphomas. 192 cases from the National Cancer Institute. Cancer 1983;52:393–8.

5. Hubbard SM, Chabner BA, DeVita VJ, et al. Histologic progression in non-Hodgkin's lymphoma. Blood 1982;59:258–64.
6. Swerdlow SH. Pediatric follicular lymphomas, marginal zone lymphomas, and marginal zone hyperplasia. Am J Clin Pathol 2004;122(Suppl):S98–109.
7. Damaj G, Verkarre V, Delmer A, et al. Primary follicular lymphoma of the gastrointestinal tract: a study of 25 cases and a literature review. Ann Oncol 2003;14:623–9.
8. López-Guillermo A, Montserrat E, Bosch F, et al. Applicability of the international index for aggressive lymphomas to patients with low-grade lymphoma [see comments]. J Clin Oncol 1994;12:1343–8.
9. Solal-Celigny P, Roy P, Colombat P, et al. Follicular Lymphoma International Prognostic Index. Blood 2004;104:1258–65.
10. Buske C, Hoster E, Dreyling M, et al. The Follicular Lymphoma International Prognostic Index (FLIPI) separates high-risk from intermediate- or low-risk patients with advanced-stage follicular lymphoma treated front-line with rituximab and the combination of cyclophosphamide, doxorubicin, vincristine, and prednisone (R-CHOP) with respect to treatment outcome. Blood 2006;108:1504–8.
11. Marcus R, Imrie K, Belch A, et al. CVP chemotherapy plus rituximab compared with CVP as first-line treatment for advanced follicular lymphoma. Blood 2005;105:1417–23.
12. Hiddemann W, Kneba M, Dreyling M, et al. Frontline therapy with rituximab added to the combination of cyclophosphamide, doxorubicin, vincristine, and prednisone (CHOP) significantly improves the outcome for patients with advanced-stage follicular lymphoma compared with therapy with CHOP alone: results of a prospective randomized study of the German Low-Grade Lymphoma Study Group. Blood 2005;106:3725–32.
13. Federico M, Bellei M, Pro B, et al. Revalidation of FLIPI in patients with follicular lymphoma (FL) registered in the F2 study and treated upfront with immunochemotherapy. J Clin Oncol 2006;25. [abstract 8008].
14. Brice P, Bastion Y, Lepage E, et al. Comparison in low-tumor-burden follicular lymphomas between an initial no-treatment policy, prednimustine, or interferon alfa: a randomized study from the Groupe d'Etude des Lymphomes Folliculaires. Groupe d'Etude des Lymphomes de l'Adulte. J Clin Oncol 1997;15:1110–7.
15. Salles G, Mounier N, De Guibert S, et al. Final analysis of the GELA-GOELAMS FL2000 study with a 5-year follow-up. Blood 2007;110:792A.
16. Harris NL, Jaffe ES, Diebold J, et al. World Health Organization classification of neoplastic diseases of the hematopoietic and lymphoid tissues: report of the Clinical Advisory Committee meeting, Airlie House, Virginia, November 1997. J Clin Oncol 1999;17:3835–49.
17. Hans CP, Weisenburger DD, Vose JM, et al. A significant diffuse component predicts for inferior survival in grade 3 follicular lymphoma, but cytologic subtypes do not predict survival. Blood 2003;101:2363–7.
18. Horsman DE, Connors JM, Pantzar T, et al. Analysis of secondary chromosomal alterations in 165 cases of follicular lymphoma with t(14;18). Genes Chromosomes Cancer 2001;30:375–82.
19. Dave SS, Wright G, Tan B, et al. Prediction of survival in follicular lymphoma based on molecular features of tumor-infiltrating immune cells. N Engl J Med 2004;351:2159–69.
20. Farinha P, Masoudi H, Skinnider BF, et al. Analysis of multiple biomarkers shows that lymphoma-associated macrophage (LAM) content is an independent predictor of survival in follicular lymphoma (FL). Blood 2005;106:2169–74.

21. Lee AM, Clear AJ, Calaminici M, et al. Number of CD4+ cells and location of forkhead box protein P3-positive cells in diagnostic follicular lymphoma tissue microarrays correlates with outcome. J Clin Oncol 2006;24:5052–9.

22. Glas AM, Knoops L, Delahaye L, et al. Gene-expression and immunohistochemical study of specific T-cell subsets and accessory cell types in the transformation and prognosis of follicular lymphoma. J Clin Oncol 2007;25:390–8.

23. Cerhan J, Wang S, Maurer M, et al. Prognostic significance of host immune gene polymorphisms in follicular lymphoma survival. Blood 2007;109:5439–46.

24. Johnson PW, Rohatiner AZ, Whelan JS, et al. Patterns of survival in patients with recurrent follicular lymphoma: a 20-year study from a single center. J Clin Oncol 1995;13:140–7.

25. Horning SJ. Natural history of and therapy for the indolent non-Hodgkin's lymphomas. Semin Oncol 1993;20:75–88.

26. Fisher RI, LeBlanc M, Press OW, et al. New treatment options have changed the survival of patients with follicular lymphoma. J Clin Oncol 2005;23:8447–52.

27. Swenson WT, Wooldridge JE, Lynch CF, et al. Improved survival of follicular lymphoma patients in the United States. J Clin Oncol 2005;23:5019–26.

28. Liu Q, Fayad L, Cabanillas F, et al. Improvement of overall and failure-free survival in stage IV follicular lymphoma: 25 years of treatment experience at The University of Texas M.D. Anderson Cancer Center. J Clin Oncol 2006;24:1582–9.

29. Tan D, Rosenberg SA, Levy R, et al. Survival in follicular lymphoma: the Stanford experience, 1960–2003. Blood 2007;110:3428A.

30. Yuen AR, Kamel OW, Halpern J, et al. Long-term survival after histologic transformation of low-grade follicular lymphoma. J Clin Oncol 1995;13:1726–33.

31. Montoto S, Davies AJ, Matthews J, et al. Risk and clinical implications of transformation of follicular lymphoma to diffuse large B-cell lymphoma. J Clin Oncol 2007;25:2426–33.

32. Tan D, Rosenberg SA, Lavori P, et al. Improved prognosis after histologic transformation of follicular lymphoma: the Stanford experience 1960–2003. Programs and abstracts of the 10th International Conference on Malignant Lymphoma. Lugano; 2008. p. 111.

33. Al-Tourah AJ, Savage KJ, Gill KK, et al. Addition of rituximab to CHOP chemotherapy significantly improves survival of patients with transformed lymphoma. ASH Annual Meeting Abstracts 2007;110:790.

34. Portlock CS, Rosenberg SA. No initial therapy for stage III and IV non-Hodgkin's lymphomas of favorable histologic types. Ann Intern Med 1979;90:10–3.

35. Ardeshna KM, Smith P, Norton A, et al. Long-term effect of a watch and wait policy versus immediate systemic treatment for asymptomatic advanced-stage non-Hodgkin lymphoma: a randomised controlled trial. Lancet 2003;362:516–22.

36. Young RC, Longo DL, Glatstein E, et al. The treatment of indolent lymphomas: watchful waiting v aggressive combined modality treatment. Semin Hematol 1988;25:11–6.

37. Portlock CS, Rosenberg SA. Combination chemotherapy with cyclophosphamide, vincristine, and prednisone in advanced non-Hodgkin's lymphomas. Cancer 1976;37:1275–82.

38. Gallagher CJ, Gregory WM, Jones AE, et al. Follicular lymphoma: prognostic factors for response and survival. J Clin Oncol 1986;4:1470–80.

39. Kimby E, Björkholm M, Gahrton G, et al. Chlorambucil/prednisone vs. CHOP in symptomatic low-grade non-Hodgkin's lymphomas: a randomized trial from the Lymphoma Group of Central Sweden. Ann Oncol 1994;5(Suppl 2):67–71.

40. Peterson BA, Petroni GA, Frizzera G. Prolonged single agent versus combination chemotherapy in indolent follicular lymphomas. A study of the Cancer and Leukemia Group B. J Clin Oncol 2002;21:5–15.
41. Solal-Céligny P, Brice P, Brousse N, et al. Phase II trial of fludarabine monophosphate as first-line treatment in patients with advanced follicular lymphoma: a multicenter study by the Groupe d'Etude des Lymphomes de l'Adulte. J Clin Oncol 1996;14:514–9.
42. McLaughlin P, Hagemeister FB, Romaguera JE, et al. Fludarabine, mitoxantrone, and dexamethasone: an effective new regimen for indolent lymphoma. J Clin Oncol 1996;14:1262–8.
43. Velasquez WS, Lew D, Grogan TM, et al. Combination of fludarabine and mitoxantrone in untreated stages III and IV low-grade lymphoma: S9501. J Clin Oncol 2003;21:1996–2003.
44. Forstpointner R, Dreyling M, Repp R, et al. The addition of rituximab to a combination of fludarabine, cyclophosphamide, mitoxantrone (FCM) significantly increases the response rate and prolongs survival as compared with FCM alone in patients with relapsed and refractory follicular and mantle cell lymphomas: results of a prospective randomized study of the German Low-Grade Lymphoma Study Group. Blood 2004;104:3064–71.
45. Hagenbeek A, Eghbali H, Monfardini S, et al. Phase III intergroup study of fludarabine phosphate compared with cyclophosphamide, vincristine, and prednisone chemotherapy in newly diagnosed patients with stage III and IV low-grade malignant non-Hodgkin's lymphoma. J Clin Oncol 2006;24:1590–6.
46. Maloney DG, Grillo-López AJ, Bodkin DJ, et al. IDEC-C2B8: results of a phase I multiple-dose trial in patients with relapsed non-Hodgkin's lymphoma. J Clin Oncol 1997;15:3266–74.
47. McLaughlin P, Grillo-Lopez AJ, Link BK, et al. Rituximab chimeric anti-CD20 monoclonal antibody therapy for relapsed indolent lymphoma: half of patients respond to a four-dose treatment program. J Clin Oncol 1998;16:2825–33.
48. Hainsworth JD, Litchy S, Burris HA 3rd, et al. Rituximab as first-line and maintenance therapy for patients with indolent non-Hodgkin's lymphoma. J Clin Oncol 2002;20:4261–7.
49. Colombat P, Salles G, Brousse N, et al. Rituximab (anti-CD20 monoclonal antibody) as single first-line therapy for patients with follicular lymphoma with a low tumor burden: clinical and molecular evaluation. Blood 2001;97:101–6.
50. Colombat P, Brousse N, Morschhauser F, et al. Single treatment with rituximab monotherapy for low-tumor burden follicular lymphoma (FL): survival analyses with extended follow-up (F/Up) of 7 years. ASH Annual Meeting Abstracts 2006;108:486.
51. Ghielmini M, Schmitz SF, Cogliatti SB, et al. Prolonged treatment with rituximab in patients with follicular lymphoma significantly increases event-free survival and response duration compared with the standard weekly × 4 schedule. Blood 2004;103:4416–23.
52. Kahl BS. Eastern Cooperative Oncology Group 4402: Rituximab Extended Schedule or Retreatment Trial (RESORT). Clin Lymphoma Myeloma 2006;6:423–6.
53. Herold M, Haas A, Srock S, et al. Rituximab added to first-line mitoxantrone, chlorambucil, and prednisolone chemotherapy followed by interferon maintenance prolongs survival in patients with advanced follicular lymphoma: an East German study group hematology and oncology study. J Clin Oncol 2007;25:1986–92.

54. Marcus R, Solal-Celigny P, Imrie K, et al. MabThera (rituximab) plus cyclophosphamide, vincristine and prednisone (CVP) chemotherapy improves survival in previously untreated patients with advanced follicular non-Hodgkins lymphoma. [abstract]. Blood 2006;108:481.

55. Hochster HS, Weller E, Gascoyne RD, et al. Maintenance rituximab after CVP results in superior clinical outcome in advanced follicular lymphoma (FL): results of the E1496 phase III trial. [abstract]. Blood 2005;106:349.

56. van Oers MH, Klasa R, Marcus RE, et al. Rituximab maintenance improves clinical outcome of relapsed/resistant follicular non-Hodgkin lymphoma in patients both with and without rituximab during induction: results of a prospective randomized phase 3 intergroup trial. Blood 2006;108:3295–301.

57. Kaminski MS, Zelenetz AD, Press OW, et al. Pivotal study of iodine I 131 tositumomab for chemotherapy-refractory low-grade or transformed low-grade B-cell non-Hodgkin's lymphomas. J Clin Oncol 2001;19:3918–28.

58. Witzig TE, Gordon LI, Cabanillas F, et al. Randomized controlled trial of yttrium-90-labeled ibritumomab tiuxetan radioimmunotherapy versus rituximab immunotherapy for patients with relapsed or refractory low-grade, follicular, or transformed B-cell non-Hodgkin's lymphoma. J Clin Oncol 2002;20:2453–63.

59. Witzig TE, White CA, Wiseman GA, et al. Phase I/II trial of IDEC-Y2B8 radioimmunotherapy for treatment of relapsed or refractory CD20(+) B-cell non-Hodgkin's lymphoma. J Clin Oncol 1999;17:3793–803.

60. Vose JM, Wahl RL, Saleh M, et al. Multicenter phase II study of iodine-131 tositumomab for chemotherapy-relapsed/refractory low-grade and transformed low-grade B-cell non-Hodgkin's lymphomas. J Clin Oncol 2000;18:1316–23.

61. Witzig TE, Flinn IW, Gordon LI, et al. Treatment with ibritumomab tiuxetan radioimmunotherapy in patients with rituximab-refractory follicular non-Hodgkin's lymphoma. J Clin Oncol 2002;20:3262–9.

62. Horning SJ, Lucas JB, Younes A, et al. Iodine-131 tositumomab for non-Hodgkin's lymphoma (NHL) patients who progressed after treatment with rituximab: results of a multi-center phase II study. Blood 2000;96:2184A.

63. Kaminski MS, Tuck M, Estes J, et al. 131I-tositumomab therapy as initial treatment for follicular lymphoma. N Engl J Med 2005;352:441–9.

64. Press OW, Unger JM, Braziel RM, et al. A phase 2 trial of CHOP chemotherapy followed by tositumomab/iodine I 131 tositumomab for previously untreated follicular non-Hodgkin lymphoma: Southwest Oncology Group Protocol S9911. Blood 2003;102:1606–12.

65. Leonard JP, Coleman M, Kostakoglu L, et al. Abbreviated chemotherapy with fludarabine followed by tositumomab and iodine I 131 tositumomab for untreated follicular lymphoma. J Clin Oncol 2005;23:5696–704.

66. Hagenbeek A, Bischof-Delaloye A, Radford JA, et al. 90Y-Ibritumomab tiuxetan (Zevalin(R)) consolidation of first remission in advanced stage follicular non-Hodgkin's lymphoma: first results of the international randomized phase 3 First-Line Indolent Trial (FIT) in 414 patients. Blood 2007;110:643.

67. Freedman AS, Gribben JG, Neuberg D, et al. High-dose therapy and autologous bone marrow transplantation in patients with follicular lymphoma during first remission. Blood 1996;88:2780–6.

68. Horning SJ, Negrin RS, Hoppe RT, et al. High-dose therapy and autologous bone marrow transplantation for follicular lymphoma in first complete or partial remission: results of a phase II clinical trial. Blood 2001;97:404–9.

69. Colombat P, Cornillet P, Deconinck E, et al. Value of autologous stem cell transplantation with purged bone marrow as first-line therapy for follicular lymphoma

with high tumor burden: a GOELAMS phase II study. Bone Marrow Transplant 2000;26:971–7.

70. Corradini P, Ladetto M, Zallio F, et al. Long-term follow-up of indolent lymphoma patients treated with high-dose sequential chemotherapy and autografting: evidence that durable molecular and clinical remission frequently can be attained only in follicular subtypes. J Clin Oncol 2004;22:1460–8.

71. Sebban C, Mounier N, Brousse N, et al. Standard chemotherapy with interferon compared with CHOP followed by high-dose therapy with autologous stem cell transplantation in untreated patients with advanced follicular lymphoma: the GELF-94 randomized study from the Groupe d'Etude des Lymphomes de l'Adulte (GELA). Blood 2006;108:2540–4.

72. Deconinck E, Foussard C, Milpied N, et al. High-dose therapy followed by autologous purged stem-cell transplantation and doxorubicin-based chemotherapy in patients with advanced follicular lymphoma: a randomized multicenter study by GOELAMS. Blood 2005;105:3817–23.

73. Lenz G, Dreyling M, Schiegnitz E, et al. Myeloablative radiochemotherapy followed by autologous stem cell transplantation in first remission prolongs progression-free survival in follicular lymphoma: results of a prospective, randomized trial of the German Low-Grade Lymphoma Study Group. Blood 2004;104:2667–74.

74. Hsu FJ, Caspar CB, Czerwinski D, et al. Tumor-specific idiotype vaccines in the treatment of patients with B-cell lymphoma—long-term results of a clinical trial. Blood 1997;89:3129–35.

75. Levy R, Robertson MJ, Leonard J, et al. Results of a phase 3 trial evaluating safety and efficacy of specific immunotherapy, recombinant idiotype conjugated to KLH with GM-CSF compared to non-specific immunotherapy, KLH, with GM-CSF in patients with follicular non-Hodgkin's lymphoma. Programs and abstracts of the 10th International Conference on Malignant Lymphoma. Lugano; 2008. p. 101.

76. Favrille announces results from phase 3 registration trial of Specifid in patients with follicular B-cell non-Hodgkin's lymphoma, 2008. Available at: http://www.favrille.com/trials/phase-3-clinical-trial-summary.htm.

77. Ai WZ, Tibshirani R, Taidi B, et al. Anti-idiotype antibody response after vaccination correlates with better overall survival in follicular lymphoma. ASH Annual Meeting Abstracts 2007;110:647.

78. Anderson T, Chabner BA, Young RC, et al. Malignant lymphoma. 1. The histology and staging of 473 patients at the National Cancer Institute. Cancer 1982;50:2699–707.

79. Mac Manus MP, Hoppe RT. Is radiotherapy curative for stage I and II low-grade follicular lymphoma? Results of a long-term follow-up study of patients treated at Stanford University. J Clin Oncol 1996;14:1282–90.

80. Wilder RB, Jones D, Tucker SL, et al. Long-term results with radiotherapy for stage I-II follicular lymphomas. Int J Radiat Oncol Biol Phys 2001;51:1219–27.

81. Pendlebury S, el Awadi M, Ashley S, et al. Radiotherapy results in early stage low grade nodal non-Hodgkin's lymphoma. Radiother Oncol 1995;36:167–71.

82. Guadagnolo BA, Li S, Neuberg D, et al. Long-term outcome and mortality trends in early-stage, grade 1-2 follicular lymphoma treated with radiation therapy. Int J Radiat Oncol Biol Phys 2006;64:928–34.

83. Peterson PM, Gaspodarowicz M, Tsang R. Long term outcome in stage I and II follicular lymphoma following treatment with involved field radiation therapy alone. J Clin Oncol 2004;22(14S):653s.

84. Seymour JF, Pro B, Fuller LM, et al. Long-term follow-up of a prospective study of combined modality therapy for stage I-II indolent non-Hodgkin's lymphoma. J Clin Oncol 2003;21:2115–22.

85. Wirth A, Foo M, Seymour JF, et al. Impact of [18F] fluorodeoxyglucose positron emission tomography on staging and management of early-stage follicular non-Hodgkin lymphoma. Int J Radiat Oncol Biol Phys 2008;71:213–9.
86. Davis TA, Grillo-Lopez AJ, White CA, et al. Rituximab anti-CD20 monoclonal antibody therapy in non-Hodgkin's lymphoma: safety and efficacy of re-treatment. J Clin Oncol 2000;18:3135–43.
87. Horning SJ, Younes A, Jain V, et al. Efficacy and safety of tositumomab and iodine-131 tositumomab (Bexxar) in B-cell lymphoma, progressive after rituximab. J Clin Oncol 2005;23:712–9.
88. Bennett JM, Kaminski MS, Leonard JP, et al. Assessment of treatment-related myelodysplastic syndromes and acute myeloid leukemia in patients with non-Hodgkin lymphoma treated with tositumomab and I^{131} tositumomab. Blood 2005;105(12):4576–82.
89. Roboz GJ, Bennett JM, Coleman M, et al. Therapy-related myelodysplastic syndrome and acute myeloid leukemia following initial treatment with chemotherapy plus radioimmunotherapy for indolent non-Hodgkin lymphoma. Leuk Res 2007; 31:1141–4.
90. Tse WW, Lazarus HM, Van Besien K. Stem cell transplantation in follicular lymphoma: progress at last? Bone Marrow Transplant 2004;34:929–38.
91. Montoto S, Canals C, Rohatiner AZ, et al. Long-term follow-up of high-dose treatment with autologous haematopoietic progenitor cell support in 693 patients with follicular lymphoma: an EBMT registry study. Leukemia 2007;21: 2324–31.
92. Freedman AS, Neuberg D, Mauch P, et al. Long-term follow-up of autologous bone marrow transplantation in patients with relapsed follicular lymphoma. Blood 1999;94:3325–33.
93. Schouten HC, Kvaloy S, Sydes M, et al. The CUP trial: a randomized study analyzing the efficacy of high dose therapy and purging in low-grade non-Hodgkin's lymphoma (NHL). Ann Oncol 2000;11:91–4.
94. Rohatiner AZ, Nadler L, Davies AJ, et al. Myeloablative therapy with autologous bone marrow transplantation for follicular lymphoma at the time of second or subsequent remission: long-term follow-up. J Clin Oncol 2007;25:2554–9.
95. van Besien K, Loberiza FR Jr, Bajorunaite R, et al. Comparison of autologous and allogeneic hematopoietic stem cell transplantation for follicular lymphoma. Blood 2003;102:3521–9.
96. Toze CL, Barnett MJ, Connors JM, et al. Long-term disease-free survival of patients with advanced follicular lymphoma after allogeneic bone marrow transplantation. Br J Haematol 2004;127:311–21.
97. Marks DI, Lush R, Cavenagh J, et al. The toxicity and efficacy of donor lymphocyte infusions given after reduced-intensity conditioning allogeneic stem cell transplantation. Blood 2002;100:3108–14.
98. Mandigers CM, Verdonck LF, Meijerink JP, et al. Graft-versus-lymphoma effect of donor lymphocyte infusion in indolent lymphomas relapsed after allogeneic stem cell transplantation. Bone Marrow Transplant 2003;32:1159–63.
99. Khouri IF, Saliba RM, Lee MC, et al. Longer follow-up confirms a low relapse rate after non-myeloablative allogeneic transplantation for non-Hodgkin's lymphoma, including patients with PET or gallium-avid disease. Blood 2005;106:A44.
100. Khouri IF, Saliba RM, Giralt SA, et al. Nonablative allogeneic hematopoietic transplantation as adoptive immunotherapy for indolent lymphoma: low incidence of toxicity, acute graft-versus-host disease, and treatment-related mortality. Blood 2001;98:3595–9.

101. Khouri IF, Saliba RM, Korbling M, et al. Nonmyeloablative allogeneic transplantation (NMT) for relapsed follicular lymphoma (FL): continuous complete remission with longer follow-up. ASH Annual Meeting Abstracts 2007;110:485.

102. Friedberg JW, Cohen P, Chen L, et al. Bendamustine in patients with rituximab-refractory indolent and transformed non-Hodgkin's lymphoma: results from a phase II multicenter, single-agent study. J Clin Oncol 2008;26:204–10.

103. Rummel MJ, von Gruenhagen U, Niederle N, et al. Bendamustine plus rituximab versus CHOP plus rituximab in the first-line treatment of patients with indolent and mantle cell lymphomas—first interim results of a randomized phase III study of the StiL (Study Group Indolent Lymphomas, Germany). ASH Annual Meeting Abstracts 2007;110:385.

104. O'Connor OA. Marked clinical activity of the proteasome inhibitor bortezomib in patients with follicular and mantle-cell lymphoma. Clin Lymphoma Myeloma 2005;6:191–9.

105. Czuczman MS, Thall A, Witzig TE, et al. Phase I/II study of galiximab, an anti-CD80 antibody, for relapsed or refractory follicular lymphoma. J Clin Oncol 2005;23:4390–8.

106. Leonard JP, Friedberg JW, Younes A, et al. A phase I/II study of galiximab (an anti-CD80 monoclonal antibody) in combination with rituximab for relapsed or refractory, follicular lymphoma. Ann Oncol 2007;18:1216–23.

107. Leonard JP, Coleman M, Ketas JC, et al. Phase I/II trial of epratuzumab (humanized anti-CD22 antibody) in indolent non-Hodgkin's lymphoma. J Clin Oncol 2003;21:3051–9.

108. Leonard JP, Coleman M, Ketas J, et al. Combination antibody therapy with epratuzumab and rituximab in relapsed or refractory non-Hodgkin's lymphoma. J Clin Oncol 2005;23:5044–51.

109. Witzig TE, Vose JM, Moore TD, et al. Results from a phase II study of lenalidomide oral monotherapy in relapsed/refractory indolent non-Hodgkin's lymphoma. ASH Annual Meeting Abstracts 2007;110:2560.

Marginal Zone Lymphomas

Emanuele Zucca, MD*, Francesco Bertoni, MD,
Anastasios Stathis, MD, Franco Cavalli, MD, FRCP

KEYWORDS

- Marginal zone lymphoma • MALT lymphoma
- Extranodal lymphomas

DEFINITION AND CLASSIFICATION OF MARGINAL ZONE LYMPHOMAS

In the World Health Organization (WHO) classification of tumors of hematopoietic and lymphoid tissues the group of marginal zone lymphomas (MZL) comprises three different entities, namely the extranodal marginal zone B-cell lymphoma of mucosa-associated lymphoid tissue (currently named "MALT lymphoma" and previously defined as "low grade B-cell lymphoma of MALT type"), the nodal marginal zone B-cell lymphoma (previously known as "monocytoid lymphoma"), and the splenic marginal zone B-cell lymphoma (with or without circulating villous lymphocytes).[1]

The term MZL means that extranodal MZL, nodal MZL, and splenic MZL are believed to derive from B cells normally present in the marginal zone, which is the outer part of the mantle zone of B-cell follicles. Most of the marginal zone B cells are naïve B cells, with a restricted immunoglobulin repertoire. Postgerminal center memory B cells are also present in the marginal zone, as well as plasma cells, macrophages, T cells, and granulocytes.

While splenic and nodal MZL are quite rare, each comprising approximately 2% of lymphomas, the extranodal MZL of MALT type is not uncommon; in a survey of more than 1,400 non-Hodgkin's lymphomas from nine institutions in the United States, Canada, the United Kingdom, Switzerland, France, Germany, South Africa, and Hong Kong, this entity represented approximately 8% of the total number of cases, including both the most common gastrointestinal and the less usual nongastrointestinal localizations.[2] This article addresses each of these entitites.

EXTRANODAL MARGINAL ZONE LYMPHOMA OF MALT (MALT LYMPHOMA)
General Description of Histologic Features and Etiopathogenesis

Primary gastric MALT lymphoma is the most common and best-studied MALT lymphoma, but the histologic features of extranodal B-cell MZL (MALT lymphomas)

Oncology Institute of Southern Switzerland, Ospedale San Giovanni, 6500 Bellinzona, Switzerland
* Corresponding author. Oncology Institute of Southern Switzerland, Ospedale San Giovanni, 6500 Bellinzona, Switzerland.
E-mail address: ielsg@ticino.com (E. Zucca).

Hematol Oncol Clin N Am 22 (2008) 883–901
doi:10.1016/j.hoc.2008.07.011
0889-8588/08/$ – see front matter © 2008 Elsevier Inc. All rights reserved.

hemonc.theclinics.com

are largely similar, regardless of the site of origin.[3,4] The most striking feature of MALT lymphoma is the presence of a variable number of lymphoepithelial lesions defined by evident invasion and partial destruction of mucosal glands by the tumor cells. The morphology of MALT lymphoma cells is heterogeneous. Marginal-zone cells are the predominant component and are small to medium-sized cells with irregularly shaped nuclei (centrocyte-like cells). Other cell types comprise monocytoid cells and small B-lymphocytes. A variable degree of plasma cell differentiation is often present. Any of these cytologic aspects can predominate, or they can coexist within the same case. The B-cells of MALT lymphoma show the immunophenotype of the normal marginal zone B cells present in spleen, Peyer's patches, and in lymph nodes. Therefore, the tumor B-cells express surface immunoglobulins and pan-B antigens (CD19, CD20, and CD79a), express the marginal zone-associated antigens CD35 and CD21, and lack CD5, CD10, CD23, and cyclin D1 expression. A number of non-neoplastic, reactive T cells is often present. Scattered transformed large blast cells are also usually found. Their prognostic significance is not fully understood, but only when solid or sheet-like proliferations of large cells are present should the lymphoma be considered to have transformed. The resulting tumor cannot reliably be distinguished from other diffuse large B-cell lymphomas. Therefore, current recommendation is that such cases are defined as diffuse large B-cell lymphoma, avoiding the term "high-grade" MALT lymphomas.[3]

Certain histologic features appear to indicate that the MALT lymphoma B cells might be or have been involved in an immune response: the presence of tumor lymphocytes in the germinal centers of non-neoplastic follicles (follicular colonization), the presence of scattered transformed blasts, the often prominent plasma cell differentiation, and the often rich T-cell non-neoplastic component. MALT lymphoma usually arises in mucosal sites where lymphocytes are not normally present and where a MALT is acquired in response to either chronic infectious conditions or autoimmune processes: Helicobacter pylori gastritis, Hashimoto's thyroiditis, Sjögren syndrome.[5] Sequence analysis of the immunoglobulin genes expressed by the MALT lymphoma B cells shows a pattern of somatic hypermutation and intraclonal variation, suggesting that the tumor cell has undergone antigen selection in germinal centers and they continue to be at least partially driven by direct antigen stimulation.[6] In the context of this continual antigenic stimulation, abnormal B cell clones acquiring successive genetic abnormalities can progressively replace the normal B cell population of the inflammatory tissue, giving rise to the lymphoma. The acquisition of MALT is induced by a series of agents that are likely different in each organs.

H. pylori was identified by epidemiologic studies in the early 1990s as likely being involved in gastric MALT lymphomas pathogenesis, and this recognition was supported by the repeated demonstration of tumor regressions in 60% to 100% of patients with early-stage H. pylori-positive gastric MALT lymphoma treated with anti-helicobacter antibiotic therapy.[7–16] Hence, this tumor became a popular model of the pathogenetic link between chronic inflammation and lymphoma development.[5,17] Recognition of the driving sources of the antigenic stimulation in different tissues may therefore have important therapeutic implications. Indeed, other bacterial infections had later been found to be possibly implicated in the pathogenesis of marginal zone lymphomas arising in the skin (Borrelia burgdorferi),[18] in the ocular adnexa (Chlamyophila psittaci),[19] and in the small intestine (Campylobacter jejuni).[20]

Wide geographic variations have been reported in the prevalence of gastric MALT lymphoma, likely related to variations of the H. pylori incidence in the examined populations.[21] Indeed, H. pylori infection can be found in 70% to 90% of patients with primary MALT lymphoma of the stomach.[22,23]

MALT lymphoma may occur in many different anatomic locations and the gastrointestinal (GI) tract is the most common site, encompassing half of all cases.[24] Within the GI tract the disease is most frequent in the stomach, where the MALT lymphomas comprise up to 50% of all primary lymphoma.[21,25] Primary intestinal involvement is typical of a special uncommon subtype of MALT lymphoma, the immunoproliferative small intestinal disease (IPSID).[3] Extranodal MZLs may also arise in a variety of non-GI organs, mucosal or not, such as the salivary gland, thyroid, upper respiratory tract, lung, ocular adnexa (lachrymal gland, conjunctiva, eyelid, orbital soft tissue), skin, breast, liver, bladder, kidney, prostate, and even in the dura.[26]

Four recurrent chromosomal translocations have been associated with the pathogenesis of MALT lymphomas: t(11;18)(q21;q21), involving the cIAP2/MALT1 genes; t(1;14)(p22;q32), involving BCL10/IgH; t(14;18)(q32;q21), involving IgH/MALT1; and t(3;14)(p14.1;q32), involving FOXP1/IgH.[27,28]

These chromosomal translocations seem to be mutually exclusive and demonstrate site-specificity in terms of their incidence. Interestingly, three seemingly disparate translocations—t(11;18)(q21;q21), t(1;14)(p22;q32) and t(14;18)(q32;q21)—despite involving different genes, all appear to affect the same signaling pathway, resulting in the activation of nuclear factor kappa B (NF-κB), a transcription factor with a central role in immunity, inflammation, and apoptosis.[27,28] The most common is the translocation t(11;18)(q21;q21), which results in a fusion of the cIAP2 region on chromosome 11q21 with the *MALT1* gene on chromosome 18q21, and is present in more than one-third of cases. The frequency of this translocation is site-related: common in the gastrointestinal tract and lung, rare in conjunctiva and orbit, and almost absent in salivary glands, thyroid, liver, and skin. It can be speculated that there are site-specific pathogenetic pathways, however, whether the presence of different infection at different sites can lead not only to chronic B-cell proliferation but also to the specific translocations that characterize most MALT lymphomas remains to be demonstrated. Nevertheless, these translocations may have a significant clinical relevance. For instance, the t(11;18) is present in only 10% of tumors confined to the gastric wall but is common in those disseminated beyond the stomach; moreover, the presence of this translocation can predict a poor therapeutic response of gastric MALT lymphoma to *H. pylori* eradication[29] but not necessarily to other therapeutic approaches.[30,31]

The pathogenetic relevance of the t(3;14)(p14.1;q32) is not completely clear; it involves the immunoglobulin heavy-chain gene on chromosome 14 and the forkhead box protein P1 (*FOXP1*) gene on chromosome 3.[27,28,32] Nuclear FOXP1 expression has been shown in 30% of MALT lymphomas, apparently associated with poor clinical outcome, especially in cases with trisomies 3 or 18 or with increased number of scattered large activated B cells.[33]

Clinical Features

MALT lymphoma is a tumor of adults, with a median age at presentation near 60 years and a slightly higher proportion of females.[2,24] The clinical features and presenting symptoms are mainly related to the primary location,[5,12,26] but some general characteristics can be described.[24,34,35] Few patients present with elevated lactate dehydrogenase (LDH) or beta-2-microglobulin levels. Constitutional B symptoms are extremely uncommon. MALT lymphoma usually remains localized for a prolonged period within the tissue of origin, but dissemination at multiple sites seems not uncommon, occurring in up to one-fourth of cases, with either synchronous or metachronous involvement of multiple mucosal sites or nonmucosal sites, such as spleen, bone marrow, or liver; regional lymph nodes can also be infiltrated.[24,34,36]

Disseminated disease appears to be more common in non-GI MALT lymphomas.[26] Bone marrow involvement is reported in up to 20% of cases.[37] Within the stomach, MALT lymphoma is often multifocal, which may explain the report of relapses in the gastric stump after surgical excision.[5] Gastric MALT lymphoma can disseminate to the intestine[38] and to the spleen.[39] A concomitant GI and non-GI involvement can be detected in approximately 10% of cases. It has been postulated that dissemination of MALT lymphoma may be because of specific expression of special homing receptors or adhesion molecules on the surface of most B-cells of MALT, either normal or transformed.[40]

Most patients with MALT lymphoma have a favorable outcome with prolonged overall survival (usually higher than 85% at 5 years).[24,34] Patients with unfavorable international prognostic index (IPI) and those with lymph node or bone marrow involvement at presentation, but not those with involvement of multiple mucosal sites, may have a worse prognosis. If initially localized, the disease is generally slow to disseminate. Recurrences may involve either extra-nodal sites or nodal sites. The median time-to-progression is apparently better for the GI compared with the non-GI lymphomas (9 versus 5 years, respectively),[35] but no significant differences in overall survival have been shown. Localization may have prognostic relevance because of organ-specific clinical problems, which result in particular management strategies but, as different genetic lesions have been reported at different anatomic locations, it may also be possible that different sites have a distinct natural history. However, the frequency of involvement of any particular site, even in large multicenter series, is not high enough to clearly determine whether patients with MALT lymphomas arising at some specific sites have a significantly different survival. In a radiotherapy study from Toronto, gastric and thyroid MALT lymphomas had the best outcome, whereas distant failures were more common for other sites.[41] In the multicenter series from the International Extranodal Lymphoma Study Group (IELSG), the patients with the disease initially presenting in the upper airways appeared to include a higher number of patients with advanced disease and had slightly poorer outcome (**Table 1**). In general, despite frequent relapses, MALT lymphomas most often maintain an indolent

Table 1
Clinical features and outcome of MALT lymphomas according to the main presentation site

Extranodal Site	Stage I$_E$	Elevated LDH	Bone Marrow Involvement	5-Year OS (95% CI)
Stomach	88%	1%	7.5%	82% (67%–91%)
Intestine	56%	11%	0	100%
Lung	60%	27%	7%	100%
Breast	100%	33%	0	100%
Thyroid	60%	10%	0	100%
Ocular adnexa[a]	84%	26%	13%	94% (77%–98%)
Salivary glands	83%	17%	9%	97% (81%–100%)
Upper airways	50%	42%	33%	46% (7%–80%)
Skin	82%	9%	9%	100%
Multi-organ[b]	NA	26	33%	77% (43%–93%)

Abbreviations: CI, confidence intervals; NA, not applicable; OS, overall survival.
[a] Recalculated from the published[34] split data on orbital and conjuntival MALT lymphomas.
[b] Patients with multiple MALT sites with or without nodal or bone marrow (or both) involvement.
Data from Pinotti G, Zucca E, Roggero E, et al. Clinical features, treatment and outcome in a series of 93 patients with low-grade gastric MALT lymphoma. Leuk Lymphoma 1997;26:529; Zucca E, Conconi A, Pedrinis E, et al. Nongastric marginal zone B-cell lymphoma of mucosa-associated lymphoid tissue. Blood 2003;101:2490–1.

course. Histologic transformation to large cell lymphoma is reported in about 10% of the cases, usually as a late event and independently from dissemination.[24]

Recommended staging procedures

The traditional Ann Arbor staging system, which is based on lymph node involvement, can be misleading in MALT lymphomas. Alternative staging systems for extranodal lymphomas had been proposed in the 1970s,[42] but still a general consensus has not been achieved.[43,44] The presence of asymptomatic dissemination in patients with apparently localized disease[38] and the relatively common presentation with early dissemination[24,34,36] appear valid reasons to suggest extensive staging procedures in all patients with MALT lymphoma.[36]

On the other hand, however, many patients with disseminated disease seem to have the same long-term outcome of those with localized disease. Moreover, in retrospective comparisons of different therapeutic approaches, in spite of higher complete response rate with surgery, no difference in survival was found between the treatment subsets (local treatment with surgery or radiotherapy versus systemic treatment with chemotherapy versus combined modality).[12,45]

Thus, outside clinical trials, it is the authors' opinion that aggressive staging procedures should be tailored to the individual patient according to the clinical conditions (presenting localization, age, intended treatment, performance status, and symptoms). In general, the staging procedures for all locations of MALT lymphoma should comprise a complete clinical history and the physical examination with a careful evaluation of all lymph nodes regions, inspection of the upper airways and tonsils, thyroid examination, and clinical evaluation of the size of liver and spleen. Standard poster anterior and lateral chest radiographs and a computed tomography scan of thorax, abdomen, and pelvis should be performed. Bone marrow biopsy must be performed at diagnosis. Laboratory tests should include complete blood counts with cytologic examination, LDH and beta-2-microglobulin levels, evaluation of renal and liver function, serology for hepatitis C virus (HCV) and HIV infections. Utility of positron emission tomography scan is controversial.[46–48] Then, according to the particular clinical presentation, the investigations may focus on specific organs. Endoscopy and endoscopic ultrasound are indicated in GI presentations, bronchoscopy with bronchoalveolar lavage may be useful in lung lesions, and mammography and MRI in cases presenting in the breast. Particular attention should finally be paid to the demonstration of certain chronic infections that may have a pathogenetic role (*H. pylori, B. burgdorferi, C. psittaci, C. jejuni*).

Staging procedures and risk assessment in gastric MALT lymphoma

Because the stomach is the most common and best-studied site of MALT lymphoma and has peculiar therapeutic strategies, it is convenient to discuss separately the main diagnostic and clinical aspects of the gastric presentation.

Non-specific upper GI complaints (dyspepsia, epigastric pain, nausea, and chronic manifestations of GI bleeding, such as anemia) are the most common presenting symptoms of gastric MALT lymphoma that often lead to an endoscopic evaluation. Gastroscopy usually reveals nonspecific gastritis or peptic ulcer, with mass lesions being unusual. Diagnosis is based on the histopathologic evaluation of the gastric biopsies.[5,26]

Which is the best staging system is still controversial[26,43] and a variety of alternative systems have been proposed. The authors have largely used the modification of the Blackledge staging system, known as the "Lugano staging system."[49] However, this system was proposed before the wide use of endoscopic ultrasound and does not accurately describe the depth of infiltration in the gastric wall, a parameter that is highly predictive for the MALT lymphoma response to anti-*Helicobacter* therapy. Indeed, there is a general consensus that initial staging procedures should include a gastroduodenal endoscopy, with multiple biopsies from each region of the stomach, duodenum, gastro-esophageal junction, and from any abnormal-appearing site. Fresh biopsy and washing material should be available for cytogenetic studies in addition to routine histology and immunohistochemistry. A molecular genetic or a fluorescence in situ hybridization analysis for detection of t(11;18) may be useful for identifying disease that is unlikely to respond to antibiotic therapy.[50] The presence of active *H. pylori* infection must be determined by histochemistry (Genta stain or Warthin-Starry stain) and breath test; serology studies are recommended when the results of histology are negative. Endoscopic ultrasound is recommended in the initial follow-up for evaluation of depth of infiltration and presence of perigastric lymph nodes. Indeed, patients with deep infiltration of the gastric wall carry a higher risk of lymph node involvement, and show a lower response rate after antibiotic therapy.[13–15] Although the disease remains usually localized in the stomach, systemic dissemination and bone marrow involvement should be excluded at presentation because prognosis is worse with advanced stage or adverse IPI.[5]

Management and Follow-up

H. pylori eradication in gastric MALT lymphoma

More than 20 reported (nonrandomized) studies repeatedly confirmed that remission of the lymphoma could be obtained in the majority of patients treated with anti-helicobacter therapy,[17,51–53] with high probabilities of long-term disease control.[54–56] Therefore, *H. Pylori* eradication with antibiotics is today the widely accepted initial standard treatment for stage I gastric lymphoma of MALT type.[57,58] The histologic remission can usually be documented within 6 months from the *H. pylori* eradication but sometimes the period required is more prolonged and the therapeutic response may be delayed up to more than 1 year.[5] Several effective anti-*H. pylori* programs are available and any of them can be employed.[59] The choice should be based on the epidemiology of the infection in the different countries, taking into account the locally expected antibiotic resistance. The most commonly used regimen is triple therapy with a proton pump inhibitor (eg, omeprazole, lansoprazole, pantoprazole, or esomeprazole), in association with amoxicillin, and clarithromycin. Metronidazole can be substituted for amoxicillin in penicillin-allergic individuals. Other regimens that include bismuth, or H2-receptor antagonists (rather than proton pump inhibitors) with antibiotics are also effective.

A number of molecular follow-up studies showed that postantibiotic histologic and endoscopic remission does not necessarily mean a cure; the authors and others described a frequent long-term persistence of monoclonal B-cell after histologic regression of the lymphoma.[60–63] In these cases, watchful waiting is recommended.[57] Indeed, most of the patients with molecular residual disease did not have a frank lymphoma relapse and the clinical relevance of the detection of monoclonality remains unclear. The need of molecular studies as a part of the routine follow-up procedures is, therefore, questionable. Transient histologic relapses have also been described, suggesting that the neoplastic clone can again temporarily expand, but without the growth stimulus from *H. pylori* this may usually remain a self-limiting event.[64] A strict follow-up is nevertheless advisable, and histologic evaluation of repeated biopsies is the fundamental follow-up procedure.[57] There is growing evidence that in case of persistent but stable residual histologic MALT lymphoma infiltrates, a "wait-and-see" policy may be safe.[55,56,64,65]

Anti-Helicobacter therapy in diffuse large B-cell lymphoma of the stomach

Gastric lymphoma with diffuse large cell infiltration should be treated according to the recommendations for diffuse large cell lymphomas. Nevertheless, the efficacy of anti-*Helicobacter* therapy has been reported in some localized cases of diffuse large B-cell lymphoma of the stomach, suggesting that high-grade transformation is not necessarily associated with the loss of *H. pylori* dependence.[66] At present, however, this approach has not yet been validated by prospective studies and the sole antibiotic therapy for gastric large cell lymphoma cannot be advised outside clinical trials.

Posttreatment histologic evaluation

The interpretation of residual lymphoid infiltrate in gastric biopsies after antibiotic treatment can be very difficult and there are no uniform criteria for the definition of histologic remission. The histologic score proposed by Wotherspoon in 1993.[7] is very useful to express the degree of confidence in the MALT lymphoma diagnosis, but it is often difficult to use in the evaluation of the response to therapy on small gastric biopsies and other criteria have also been proposed (**Table 2**).[11,67] This lack of standard reproducible criteria can affect the comparison of the results of the different clinical trials and may explain the relatively wide range of complete responses in the literature reports.

Factors predicting the lymphoma response to H. pylori eradication

The large majority of gastric MALT lymphomas can be cured by *H. pylori* eradication; nevertheless, it would be very useful to identify, at the time of diagnosis, the cases that will not respond to *H pylori* eradication. In general, lymphomas at stage II or above do not respond to *H pylori* eradication because a response to antibiotic therapy is unlikely in the cases with documented nodal involvement.[14,15,68] However, the majority of gastric MALT lymphomas at diagnosis are at stage I_E and the prognostic value of staging in these cases is limited. In this setting, endoscopic ultrasound can be useful to predict the lymphoma response to *H. pylori* eradication. Several studies showed that there is a significant difference between the response rates of lymphomas restricted to the gastric mucosa and those with less superficial lesions.[13,16] The response rate is highest for the mucosa-confined lymphomas (approximately 70%–90%) and then decreases markedly and progressively for the tumors infiltrating the submucosa, the muscularis propria, and the serosa.

Liu and colleagues[50,69] have shown that the t(11;18) was present in only 10% of tumors confined to the gastric wall but in 78% of those disseminated beyond the stomach. As stated before, the presence of the t(11;18) translocation can predict the therapeutic response of gastric MALT lymphoma to *H. pylori* eradication but not necessarily to other therapeutic approaches.[30,31] *H. pylori*-independent status is often associated with nuclear translocation of BCL10 and gastric MALT lymphomas with strong BCL10 nuclear expression or t(1;14) are also usually resistant to *H. pylori* eradication.[70] Indeed, the frequencies of t(11;18)(q21;q21) and BCL10 nuclear expression are significantly higher in the *H. pylori*-negative than in the *H. pylori*-positive cases.[71]

Management of H. pylori-negative or antibiotic-resistant cases

No definite guidelines exist for the management of the subset of *H. pylori*-negative cases and for the patients who fail antibiotic therapy.[57] In two retrospective series of patients with gastric low-grade MALT lymphoma, no statistically significant difference was apparent in survival between patients who received different initial treatments (including chemotherapy alone, surgery alone, surgery with additional chemotherapy or radiation therapy or antibiotics against *H. pylori*).[12,45] Patients with a negative *H. pylori* status and those with persistant gastric lymphoma infiltrates

Table 2
Different reported criteria to define histologic lymphoma remission in gastric MALT lymphoma endoscopic biopsies after anti-*Helicobacter* treatment

Response	Definition	Histologic Features
Wotherspoon's score[7]		
Score 0	Complete histologic remission	Normal gastric mucosa with scattered plasma cells in LP.
Score 1	Complete histologic remission	Chronic active gastritis with small clusters of lymphocytes in LP, no lymphoid follicles; no LEL
Score 2	Complete histologic remission	Chronic active gastritis with prominent lymphoid follicles with surrounding mantle zone and plasma cells; no LEL
Score 3	Partial histologic remission	Suspicious lymphoid infiltrate, probably reactive with lymphoid follicles surrounded by small lymphocytes that infiltrate diffusely in LP and occasionally into epithelium
Score 4	No change (persistent lymphoma)	Suspicious lymphoid infiltrate, probably lymphoma with lymphoid follicles surrounded by centrocyte-like cells that infiltrate diffusely in LP and into epithelium in small groups
Score 5	No change (persistent lymphoma)	MALT lymphoma with dense diffuse infiltrate of centrocyte-like cells in LP and prominent LEL
German system[9,11]		
CR	Complete histologic regression	No remnant lymphoma cells detectable in the post-treatment biopsy specimens and "empty" LP with small basal clusters of lymphocytes and scattered plasma cells
PR	Partial histologic regression	Only partial depletion of atypical lymphoid cells from the LP or focal LEL
NC	No change (low-grade gastric MALT lymphoma)	Unequivocal evidence of LEL and replacement of the gastric glands by uniform centrocyte-like cells
Groupe d'Etudes des Lymphomes de L'Adulte grading system[67]		
CR	Complete histologic remission	Normal or empty LP or fibrosis with absent or scattered plasma cells and small lymphoid cells in the LP, no LEL
pMRD	Probable minimal residual disease	Empty LP or fibrosis with aggregates of lymphoid cells or lymphoid nodules in the LP/MM or SM, no LEL
rRD	Responding residual disease	Focal empty LP or fibrosis with dense, diffuse or nodular lymphoid infiltrate, extending around glands in the LP, focal LEL or absent
NC	No change	Dense, diffuse or nodular lymphoid infiltrate, LEL usually present

Abbreviations: LEL, lymphoepithelial lesions; LP, lamina propria; MM, muscolaris mucosa; SM, submucosa.
Data from Refs.[7,11,67]

following effective anti-*Helicobacter* treatment are usually referred for oncologic treatments (irradiation, surgery, chemotherapy, immunotherapy or a combination of these).[72] However, these patients do not necessarily need prompt aggressive lymphoma therapy. Indeed, response to antibiotic treatment can sometimes be observed also in *H. pylori*-negative patients, especially if they are not carrying t(11;18)(q21;q21).[71] Moreover, most patients with persistent but stable minimal histologic residuals of gastric MALT lymphoma after successful eradication of *H. pylori* appear to have a favorable disease course without oncologic treatment.[56,65] Thus, a "wait-and-see" strategy with regular endoscopies and biopsies appears to be safe and should be considered in this situation.

There are no published randomized studies to help the treatment choice when treatment is needed. Surgery has been widely and successfully used in the past, but the precise role for surgical resection should be redefined in view of the promising results of the conservative approach.[5] Excellent disease control using radiation therapy has been reported by several institutions, supporting the approach that involved-field radiotherapy (30–36 Gy given in 4 weeks of radiation to the stomach and perigastric nodes) is the treatment of choice for patients with stage I-II MALT lymphoma of the stomach without evidence of *H. pylori* infection or with persistent lymphoma after antibiotics.[41,73,74]

Patients with systemic disease should be considered for systemic treatment with chemotherapy or immunotherapy with anti CD20 monoclonal antibodies.[17,75] In the presence of disseminated or advanced disease, chemotherapy is an obvious choice, but only few compounds and regimens have been tested specifically in MALT lymphomas. Oral alkylatyng agents (either cyclophosphamide or chlorambucil, with median treatment duration of 1 year) can result in a high rate of disease control.[68,76] More recent phase II studies demonstrated the antitumor activity of the purine analogs fludarabine[77] and cladribine (2-CDA),[78] which might however be associated with an increased risk of secondary myelodysplasic syndrome,[79] and of a combination regimen of chlorambucil/mitoxantrone/prednisone.[80] Aggressive anthracycline-containing chemotherapy should be reserved for patients with high tumor burden (bulky masses, high IPI score).[81] The activity of rituximab has been shown in a phase II studies (with response rate of about 70%) and may represent an additional option.[30,82,83] The efficacy of the combination of rituximab with chemotherapy is being explored in a phase III study of the IELSG.

Management of nongastric localizations

Nongastric MALT lymphomas have been difficult to characterize because these tumors are widely distributed throughout the body and it is difficult to assemble adequate series of any single site. At least one-fourth of non-GI MALT lymphomas has been reported to present with involvement of multiple mucosal sites with or without the participation of nonmucosal sites, such as bone marrow and lymph nodes.[24,34,36] Non-GI MALT lymphomas, despite presenting with stage IV disease more often than the gastric variant, usually have a quite indolent course. In a multicenter retrospective survey of 180 nongastric cases observed over a long period, subjects were treated according to the current policy of each institution at the time of diagnosis. This study showed no evidence of a clear advantage for any type of therapy and, despite the high proportion of cases with disseminated disease, which should require a systemic approach, no clear advantage was associated with a chemotherapy program.[34]

In general, the consideration previously done regarding the treatment of *H. pylori*-negative cases can be applied to nongastric MALT lymphoma. Radiation therapy is the best studied approach and is considered the treatment of choice for localized lesions.[74] The finding that *C. psittaci* is associated with MALT lymphoma of the ocular adnexa may provide the rationale for the antibiotic treatment of localized lesions. Preliminary encouraging results have been reported but need to be confirmed by additional prospective studies and at present this approach should be considered investigational.[84]

In general, the optimal management of disseminated MALT lymphomas is less clearly defined and should take into account the site, the stage, and the clinical characteristics of the individual patient.

Immunoproliferative small intestinal disease

IPSID, also known as Mediterranean lymphoma or alpha-heavy-chain disease, is today considered a special variant of MALT lymphoma.[3,85] It is characterized by a diffuse lymphoplasmacytic/plasmacytic infiltrate in the proximal small intestine.[86] The distinguishing feature of IPSID is the synthesis of alpha-heavy chain. Most of the cases have been described in the Middle East, especially in the Mediterranean area where the disease is endemic, affecting young adults of both sexes but predominantly the males. A few cases have been reported from industrialized Western countries, usually among immigrants from the endemic area.[85] The IPSID natural course is usually prolonged, often over many years, including a potentially reversible early phase, with the disease usually confined to the abdomen. It was already known in the 1970s that in the early phases of IPSID, durable remissions can be obtained with sustained treatment with antibiotics, but only in 2004 Lecuit and colleagues[20] demonstrated the presence of a specific pathogen, linking this lymphoma to *C. jejuni*. In early-stage disease antibiotic treatment directed against *C. jejuni* may lead to lymphoma regression.[20] However, there is no clear evidence that antibiotics alone are of benefit in the advanced phases. Surgery has a diagnostic but no therapeutic role because intestinal involvement is generally diffuse. Although the early studies reported that aggressive chemotherapy is not well tolerated by patients with advanced disease and severe malabsorption who then have poor survival rates, more recent data suggest that anthracycline-containing regimens, combined with nutritional support plus antibiotics to control diarrhea and malabsorption, may offer the best chance of cure.[85,86]

PRIMARY SPLENIC MARGINAL ZONE LYMPHOMA (WITH OR WITHOUT CIRCULATING VILLOUS LYMPHOCYTES)

Splenic MZL (SMZL) is a very rare disorder, comprising less than 2% of all lymphoid malignancies.[87] The term SMZL was first used in 1992 to describe a primary splenic indolent lymphoma with the morphology and immunophenotype of splenic marginal zone lymphocytes and a micronodular pattern of spleen involvement.[88] Up to two-thirds of the patients with SMZL present circulating villous lymphocytes with characteristic fine cytoplasm polar projections. When these are more than 20% of the lymphocyte count, the term "splenic lymphoma with villous lymphocytes" is commonly used. In the WHO classification, SMZL with or without villous lymphocytes is considered as a separate entity.[89] cDNA microarray expression profiling and tissue microarray immunohistochemical studies showed a largely homogenous signature of SMZLs, suggesting the existence of a single molecular entity.[90,91] Revised guidelines for its diagnosis, staging, and treatment was proposed by a panel of experts in 2007.[87] In series from southern Europe, HCV seems to be involved in lymphomagenesis, but there are relevant geographic variations.[92–99] Very interesting is the observation that some patients with splenic lymphoma with villous lymphocyes and HCV infection obtained a complete remission after treatment with interferon alfa.[100] Interferon treatment had no antitumor effect on HCV-negative SMZL. These data, confirmed also by other groups,[99] suggest a pathogenetic relationship between HCV and some cases of SMZL.

Most patients with primary SMZL are over 60, with a similar incidence in males and females.[87] The disease usually presents with massive splenomegay, which produces abdominal discomfort and pain. Diagnosis is often made at splenectomy performed to establish the cause of unexplained spleen enlargement.

According to the WHO classification, the peripheral lymph node involvement is typically absent,[101] but some reports refer to SMZL even with some evidence of peripheral nodal or extranodal involvement.[102] Patients with disseminated marginal zone lymphomas can be observed in advanced stages of either SMZL or nodal MZL or extranodal MZL,[103] and a precise diagnosis can be very difficult in cases presenting with concomitant splenic, extranodal, and nodal involvement. In a retrospective French series of 124 patients with non-MALT type MZL,[104] four clinical subtypes were observed: splenic (48% of cases), nodal (30%), disseminated (splenic and nodal, 16%), and leukemic (not splenic nor nodal, 6%). Even when the disease is restricted to the cases presenting with splenomegaly, nearly all patients have bone marrow involvement, often accompanied by involvement of peripheral blood (defined as the present of absolute lymphocytosis of more than 5%),[102] Because of the high frequency of bone marrow or liver involvement, about 95% of cases are classified as Ann Arbor stage IV. The clinical course is most usually indolent, with 5-year overall survival ranging from 65% to 80%. Histologic transformation is rare, often associated with B-symptoms, disease dissemination and poorer outcome.[81]

Most patients can be initially managed with a "wait-and-see" policy, and they did not seem to have a worst outcome.[87,102–106] All the cases should be tested for HCV infection and antiviral therapy should be considered in the positive cases before any decision about more aggressive therapeutic approaches. Interferon-alpha (or pegylated interferon) alone or in combination with Ribavirine could be used according to the HCV genotype.[87]

When treatment is needed, this is usually because of large symptomatic splenomegaly or cytopenias. Splenectomy appears to be the treatment of choice in patients with bulky spleen or hypersplenism and no evidence of HCV infection;[87] it allows a reduction or disappearance of circulating tumor lymphocytes and recover of the lymphoma-associated cytopenia.[103,105–107] The benefit of splenectomy often persists for several years and time to next treatment can be longer than 5 years. Adjuvant chemotherapy after splenectomy may result in higher rate of complete responses; however, there is no evidence of a survival benefit.[103]

Chemotherapy alone may be considered for patients who require treatment but have contraindication to splenectomy and for the patient with clinical progression after spleen removal. Alkylating agents (chlorambucil or cyclophosphamide) have been reported to be active and can be used as single agent or in combination (as in the cyclophosphamide, vincristine, prednisone or CVP and cyclophosphamide-hydroxydaunomycin oncovin prednisone or CHOP regimens). Among the purine analogs, Fludarabine has been shown to be effective[108] and can be used alone or in combination with cyclophosphamide.[87] Rituximab, alone or in combination with chemotherapy is very active[109–111] and rituximab alone can be the treatment of choice in elderly patients and in those with impaired renal function.[87]

NODAL MARGINAL ZONE LYMPHOMA (MONOCYTOID LYMPHOMA)

Nodal MZL is very rare and accounts for less than 1% of all lymphomas.[2,81] It also has been associated with HCV infection in some epidemiologic studies.[98,99] This type of lymphoma is a disease of older people, with the median age at presentation in the sixth decade, and affects both sexes, with a slight female predominance. In contrast with mucosa-based extranodal MALT lymphoma, nodal marginal zone (nodal MZL) lymphoma typically affects the lymph-nodes.[112] A common presenting feature is a localized adenopathy, most often in the neck. Concurrent extranodal involvement, most often of the salivary gland, is not rare, and some patients have a history of Sjögren's syndrome or other autoimmune diseases, suggesting a possible overlap with extranodal MALT lymphomas. Many patients present with generalized adenopathy. Bone marrow is involved at presentation in less than half of the cases. Transformation to high-grade lymphoma has been described in some cases.

There is at present no consensus about the best treatment, individual cases being managed differently according to site and stage. In the above-mentioned French series of non-MALT marginal zone B-cell lymphomas,[104] the nodal cases comprised 30% of patients and showed a more aggressive behavior. Nodal and disseminated subtypes had shorter median time-to-progression (about 1 year) in comparison with the splenic and leukemic subtypes (median time to progression longer than 5 years). The cases with disseminated disease more often presented with poor prognosis parameters (high LDH and beta 2 microglobulin, poor performance status, bulky disease) and might represent the end-stage of the other subtypes.[103,104] However, in all subsets, even if the median time-to-progression was short, a prolonged overall survival was observed (splenic, 9 years; nodal, 5.5 years; disseminated 15 years; leukemic 7 years). The retrospective nature of the published studies precludes any conclusion on the therapeutic aspects and treatment decision should be based on the histologic and clinical features of the individual patient.[98,113] Conservative treatments seem recommended for leukemic and splenic subtypes, while in nodal and disseminated subtypes front-line chemotherapy may be considered. Treatment options may include single agent chlorambucil or fludarabine or combination chemotherapy regimens (such as the CVP or CHOP). Rituximab may also have some efficacy[114] and can be combined with chemotherapy;[81] anti-HCV treatment may induce lymphoma regression in some HCV-infected patients.[115] Autologous transplantation has been used in younger patients with adverse prognostic factors or increased large cell number.[104]

REFERENCES

1. Jaffe ES, Harris NL, Stein H, et al. World Health Organization classification of tumours. Pathology and genetics of tumours of haematopoietic and lymphoid tissues. Lyon (France): IARC Press; 2001. p. 1–351.
2. The Non-Hodgkin's Lymphoma Classification project: a clinical evaluation of the International Lymphoma Study Group classification of non-Hodgkin's lymphoma. Blood 1997;89:3909–18.
3. Isaacson PG, Muller-Hermelink HK, Piris MA, et al. Extranodal marginal zone B-cell lymphoma of mucosa-associated lymphoid tissue (MALT lymphoma). In: Jaffe ES, Harris NL, Stein H, et al, editors. World Health Organization classification of tumours. Pathology and genetics of tumours of haematopoietic and lymphoid tissues. Lyon (France): IARC Press; 2001. p. 157–60.
4. Pozzi B, Cerati M, Capella C. MALT lymphoma: pathology. In: Bertoni F, Zucca E, editors. MALT lymphomas. Georgetown (TX): Landes Bioscience/Kluwer Academic; 2004. p. 17–45.
5. Zucca E, Bertoni F, Roggero E, et al. The gastric marginal zone B-cell lymphoma of MALT type. Blood 2000;96:410–9.

6. Bertoni F, Cazzaniga G, Bosshard G, et al. Immunoglobulin heavy chain diversity genes rearrangement pattern indicates that MALT-type gastric lymphoma B cells have undergone an antigen selection process. Br J Haematol 1997;97:830–6.

7. Wotherspoon AC, Doglioni C, Diss TC, et al. Regression of primary low-grade B-cell gastric lymphoma of mucosa- associated lymphoid tissue type after eradication of *Helicobacter pylori*. Lancet 1993;342:575–7.

8. Roggero E, Zucca E, Pinotti G, et al. Eradication of *Helicobacter pylori* infection in primary low-grade gastric lymphoma of mucosa-associated lymphoid tissue. Ann Intern Med 1995;122:767–9.

9. Bayerdorffer E, Neubauer A, Rudolph B, et al. Regression of primary gastric lymphoma of mucosa-associated lymphoid tissue type after cure of *Helicobacter pylori* infection. MALT Lymphoma Study Group. Lancet 1995;345:1591–4.

10. Montalban C, Manzanal A, Boixeda D, et al. *Helicobacter pylori* eradication for the treatment of low-grade gastric MALT lymphoma: follow-up together with sequential molecular studies. Ann Oncol 1997;8(Suppl 2):37–9.

11. Neubauer A, Thiede C, Morgner A, et al. Cure of *Helicobacter pylori* infection and duration of remission of low-grade gastric mucosa-associated lymphoid tissue lymphoma. J Natl Cancer Inst 1997;89:1350–5.

12. Pinotti G, Zucca E, Roggero E, et al. Clinical features, treatment and outcome in a series of 93 patients with low-grade gastric MALT lymphoma. Leuk Lymphoma 1997;26:527–37.

13. Sackmann M, Morgner A, Rudolph B, et al. Regression of gastric MALT lymphoma after eradication of *Helicobacter pylori* is predicted by endosonographic staging. MALT Lymphoma Study Group. Gastroenterology 1997;113:1087–90.

14. Steinbach G, Ford R, Glober G, et al. Antibiotic treatment of gastric lymphoma of mucosa-associated lymphoid tissue. An uncontrolled trial. Ann Intern Med 1999; 131:88–95.

15. Ruskone-Fourmestraux A, Lavergne A, Aegerter PH, et al. Predictive factors for regression of gastric MALT lymphoma after anti-*Helicobacter pylori* treatment. Gut 2001;48:297–303.

16. Nakamura S, Matsumoto T, Suekane H, et al. Predictive value of endoscopic ultrasonography for regression of gastric low grade and high grade MALT lymphomas after eradication of *Helicobacter pylori*. Gut 2001;48:454–60.

17. Zucca E, Cavalli F. Are antibiotics the treatment of choice for gastric lymphoma? Curr Hematol Rep 2004;3:11–6.

18. Roggero E, Zucca E, Mainetti C, et al. Eradication of *Borrelia burgdorferi* infection in primary marginal zone B-cell lymphoma of the skin. Hum Pathol 2000;31: 263–8.

19. Ferreri AJ, Guidoboni M, Ponzoni M, et al. Evidence for an association between *Chlamydia psittaci* and ocular adnexal lymphomas. J Natl Cancer Inst 2004;96: 586–94.

20. Lecuit M, Abachin E, Martin A, et al. Immunoproliferative small intestinal disease associated with *Campylobacter jejuni*. N Engl J Med 2004;350:239–48.

21. Doglioni C, Wotherspoon AC, Moschini A, et al. High incidence of primary gastric lymphoma in northeastern Italy. Lancet 1992;339:834–5.

22. Nakamura S, Yao T, Aoyagi K, et al. *Helicobacter pylori* and primary gastric lymphoma. A histopathologic and immunohistochemical analysis of 237 patients. Cancer 1997;79:3–11.

23. Wotherspoon AC, Ortiz-Hidalgo C, Falzon MR, et al. *Helicobacter pylori*-associated gastritis and primary B-cell gastric lymphoma. Lancet 1991;338: 1175–6.

24. Thieblemont C, Berger F, Dumontet C, et al. Mucosa-associated lymphoid tissue lymphoma is a disseminated disease in one third of 158 patients analyzed. Blood 2000;95:802–6.

25. Radaszkiewicz T, Dragosics B, Bauer P. Gastrointestinal malignant lymphomas of the mucosa-associated lymphoid tissue: factors relevant to prognosis. Gastroenterology 1992;102:1628–38.

26. Thieblemont C, Coiffier B. MALT lymphoma: sites of presentations, clinical features and staging procedures. In: Zucca E, Bertoni F, editors. MALT lymphomas. Georgetown (TX): Landes Bioscience/Kluwer Academic; 2004. p. 60–80.

27. Bertoni F, Zucca E. Delving deeper into MALT lymphoma biology. J Clin Invest 2006;116:22–6.

28. Farinha P, Gascoyne RD. Molecular pathogenesis of mucosa-associated lymphoid tissue lymphoma. J Clin Oncol 2005;23:6370–8.

29. Liu H, Ye H, Dogan A, et al. T(11;18)(q21;q21) is associated with advanced mucosa-associated lymphoid tissue lymphoma that expresses nuclear BCL10. Blood 2001;98:1182–7.

30. Martinelli G, Laszlo D, Ferreri AJ, et al. Clinical activity of Rituximab in gastric marginal zone Non-Hodgkin's lymphoma resistant to or not eligible for anti-*Helicobacter pylori* therapy. J Clin Oncol 2005;23:1979–83.

31. Streubel B, Ye H, Du MQ, et al. Translocation t(11;18)(q21;q21) is not predictive of response to chemotherapy with 2CdA in patients with gastric MALT lymphoma. Oncology 2004;66:476–80.

32. Streubel B, Vinatzer U, Lamprecht A, et al. T(3;14)(p14.1;q32) involving IGH and FOXP1 is a novel recurrent chromosomal aberration in MALT lymphoma. Leukemia 2005;19:652–8.

33. Sagaert X, de Paepe P, Libbrecht L, et al. Forkhead box protein P1 expression in mucosa-associated lymphoid tissue lymphomas predicts poor prognosis and transformation to diffuse large B-cell lymphoma. J Clin Oncol 2006;24:2490–7.

34. Zucca E, Conconi A, Pedrinis E, et al. Nongastric marginal zone B-cell lymphoma of mucosa-associated lymphoid tissue. Blood 2003;101:2489–95.

35. Thieblemont C, Bastion Y, Berger F, et al. Mucosa-associated lymphoid tissue gastrointestinal and nongastrointestinal lymphoma behavior: analysis of 108 patients. J Clin Oncol 1997;15:1624–30.

36. Raderer M, Vorbeck F, Formanek M, et al. Importance of extensive staging in patients with mucosa-associated lymphoid tissue (MALT)-type lymphoma. Br J Cancer 2000;83:454–7.

37. Cavalli F, Isaacson PG, Gascoyne RD, et al. MALT Lymphomas. Hematology Am Soc Hematol Educ Program 2001;241–58.

38. Du MQ, Xu CF, Diss TC, et al. Intestinal dissemination of gastric mucosa-associated lymphoid tissue lymphoma. Blood 1996;88:4445–51.

39. Du MQ, Peng HZ, Dogan A, et al. Preferential dissemination of B-cell gastric mucosa-associated lymphoid tissue (MALT) lymphoma to the splenic marginal zone. Blood 1997;90:4071–7.

40. Drillenburg P, van der Voort R, Koopman G, et al. Preferential expression of the mucosal homing receptor integrin alpha 4 beta 7 in gastrointestinal non-Hodgkin's lymphomas. Am J Pathol 1997;150:919–27.

41. Tsang RW, Gospodarowicz MK, Pintilie M, et al. Localized mucosa-associated lymphoid tissue lymphoma treated with radiation therapy has excellent clinical outcome. J Clin Oncol 2003;21:4157–64.

42. Musshoff K. [Clinical staging classification of non-Hodgkin's lymphomas (author's transl]. Strahlentherapie 1977;153:218–21 [in German].

43. de Jong D, Aleman BM, Taal BG, et al. Controversies and consensus in the diagnosis, work-up and treatment of gastric lymphoma: an International survey. Ann Oncol 1999;10:275–80.
44. Ferrucci PF, Zucca E. Primary gastric lymphoma pathogenesis and treatment: what has changed over the past 10 years? Br J Haematol 2007; 136:521–38.
45. Thieblemont C, Dumontet C, Bouafia F, et al. Outcome in relation to treatment modalities in 48 patients with localized gastric MALT lymphoma: a retrospective study of patients treated during 1976–2001. Leuk Lymphoma 2003;44:257–62.
46. Beal KP, Yeung HW, Yahalom J. FDG-PET scanning for detection and staging of extranodal marginal zone lymphomas of the MALT type: a report of 42 cases. Ann Oncol 2005;16:473–80.
47. Elstrom R, Guan L, Baker G, et al. Utility of FDG-PET scanning in lymphoma by WHO classification. Blood 2003;101:3875–6.
48. Hoffmann M, Kletter K, Becherer A, et al. 18F-fluorodeoxyglucose positron emission tomography (18F-FDG-PET) for staging and follow-up of marginal zone B-cell lymphoma. Oncology 2003;64:336–40.
49. Rohatiner A, d'Amore F, Coiffier B, et al. Report on a workshop convened to discuss the pathological and staging classifications of gastrointestinal tract lymphoma. Ann Oncol 1994;5:397–400.
50. Liu H, Ye H, Ruskone-Fourmestraux A, et al. T(11;18) is a marker for all stage gastric MALT lymphomas that will not respond to *H. pylori* eradication. Gastroenterology 2002;122:1286–94.
51. Stolte M, Bayerdorffer E, Morgner A, et al. *Helicobacter* and gastric MALT lymphoma. Gut 2002;50(Suppl 3):III19–24.
52. Ahmad A, Govil Y, Frank BB. Gastric mucosa-associated lymphoid tissue lymphoma. Am J Gastroenterol 2003;98:975–86.
53. Conconi A, Cavalli F, Zucca E. Gastric MALT lymphomas: the role of antibiotics. In: Bertoni F, Zucca E, editors. MALT lymphomas. Georgetown (TX): Landes Bioscience/Kluwer Academic; 2004. p. 81–90.
54. Fischbach W, Goebeler-Kolve ME, Dragosics B, et al. Long term outcome of patients with gastric marginal zone B cell lymphoma of mucosa associated lymphoid tissue (MALT) following exclusive *Helicobacter pylori* eradication therapy: experience from a large prospective series. Gut 2004;53:34–7.
55. Wundisch T, Thiede C, Morgner A, et al. Long-term follow-up of gastric MALT lymphoma after *Helicobacter pylori* eradication. J Clin Oncol 2005;23:8018–24.
56. Chini C, Pinotti G, Stathis A, et al. Long term outcome of gastric MALT lymphoma patients treated with Anti-Helicobacter (antibiotic and proton-pump inhibitor) regimens. Blood (presented at the ASH Annual Meeting Abstracts) 110:110:Abstract 2583, 2007.
57. Zucca E, Dreyling M. Gastric marginal zone lymphoma of MALT type: ESMO clinical recommendations for diagnosis, treatment and follow-up. Ann Oncol 2008;19(Suppl 2):ii70–1.
58. Bertoni F, Zucca E. State-of-the-art therapeutics: marginal-zone lymphoma. J Clin Oncol 2005;23:6415–20.
59. Howden CW, Hunt RH. Guidelines for the management of *Helicobacter pylori* infection. Ad Hoc Committee on Practice Parameters of the American College of Gastroenterology. Am J Gastroenterol 1998;93:2330–8.
60. Bertoni F, Conconi A, Capella C, et al. Molecular follow-up in gastric mucosa-associated lymphoid tissue lymphomas: early analysis of the LY03 cooperative trial. Blood 2002;99:2541–4.

61. Thiede C, Wundisch T, Alpen B, et al. Persistence of monoclonal B cells after cure of *Helicobacter pylori* infection and complete histologic remission in gastric mucosa- associated lymphoid tissue B-cell lymphoma. Journal of Clinical Oncology 2001;19:1600–9.

62. Montalban C, Santon A, Redondo C, et al. Long-term persistence of molecular disease after histological remission in low-grade gastric MALT lymphoma treated with *H. pylori* eradication. Lack of association with translocation t(11;18): a 10-year updated follow-up of a prospective study. Ann Oncol 2005;16:1539–44.

63. de Mascarel A, Ruskone-Fourmestraux A, Lavergne-Slove A, et al. Clinical, histological and molecular follow-up of 60 patients with gastric marginal zone lymphoma of mucosa-associated lymphoid tissue. Virchows Arch 2005;446: 219–24.

64. Isaacson PG, Diss TC, Wotherspoon AC, et al. Long-term follow-up of gastric MALT lymphoma treated by eradication of *H. pylori* with antibiotics. Gastroenter-ology 1999;117:750–1.

65. Fischbach W, Goebeler ME, Ruskone-Fourmestraux A, et al. Most patients with minimal histological residuals of gastric MALT lymphoma after successful eradication of *Helicobacter pylori* can be managed safely by a watch and wait strategy: experience from a large international series. Gut 2007;56:1685–7.

66. Chen LT, Lin JT, Tai JJ, et al. Long-term results of anti-*Helicobacter pylori* therapy in early-stage gastric high-grade transformed MALT lymphoma. J Natl Cancer Inst 2005;97:1345–53.

67. Copie-Bergman C, Gaulard P, Lavergne-Slove A, et al. Proposal for a new histo-logical grading system for post-treatment evaluation of gastric MALT lymphoma. Gut 2003;52:1656.

68. Levy M, Copie-Bergman C, Traulle C, et al. Conservative treatment of primary gastric low-grade B-cell lymphoma of mucosa-associated lymphoid tissue: predictive factors of response and outcome. Am J Gastroenterol 2002;97:292–7.

69. Alpen B, Neubauer A, Dierlamm J, et al. Translocation t(11;18) absent in early gastric marginal zone B-cell lymphoma of MALT type responding to eradication of *Helicobacter pylori* infection. Blood 2000;95:4014–5.

70. Ye H, Gong L, Liu H, et al. Strong BCL10 nuclear expression identifies gastric MALT lymphomas that do not respond to *H. pylori* eradication. Gut 2006;55: 137–8.

71. Nakamura S, Matsumoto T, Ye H, et al. *Helicobacter pylori*-negative gastric mucosa-associated lymphoid tissue lymphoma: a clinicopathologic and molec-ular study with reference to antibiotic treatment. Cancer 2006;107:2770–8.

72. Cohen SM, Petryk M, Varma M, et al. Non-Hodgkin's lymphoma of mucosa-associated lymphoid tissue. Oncologist 2006;11:1100–17.

73. Schechter NR, Portlock CS, Yahalom J. Treatment of mucosa-associated lymphoid tissue lymphoma of the stomach with radiation alone. J Clin Oncol 1998;16:1916–21.

74. Gospodarowicz M, Tsang R. Radiation therapy of mucosa-associated lymphoid tissue (MALT) lymphomas. In: Bertoni F, Zucca E, editors. MALT lymphomas. Georgetown (TX): Landes Bioscience/Kluwer Academic; 2004. p. 104–29.

75. Conconi A, Cavalli F, Zucca E. MALT lymphomas: the role of chemotherapy. In: Bertoni F, Zucca E, editors. MALT lymphomas. Georgetown (TX): Landes Biosci-ence/Kluwer Academic; 2004. p. 99–103.

76. Hammel P, Haioun C, Chaumette MT, et al. Efficacy of single-agent chemother-apy in low-grade B-cell mucosa- associated lymphoid tissue lymphoma with prominent gastric expression. J Clin Oncol 1995;13:2524–9.

77. Zinzani PL, Stefoni V, Musuraca G, et al. Fludarabine-containing chemotherapy as frontline treatment of nongastrointestinal mucosa-associated lymphoid tissue lymphoma. Cancer 2004;100:2190–4.
78. Jager G, Neumeister P, Brezinschek R, et al. Treatment of extranodal marginal zone B-Cell lymphoma of mucosa- associated lymphoid tissue type with cladribine: a phase II study. J Clin Oncol 2002;20:3872–7.
79. Jager G, Hofler G, Linkesch W, et al. Occurence of a myelodysplastic syndrome (MDS) during first-line 2-chloro-deoxyadenosine (2-CDA) treatment of a low-grade gastrointestinal MALT lymphoma. Case report and review of the literature. Haematologica 2004;89:ECR01.
80. Wohrer S, Drach J, Hejna M, et al. Treatment of extranodal marginal zone B-cell lymphoma of mucosa-associated lymphoid tissue (MALT lymphoma) with mitoxantrone, chlorambucil and prednisone (MCP). Ann Oncol 2003;14:1758–61.
81. Thieblemont C. Clinical presentation and management of marginal zone lymphomas. Hematology Am Soc Hematol Educ Program 2005;307–13.
82. Conconi A, Martinelli G, Thieblemont C, et al. Clinical activity of rituximab in extranodal marginal zone B-cell lymphoma of MALT type. Blood 2003;102:2741–5.
83. Raderer M, Jager G, Brugger S, et al. Rituximab for treatment of advanced extranodal marginal zone B cell lymphoma of the mucosa-associated lymphoid tissue lymphoma. Oncology 2003;65:306–10.
84. Ferreri AJ, Dolcetti R, Du MQ, et al. Ocular adnexal MALT lymphoma: an intriguing model for antigen-driven lymphomagenesis and microbial-targeted therapy. Ann Oncol 2008;19:835–46.
85. Al-Saleem T, Al-Mondhiry H. Immunoproliferative small intestinal disease (IPSID): a model for mature B-cell neoplasms. Blood 2005;105:2274–80.
86. Zucca E, Roggero E, Bertoni F, et al. Primary extranodal non-Hodgkin's lymphomas. Part 1: gastrointestinal, cutaneous and genitourinary lymphomas. Ann Oncol 1997;8:727–37.
87. Matutes E, Oscier D, Montalban C, et al. Splenic marginal zone lymphoma proposals for a revision of diagnostic, staging and therapeutic criteria. Leukemia 2008;22:487–95.
88. Schmid C, Kirkham N, Diss T, et al. Splenic marginal zone cell lymphoma. Am J Surg Pathol 1992;16:455–66.
89. Isaacson PI, Piris MA, Catovsky D, et al. Splenic marginal zone lymphoma. In: Jaffe ES, Harris NL, Stein H, editors. World Health Organization classification of tumours. Pathology and genetics of tumours of haematopoietic and lymphoid tissues. Lyon (France): IARC Press; 2001. p. 135–7.
90. Ruiz-Ballesteros E, Mollejo M, Rodriguez A, et al. Splenic marginal zone lymphoma: proposal of new diagnostic and prognostic markers identified after tissue and cDNA microarray analysis. Blood 2005;106:1831–8.
91. Mollejo M, Camacho FI, Algara P, et al. Nodal and splenic marginal zone B cell lymphomas. Hematol Oncol 2005;23:108–18.
92. Gisbert JP, Garcia-Buey L, Pajares JM, et al. Prevalence of hepatitis C virus infection in B-cell non-Hodgkin's lymphoma: systematic review and meta-analysis. Gastroenterology 2003;125:1723–32.
93. Chan CH, Hadlock KG, Foung SK, et al. V(H)1-69 gene is preferentially used by hepatitis C virus-associated B cell lymphomas and by normal B cells responding to the E2 viral antigen. Blood 2001;97:1023–6.
94. Karavattathayyil SJ, Kalkeri G, Liu HJ, et al. Detection of hepatitis C virus RNA sequences in B-cell non-Hodgkin lymphoma. Am J Clin Pathol 2000;113:391–8.

95. Zucca E, Roggero E, Maggi-Solca N, et al. Prevalence of *Helicobacter pylori* and hepatitis C virus infections among non-Hodgkin's lymphoma patients in Southern Switzerland. Haematologica 2000;85:147–53.

96. Thalen DJ, Raemaekers J, Galama J, et al. Absence of hepatitis C virus infection in non-Hodgkin's lymphoma. Br J Haematol 1997;96:880–1.

97. Luppi M, Negrini R. MALT lymphoma: epidemiology and infectious agents. In: Bertoni F, Zucca E, editors. MALT lymphomas. Georgetown (TX): Landes Bioscience/Kluwer Academic; 2004. p. 1–16.

98. Arcaini L, Paulli M, Boveri E, et al. Marginal zone-related neoplasms of splenic and nodal origin. Haematologica 2003;88:80–93.

99. Arcaini L, Paulli M, Boveri E, et al. Splenic and nodal marginal zone lymphomas are indolent disorders at high hepatitis C virus seroprevalence with distinct presenting features but similar morphologic and phenotypic profiles. Cancer 2004; 100:107–15.

100. Hermine O, Lefrere F, Bronowicki JP, et al. Regression of splenic lymphoma with villous lymphocytes after treatment of hepatitis C virus infection. N Engl J Med 2002;347:89–94.

101. Isaacson PG. Splenic marginal zone B cell lymphoma. In: Mason DY, Harris NL, editors. Human lymphoma: clinical implications of the REAL classification. London: Springer-Verlag; 1999. p. 7.1–6.

102. Chacon JI, Mollejo M, Munoz E, et al. Splenic marginal zone lymphoma: clinical characteristics and prognostic factors in a series of 60 patients. Blood 2002; 100:1648–54.

103. Thieblemont C, Felman P, Callet-Bauchu E, et al. Splenic marginal-zone lymphoma: a distinct clinical and pathological entity. Lancet Oncol 2003;4:95–103.

104. Berger F, Felman P, Thieblemont C, et al. Non-MALT marginal zone B-cell lymphomas: a description of clinical presentation and outcome in 124 patients. Blood 2000;95:1950–6.

105. Troussard X, Valensi F, Duchayne E, et al. Splenic lymphoma with villous lymphocytes: clinical presentation, biology and prognostic factors in a series of 100 patients. Groupe Francais d'Hematologie Cellulaire (GFHC). Br J Haematol 1996;93:731–6.

106. Catovsky D, Matutes E. Splenic lymphoma with circulating villous lymphocytes/splenic marginal-zone lymphoma. Semin Haematol 1999;36:148–54.

107. Mulligan SP, Matutes E, Dearden C, et al. Splenic lymphoma with villous lymphocytes: natural history and response to therapy in 50 cases. Br J Haematol 1991; 78:206–9.

108. Lefrere F, Hermine O, Belanger C, et al. Fludarabine: an effective treatment in patients with splenic lymphoma with villous lymphocytes. Leukemia 2000;14: 573–5.

109. Arcaini L, Orlandi E, Scotti M, et al. Combination of rituximab, cyclophosphamide, and vincristine induces complete hematologic remission of splenic marginal zone lymphoma. Clin Lymphoma 2004;4:250–2.

110. Kalpadakis C, Pangalis GA, Dimopoulou MN, et al. Rituximab monotherapy is highly effective in splenic marginal zone lymphoma. Hematol Oncol 2007;25: 127–31.

111. Bennett M, Yegena S, Dave HP, et al. Rituximab monotherapy is highly effective in splenic marginal zone lymphoma. Hematol Oncol 2008;26:114.

112. Nathwani BN, Anderson JR, Armitage JO, et al. Marginal zone B-cell lymphoma: a clinical comparison of nodal and mucosa-associated lymphoid tissue types. Non-Hodgkin's Lymphoma Classification Project. J Clin Oncol 1999;17:2486–92.

113. Berger F, Traverse-Glehen A, Salles G. Nodal marginal zone B-Cell lymphoma. In: Mauch PM, Armitage J, Coiffier B, et al, editors. Non-Hodgkin's lymphomas. Philadelphia: Lippincott Williams & Wilkins; 2004. p. 361–5.

114. Koh LP, Lim LC, Thng CH. Retreatment with chimeric CD 20 monoclonal antibody in a patient with nodal marginal zone B-cell lymphoma. Med Oncol 2000;17:225–8.

115. Vallisa D, Bernuzzi P, Arcaini L, et al. Role of Anti-Hepatitis C Virus (HCV) Treatment in HCV-Related, Low-Grade, B-Cell, Non-Hodgkin's Lymphoma: a multicenter Italian experience. J Clin Oncol 2005;23:468–73.

Indolent Lymphomas Other than Follicular and Marginal Zone Lymphomas

Stefan Peinert, MD[a], John F. Seymour, MB, BS, FRACP, PhD[a,b],*

KEYWORDS

- Lymphoma • Indolent • Management

This article addresses two of the less common entities among clinically indolent B-cell non-Hodgkin lymphomas (NHL): small lymphocytic lymphoma (SLL) and lymphoplasmacytic lymphoma (LPL), also known as Waldenstrom's macroglobulinemia (WM).

SLL is a very rare disease closely related to the more common chronic lymphocytic leukemia (CLL). Localized SLL should be treated with radiotherapy with curative intent, but most cases of SLL cases are disseminated and are managed in the same manner as CLL. The management strategy depends greatly on the individual case and can range from watchful waiting or single-agent treatment (eg, chlorambucil, rituximab) to intensive chemoimmunotherapy with fludarabine and cyclophosphamide plus rituximab (FCR) or even stem cell transplantation in selected patients. New agents such as the immunologically active lenalidomide have shown promising results in relapsed disease and currently are being explored in studies for first-line treatment of SLL and CLL. For patients who have LPL/WM, treatment is required only for symptomatic disease. Intensive chemoimmunotherapy (eg, FCR) results in improved response rates and progression-free survival (PFS) but so far has failed to achieve an improvement in overall survival (OS) compared with treatment using alkylators or rituximab alone. High-dose chemotherapy and stem cell transplantation should be considered in younger patients to achieve prolonged remissions (with autologous stem cell transplantation, ASCT) or even potential cure (with allogeneic stem cell transplantation, alloSCT). Proteasome inhibitors and immunomodulatory agents have shown some activity in recent studies of LPL/WM.

[a] Department of Haematology, Peter MacCallum Cancer Centre, Locked Bag 1, A'Beckett St, East Melbourne, Victoria 8006, Australia
[b] University of Melbourne, Parkville, Victoria, Australia
* Corresponding author. Department of Haematology, Peter MacCallum Cancer Centre, Locked Bag 1, A'Beckett St, Victoria 8006, Australia.
E-mail address: john.seymour@petermac.org (J.F. Seymour).

Hematol Oncol Clin N Am 22 (2008) 903–940
doi:10.1016/j.hoc.2008.07.005   hemonc.theclinics.com
0889-8588/08/$ – see front matter. Crown Copyright © 2008 Elsevier Inc. All rights reserved.

SMALL LYMPHOCYTIC LYMPHOMA

SLL is histologically and (using routine diagnostic antibody panels) immunophenotypically identical to the much more common CLL, and both entities are subsumed in one category of B-cell-lymphomas in the World Health Organization (WHO) classification.[1] By definition, SLL is characterized by lymphadenopathy and/or hepatosplenomegaly or other organ infiltration and by an absolute peripheral blood lymphocyte count lower than required for the diagnosis of CLL ($< 5 \times 10^9$/L). This threshold is arbitrary, however, and about 20% to 30% of patients have been shown to progress from SLL to CLL during a follow-up of 5 years from the time of diagnosis.[2,3] At the time of diagnosis about 25% to 50% of patients who have SLL have bone marrow involvement. Of note, disease manifestations outside lymphopoietic and hematopoietic organs is common in SLL, the most common sites being the gastrointestinal tract, lungs, and orbit.[2,4,5] If a monoclonal B-cell population of less than 5×10^9/L is found in the absence of lymphadenopathy or extranodal disease (including bone marrow biopsy, if performed), the diagnosis is monoclonal B-lymphocytosis (MBL).[6] The most recent revision of the International Workshop on Chronic Lymphocytic Leukemia (IWCLL) guidelines recommends that the presence of cytopenia resulting from marrow infiltration is adequate to establish the diagnosis of CLL, regardless of peripheral blood B-lymphocyte counts or lymph node involvement.[7] For the diagnostic criteria of MBL, SLL, and CLL, see **Table 1**.

Both SLL and CLL are diseases predominantly of the elderly, with a median age at onset in excess of 60 years and an increasing incidence with older age.[8] They also occur, although uncommonly, in younger age groups. In recent years, both entities have been diagnosed with increasing frequency in younger patients and even in adolescents.[9,10] It is not quite clear if this change results from a true rise in the incidence within these age groups or is an artifact caused by improved and more abundantly applied diagnostics such as flow cytometry. The second possibility is supported by low numbers of monoclonal B-cells with SLL/CLL phenotype that can be found in about 3.5% of healthy individuals who have normal peripheral blood counts.[11] These cases show the same male preponderance of about 1.2 to 2:1 that is found consistently in CLL and SLL,[9,10,12] possibly indicating a higher prevalence of early-stage indolent CLL/SLL in the general population than previously recognised.[11]

CLL is the most common form of leukemia in the Western Hemisphere, with approximately 15,300 new cases per year in the United States. SLL, on the other hand, is a relatively rare disease, comprising only about 4% to 7% of all NHL.[9,12,13] In a recent retrospective analysis at the MD Anderson Cancer Center including 2126 patients who had SLL or CLL, only 15% of patients had SLL. Consequently most of the published data address either CLL exclusively or both diseases with SLL comprising only

Table 1
The differential diagnosis of CLL, SLL, and MBL according to the WHO classification is made according to the extent of lymphocytosis in the peripheral blood and bone marrow

Disase	Peripheral Blood Lymphocytes	Bone Marrow Lymphocyte Infiltration[a] (%)	Extramedullary Disease
CLL	$\geq 5 \times 10^9$/L	≥ 30	Present or absent
SLL	$< 5 \times 10^9$/L	< 30	Present
MBL	$< 5 \times 10^9$/L	< 30	Absent

[a] Bone marrow (here as percentage of nucleated cells), if a bone marrow biopsy has been performed.

a minority of cases. This focus on CLL certainly has contributed to the similar manner in which SLL and CLL are managed (except for rare early-stage SLL and a few differences caused by the specific characteristics and complications of each entity).

DIAGNOSIS AND DIFFERENTIAL DIAGNOSIS OF SMALL LYMPHOCYTIC LYMPHOMA AND CHRONIC LYMPHOCYTIC LEUKEMIA

Because the management of SLL differs from that of other indolent B-cell NHL, an accurate diagnosis is important. If circulating monoclonal cells are present, as is true in most cases of SLL, the examination of peripheral blood usually is sufficient to ascertain the diagnosis SLL/CLL. Besides a complete blood cell count with differential and film, the immunophenotype of the leukemic cells in the peripheral blood should be determined.[14]

Flow cytometry analysis of the leukemic cells shows a distinct pattern of marker expression with positivity of CD5, CD19, CD20, and CD23 and weak surface immunoglobulin with light-chain restriction. Characteristically, the expression levels of immunoglobulin and of pan–B-cell markers such as CD20 and CD79b are lower than in normal B lymphocytes.[15]

If the results of the peripheral blood examinations are unequivocal, a bone marrow biopsy is not mandatory but usually is recommended for several reasons: The histologic examination enables the assessment of the extent and pattern (diffuse versus nondiffuse) of the marrow infiltration and, if the lymphocyte count in the peripheral blood is less than $5 \times 10^9/L$, distinguishes SLL from CLL (< 30% versus $\geq$ 30% lymphocytic infiltrate, respectively). Furthermore, the bone marrow examination allows the cause of cytopenia to be determined (eg, hypoplasia of hematopoietic marrow versus sufficient normal hematopoiesis, which suggests a peripheral cause for cytopenia). Also, if successful treatment leads to resolution of disease manifestations such as leukemic cells in the peripheral blood, lymphadenopathy, and other extramedullary sites of disease, a bone marrow biopsy showing absence of a leukemic infiltrate is required to establish a complete remission (CR).

Genetic analyses can be performed with malignant cells from the peripheral blood or from the bone marrow and are becoming increasingly important in prognostication, as discussed later.

Patients who have SLL often have marked lymphadenopathy; hepato- and/or splenomegaly may be present at the time of initial diagnosis or may develop as the disease progresses.

If malignant cells are absent in the peripheral blood at the time of first presentation, a tissue biopsy, usually from an enlarged lymph node, is required to establish the diagnosis. If lymphadenopathy is the most prominent manifestation of disease, and typical CLL/SLL cells are found in the peripheral blood and/or bone marrow, a lymph node core biopsy or lymph node excision still should be performed for histologic assessment to confirm the diagnosis. Fine-needle aspirations are discouraged because of the high likelihood of a false-negative result. Biopsy is especially important if any clinical or biochemical parameters (eg, a rapidly enlarging mass, B symptoms [fever, night sweats, and weight loss], or high lactate dehydrogenase levels) suggest transformation to a more aggressive form of lymphoma.

Differential expression of chemokine receptors has been suggested as an explanation for the differences in the clinical pictures of CLL and SLL and the more pronounced nodal involvement in SLL. Both CLL and SLL are positive for chemokine receptor-6 (CCR6), but CLL usually shows strong expression of CCR1, CCR3, and CCR7, whereas SLL does not (**Table 2**).[16,17] The expression of CD38, which also

Table 2 Immunophenotypes of CLL and SLL		
Chemokine Receptor	CLL	SLL
CXCR4	+	+
CCR1	+	−
CCR3	+	−
CCR6	+	+
CCR7	+	−

The chemokine receptor expression in CLL and SLL shows congruence for some receptors but differential expression for others. This variation may explain the different patterns of disease manifestation and might enable differentiation in equivocal cases.

has prognostic implications, seems to be more prevalent in SLL than in CLL.[18,19] A study investigating different hematologic malignancies for the expression of the lymphotoxin-β (*LTB*) gene, which plays an important role in the formation of germinal center reactions and the regulation of immune response and apoptosis, also assessed 32 cases of CLL and 22 samples from patients who had SLL. LTB expression generally was much lower in the malignant cells than in normal B cells and also was much lower in SLL than in CLL; this finding suggests that LTB expression could serve as a potential marker differentiating SLL from CLL.[20]

The clinical course of SLL is generally indolent, and in disseminated cases treatment often is deferred until the patient becomes symptomatic or clinical features indicate evidence of disease progression. Given the indolent natural history of SLL, concomitant diseases often influence the life expectancy in these mostly elderly patients.[21] On the other hand, SLL does occur in younger patients, and the clinical course of the disease can vary widely; therefore factors predictive of treatment response and survival have become of increasing interest.

PROGNOSTIC FACTORS IN SMALL LYMPHOCYTIC LYMPHOMA AND CHRONIC LYMPHOCYTIC LEUKEMIA

In contrast to CLL, for which specific staging systems exist, SLL belongs to the group of NHL, and therefore staging is performed according to the Ann Arbor classification.[22] The relevance of this staging system in SLL, however, is largely restricted to the distinction between localized and disseminated SLL, because localized SLL may be treated with local radiotherapy. Because of frequent extranodal manifestations (mainly bone marrow infiltration in 25%–50% of cases),[23] most SLL cases represent stage 4 disease and therefore are treated with systemic chemotherapy. The traditional staging systems for CLL according to Binet and colleagues[24] and Rai and colleagues[25] heavily reflect the extent of bone marrow infiltration and therefore are not useful for the classification of SLL, in which, by definition, the bone marrow infiltrate is below 30%. New prognostic parameters for SLL and CLL are being explored that rely more on the biologic features of the disease and therefore are more relevant for the prognostication of SLL.[10,26]

Because of SLL is much rarer than CLL and because of the similarity between the malignant cells in these diseases, most studies exploring prognostic markers have included patients who have either of the two diseases, and very few studies have enrolled only patients who have SLL. This situation is particularly true now that the WHO classification subsumes both diseases in one entity.

Genetic Alterations

Cytogenetic analysis using fluorescence in situ hybridization (FISH) identifies aberrations in more than 80% of CLL cases.[27] In prospective assessments of prognostic factors in clinical trials, the 17p deletion associated with mutation/loss of the tumor suppressor gene *p53* and deletion of the long arm of chromosome 11 have been shown to be among the strongest adverse prognostic factors associated with reduced response rates, PFS, and OS.[28,29] These adverse prognostic factors remain relevant when the anti-CD20 monoclonal antibody rituximab is included in the treatment regimen.[30] In retrospective analyses, a 6q deletion also has been found to be an independent adverse prognostic factor, similar to 17p or 11q deletions.[10,31]

Another feature of CLL/SLL with prognostic relevance is the mutational status of the immunoglobulin heavy-chain variable region genes (IgV$_H$ genes). Patients whose disease carries unmutated IgV$_H$ genes have worse outcome than those who have mutated IgV$_H$ genes.[32,33] Unmutated status of IgV$_H$ genes has been found to be associated with expression of CD38 and ZAP-70.[34–36] This correlation is not absolute, however, and the impact on response to treatment and OS is uncertain.[29,30]

Other Prognostic Factors

Not surprisingly, age has been shown to be an important prognostic factor for OS.[8,37,38] In a large retrospective analysis, advanced age was the second most important prognostic factor for OS after the previously mentioned genetic alterations.[10] Male sex has long been recognized as an adverse prognostic factor.[39,40]

Several additional routinely available laboratory parameters such as β_2-microglobulin and serum thymidine kinase have been shown to have prognostic impact.[41,42] A large retrospective study confirmed the predictive value of β_2-microglobulin and also identified serum albumin and creatinine levels as independent prognostic factors.[10] Given the relatively broad basis of these results derived from more than 2000 patients (15% of whom had SLL), the authors propose including these parameters in a score to supplement the established CLL staging systems.[10]

Recently the results of the German CLL1 study in early-stage CLL that prospectively analyzed different prognostic markers identified thymidine kinase, lymphocyte doubling time, β_2-microglobulin, absolute lymphocyte count, sex, and age as independent prognostic factors for PFS; lymphocyte doubling time, β_2-microglobulin, absolute lymphocyte count, and age were prognostic for OS.

The prognostic usefulness of other characteristics such as soluble CD23, microRNA signatures, and CD69 expression is being evaluated but is not yet established.[43–45] An increased percentage of "smudge" cells on the peripheral blood smear seems to be correlated with a favorable prognosis.[46]

Prognostic Factors Specific to Small Lymphocytic Lymphoma

As in other lymphomas, early studies in SLL have identified B symptoms as a negative prognostic factor for OS.[2,8,47] Other patient characteristics such as age, male gender, anemia, or lymphocyte count at the time of diagnosis have been found to have prognostic importance in SLL in some but not all studies. The largest retrospective analysis of prognostic factors performed exclusively in patients who had SLL showed that in patients who had leukocytosis greater than 10×10^9/L, B-symptoms, the presence of "large cells," and bone marrow involvement were independently associated with survival. In patients who did not have leukocytosis, an age of 55 years or more was the only independent prognostic factor for OS.[8]

In all these studies, histologic features of the lymph node suggestive of a more aggressive biologic behavior (ie, diffuse versus pseudofollicular nodal architecture, sinus obliteration, degree of capsular invasion, presence of "large cells," and mitotic index) were associated with shortened OS.[2,3,8,47]

In a study that retrospectively analyzed 54 patients who had SLL (excluding CLL), the 14 patients who had stage 1 or stage 2 disease who were treated with radiotherapy had a better freedom from relapse at 10 years than patients who had stage 3 or stage 4 disease, but there was no significant difference in OS.[2]

Unfortunately, the largest study of prognostic factors in CLL/SLL, which included more than 300 patients who had SLL, has not reported separate data for this subgroup.[10]

TREATMENT OF SMALL LYMPHOCYTIC LYMPHOMA

Despite the similarities between SLL and CLL, there seems to be a difference in the homing characteristics that result in CLL being a systemic disease with manifestation in peripheral blood and bone marrow, whereas SLL can present in a localized manner confined to certain lymph node areas or extranodal tissues. Thus far the underlying mechanisms for this difference have been elucidated only partly with the detection of the differential expression of certain chemokine receptors (as discussed earlier).[16,17] The dichotomy between localized and disseminated SLL has important implications for therapeutic management.

Localized Small Lymphocytic Lymphoma

Like other indolent lymphomas, SLL occurs in a truly localized stage in a minority of patients. This evidence derives from early studies in which a proportion of these patients achieved long-term remissions with involved-field or extended-field radiotherapy alone and without any systemic treatment.[2,4] In the largest cohort of these patients comprising seven patients each who had stage 1 or stage 2 SLL, the 10-year freedom from relapse was 80% and 62%, respectively, after radiotherapy with 40 to 44 Gy over 4 to 6 weeks.[2] This evidence clearly suggests the curative potential of radiotherapy, which therefore should be the treatment modality of choice in the rare cases of stage 1 or stage 2 SLL. Thus, treatment for patients who have localized SLL should not be deferred until the occurrence of disease-related symptoms or other signs of disease progression but should be initiated as soon as the diagnosis is established.

Disseminated Small Lymphocytic Lymphoma

Because of the very similar biology, the treatment of disseminated SLL principally follows that of CLL, except the often more bulky lymphadenopathy and the more common extranodal/extramedullary manifestations may require radiotherapy for local control.

The first important decision regarding treatment for disseminated SLL is when treatment should be initiated, because life expectancy often is limited by comorbidities, not by the disease itself. Some patients who have early-stage disease show rapid disease progression, however, and eventually die from the SLL. One major goal of current and future clinical trials is to characterize a patient's individual disease-related risk and, based on this risk, to stratify the therapeutic strategy. Therefore, it is highly desirable that patients be enrolled in clinical trials that can answer these questions and identify new therapeutic options. As mentioned earlier, most clinical trials performed thus far have included only patients who have CLL or both patients who have CLL and those who have SLL. The results of these trials, therefore, provide the evidence for treatment recommendations for patients who have disseminated SLL.

Several large, prospective, randomized studies have shown that chemotherapy with alkylating agents provides no OS benefit for newly diagnosed patients who have asymptomatic disease.[48–50] Therefore, the recently published IWCLL guidelines recommend a strategy of watchful waiting until any of the defined signs of disease progression occurs.[7] The criteria for initiation of first-line treatment still rely on clinical characteristics such as B-symptoms, fatigue, or symptomatic lymphadenopathy/organomegaly or on classic laboratory parameters (eg, lymphocyte doubling time and cytopenias) and do not include any of the newer prognostic factors (eg, genetic alterations or β_2-microglobulin).[7]

A thorough analysis of the disease should be performed at the time of diagnosis to estimate the patient's prognosis and to plan the timing and intensity of potential treatment. This assessment is especially relevant for younger patients, for whom stem cell transplantation should be considered.

Moreover, with new and increasingly effective therapies becoming available, the treatment paradigm has started to change. Several more recent studies were able to demonstrate that patients achieving a CR enjoy superior OS,[51–54] particularly if minimal residual disease (MRD), as shown by sensitive flow cytometric or molecular techniques, can be eradicated.[52,53,55]

Chemotherapy of Small Lymphocytic Lymphoma

Two major classes of cytostatics are used either as a single agent or in combination: alkylating agents with DNA-damaging capacity (chlorambucil, cyclophosphamide) and purine nucleoside analogues (fludarabine and cladribine) and the structurally related adenosine deaminase inhibitor, pentostatin. The anthracyclines, doxorubicin or mitoxantrone, have been used mainly in combination with any of the alkylating agents or purine nucleoside analogues.

There is a rationale for combining alkylating agents with purine analogues because synergism has been shown in vitro: fludarabine inhibits DNA damage repair caused by cyclophosphamide and is incorporated into the DNA to a greater extent after cells are exposed to cyclophosphamide.[56]

The combination of fludarabine and cyclophosphamide (FC) is the most widely studied in clinical trials, showing better response rates and remission durations than seen with chlorambucil or fludarabine alone.[57,58]

Because fludarabine is the most active single agent in SLL/CLL, numerous studies have combined fludarabine with other DNA-damaging agents such as mitoxantrone,[59,60] mitoxantrone and cytarabine,[61] or anthracyclines.[62,63] None of these regimens has been compared with FC in a prospective, randomized trial, but response rates and response durations seem to be equivalent to those achieved with FC. Studies with combinations of alternative purine analogues (eg, pentostatin or cladribine with cyclophosphamide with or without mitoxantrone) did not achieve better results than those achieved with FC.[64,65] Therefore, FC has emerged as the standard chemotherapy regimen for the intensive treatment of disseminated SLL.

Monoclonal Antibodies

During the last 10 years, monoclonal antibodies have become an important component of the treatment for disseminated SLL. The cell-surface antigen CD20 is expressed on more than 90% of mature B-cell leukemias and lymphomas.[66] The monoclonal anti-CD20 antibody rituximab has shown single-agent activity against relapsed indolent lymphomas, but with the standard regimen of four weekly infusions of rituximab at a dose of 375 mg/m^2 the response rate was considerably lower in SLL than in follicular lymphoma (12% versus 60%).[67] In fact, lower postinfusion rituximab levels were detected in patients who had CLL than in patients who had follicular lymphoma, and a dose escalation up to 2250 mg/m^2 resulted in a 75% response rate in patients who had CLL.[68]

In patients who had previously untreated SLL/CLL, the outcome with standard-dose rituximab was considerably better than in the pretreated population, with response rates greater than 50% and a PFS of 18.6 months.[69] These results still are inferior to those achievable with chemotherapy or chemoimmunotherapy, however, so treatment with single-agent rituximab is indicated primarily for frail patients who are considered unsuitable for chemotherapy but who usually can tolerate rituximab without significant side effects apart from occasional infusion-related reactions.

Another antigen that has gained clinical relevance in the treatment of disseminated SLL and CLL is CD52, which is expressed at high density on normal and malignant B and T lymphocytes but not on hematopoietic stem cells.[70] Alemtuzumab is a human-ized monoclonal antibody against CD52. In a pivotal trial alemtuzumab was adminis-tered to 93 patients who had fludarabine-refractory CLL at a dose of 30 mg administered intravenously three times a week for 12 weeks, resulting in a response rate of 33% and median time to progression and OS of 4.7 and 16 months, respectively. Of note, alemtuzumab was very successful in clearing MRD from peripheral blood and bone marrow but was less effective against lymphadenopathy, which usually is more prominent in SLL than in CLL. The main toxicities were infectious complications, mainly in the nonresponders, with 27% of patients experiencing severe episodes despite pro-phylaxis against *Pneumocystis carinii* pneumonia and herpes simplex virus.[71] These results, which were confirmed in subsequent studies,[72,73] led to alemtuzumab being approved for the treatment of relapsed, fludarabine-refractory CLL. Alemtuzumab seems to maintain moderate efficacy despite the presence of 17p deletions.[71–75]

Administration of alemtuzumab as first-line treatment for CLL in a subcutaneous schedule resulted in an response rate of 81% in the intent-to-treat population, with 19% of patients achieving CRs. Time to treatment failure had not been reached at 18 months' follow-up, and the incidence of severe infections seemed to be lower than with the intravenous schedule. Again, as in the treatment of patients who have refractory SLL/CLL, alemtuzumab is less effective against nodal disease.[76]

The combination of alemtuzumab and rituximab showed very promising response rates of up to 63% in patients who had relapsed or refractory CLL, but the reported time to progression of 6 months was relatively short.[77] Recently, it was suggested in a preclinical model that rituximab resistance in SLL/CLL may be caused in part by CD52 overexpression and potentially could be overcome by alemtuzumab.[78]

Chemo-Immunotherapy

There are several compelling arguments for combining chemotherapy with monoclo-nal antibodies: the two modalities use different mechanisms of cytotoxicity and there-fore should provide at least additive efficacy and reduced risk of resistance, whereas the side effects are only partly overlapping. Preclinical studies have shown synergistic antitumor effects (eg, of rituximab and fludarabine).[79–81] In fact, in a study of the first-line treatment of 224 patients who had CLL, the addition of rituximab, 500 mg/m^2 given intraveneously every 4 weeks on day 1 of the FC regimen, resulted in an overall re-sponse rate of 95% with 70% of patients achieving a CR. A high quality of response was demonstrated in the analysis of MRD by flow cytometry, which found no MRD in the bone marrow of 78% of the patients in CR. This response also translated into durable remissions: an updated analysis of 300 patients showed 5-year PFS and OS rates of 68% and 78%, respectively.[82]

The German CLL study group performed a phase III trial comparing FC with FCR that included 817 patients. The results have not yet been published formally, but according to a press release, the primary end point of the study, increasing the PFS by at least 35%, has been reached.[83] More detailed results and long-term outcome still are awaited.

The FCR regimen also has shown remarkable activity in patients who have previously treated CLL. A study of 177 patients, most of whom had been exposed previously to fludarabine, reported overall response and CR rates of 73% and 25%, respectively, with a median duration of response of 28 months.[54] Another study included a similar cohort of patients who had SLL/CLL for treatment with FCR at the standard rituximab dose of 375 mg/m^2. Overall, the results were very similar, with 100% of patients who had previously untreated SLL/CLL experiencing PFS at 3-year follow-up. In this study, also, the absence of MRD resulted in prolonged remissions in the entire CLL cohort, including pretreated and treatment-naïve patients.[84]

Historical comparisons adjusting for differences in prognostic factors have shown that FCR improves OS in both the first-line and the salvage settings.[53,85]

When combined only with fludarabine, rituximab also seems to improve the overall outcome. In a Cancer and Leukemia Group B study of 104 patients who had previously untreated CLL, first-line treatment with the combination of fludarabine and rituximab resulted in a CR rate of 33% compared with 15% with fludarabine alone.

Various attempts have been made to improve further the results achieved with FCR. Although a dose–response correlation has been shown for rituximab as single agent in the treatment of SLL/CLL,[68,86] tripling the rituximab dose in FCR as first-line therapy did not achieve further benefit in a study of 65 patients who had CLL.[87] Similarly, the addition of mitoxantrone to the FCR regimen did not improve the response rate, but studies with mitoxantrone-containing schedules are ongoing.[88,89]

Pentostatin has been used as an alternative purine analogue in chemoimmunotherapy combinations that were tested in smaller studies with patients who had CLL, but the results did not seem superior to those achieved with fludarabine-based regimens.[90–92]

Combinations of alemtuzumab and fludarabine have been shown to be active in patients who previously were resistant to both single agents.[93,94] A study used fludarabine, 30 mg/m^2, and alemtuzumab, 30 mg, both on days 1 through 3 every 28 days for up to six cycles in 36 patients who had relapsed or refractory CLL previously exposed to fludarabine. The results revealed overall and complete response rates of 83% and 37%, respectively; in patients who had a CR, the median duration of response was 22 months. These results were similar to those achieved with FCR in comparable patient populations.[95]

New Treatment Options for Disseminated Small Lymphocytic Lymphoma and Chronic Lymphocytic Leukemia

As in other B-cell malignancies, immunomodulatory drugs are being explored for the treatment of disseminated SLL or CLL. Thalidomide, alone or in combination with fludarabine, has been shown to have immunologic as well as antileukemic effects in previously untreated patients and in patients who have relapsed or refractory CLL and in some fludarabine-refractory cases.[96–98] In the study recently presented by Giannopoulos and colleagues,[98] thalidomide was given at 100 mg/d for 1 week; then fludarabine was added (25 mg/m^2 for 5 days every 28 days). In previously untreated patients, the response rate was 100%, with four CRs and 14 partial responses

(PRs), and in pretreated patients the response rate was 44% (all PRs). As in other studies, a flare reaction was a common side effect of thalidomide in the first cycle.

Thus far, two phase II trials have been reported that studied lenalidomide as single agent in relapsed or refractory CLL. In the study at the Roswell Park Cancer Institute, the first 29 patients were treated with 25 mg of lenalidomide on days 1 through 21 of a 28-day cycle. For the subsequent 16 patients, the starting dose was reduced to 10 mg and was titrated up to 25 mg, depending on tolerance. The overall response rate was 58%, with a CR rate of 18%. The median time to response and PFS were 5.9 months and 19.4 months, respectively.[99,100]

A similar study performed at the MD Anderson Cancer Center used a lower starting dose of 10 mg of lenalidomide with continuous administration and dose titration up to 25 mg starting after 4 weeks of treatment, but the median tolerated dose was only 10 mg. The overall response rate and CR rates in this study were 32% and 7%, respectively.[101,102] Importantly, the RRs in both studies seemed to be independent of adverse cytogenetic abnormalities (ie, 17p or 11q deletions).[103]

Administration of lenalidomide led to significant immunologic effects such as increases in levels of interleukin (IL)-6, IL-10, IL-2, and tumor necrosis factor-α, but no changes were observed in median levels of vascular endothelial growth factor.[101] The clinical correlate of this immune reaction can be a tumor flare reaction with tender swelling of disease-involved lymph nodes, low-grade fever, rash, and, rarely, a rise in the peripheral blood white cell count. In the Roswell Park study, the median duration of the flare reaction was 14 days; the reaction occurred mainly during the first treatment cycle and correlated with clinical response.[99] The flare reaction usually is easily treated with nonsteroidal anti-inflammatory agents but can be life threatening when associated with tumor lysis syndrome.[104] The other main side effects of lenalidomide were fatigue, neutropenia, and thrombocytopenia.[99,101]

The bcl-2 antisense oligonucleotide oblimersen was evaluated in a phase III trial for patients who had relapsed or refractory CLL that had been pretreated with at least one fludarabine-containing regimen. Patients were treated with a standard FC regimen or with oblimersen and FC. The addition of oblimersen resulted in a modest increase in the rate of CRs and nodal PRs, particularly in fludarabine-sensitive patients, as well as a prolongation of response durations in patients who achieved a CR or nodal PR. Oblimersen was associated frequently with thrombocytopenia and, rarely, with tumor lysis and cytokine release syndrome.[105]

Further new strategies, such as the anti-CD23 monoclonal antibody lumiliximab,[106] the fully humanized anti-CD20 monoclonal antibody ofatumumab,[107] and the semi-synthetic flavone flavopiridol,[108] have shown some activity in CLL, but the evidence is still limited.

Stem Cell Transplantation

Although most patients who have SLL/CLL are elderly, 40% are under the age of 60 years.[109] High-risk patients can be identified using a number of clinical and biologic features,[110] and the presence of these features in younger patients should prompt consideration of a stem cell transplantation, preferably within a clinical trial. So far, no trial has prospectively compared standard chemotherapy with ASCT. A matched-pair analysis comparing 66 patients who had CLL treated with ASCT and 291 patients treated with conventional chemotherapy showed a survival advantage for ASCT.[111] None of these patients, however, had received monoclonal antibodies, which have improved the efficacy of conventional treatment considerably, as part of their treatment.[71–73,83]

Several phase II studies have explored the outcome of ASCT in SLL and CLL.[112–116] Taken together, the transplantation-related mortality (TRM) was 1% to 10%, with most toxicity occurring late. Of particular concern is the induction of second malignancies. One study reported the 5-year actuarial risk of developing myelodysplastic syndrome and acute myeloid leukemia (MDS/AML) after ASCT for SLL/CLL to be 12.4%,[114] another study reported the overall incidence of second malignancies after ASCT in patients who had CLL to be 19%.[113] Chemoresistance at the time of ASCT has been shown to be associated with adverse outcome.[116] In the Medical Research Council study, only one of 65 patients died from ASCT, the CR rate was 74%, and the 5-year OS and PFS rates were 77.5% and 51.5%, respectively.[114]

A retrospective study analyzed the outcome of ASCT (mostly after conditioning with total-body irradiation and cyclophosphamide) for 72 patients who had CLL treated between 1995 and 2005 at five different centers in Finland. None of the patients died from transplant-related complications, but at a median follow-up of 28 months 37% of these moderately pretreated patients had relapsed or progressed, and the estimated median PFS and OS were 48 and 95 months, respectively.[117] These results indicate that ASCT cannot be considered curative in SLL/CLL, and in a cross-trial comparison the outcome generally does not seem superior to that of chemoimmunotherapy (eg, FCR).[82] Furthermore, the collection of hematopoietic stem cells in patients who have SLL/CLL is difficult, especially if they are pretreated with fludarabine.[118–121] A combination of stem cell factor and high-dose granulocyte colony-stimulating factor has been shown to be superior to standard mobilization regimens and more frequently enables successful stem cell collection in this patient population.[122] ASCT is the treatment of choice only in selected patients who have SLL requiring aggressive treatment for long-term disease control.

Allogeneic Stem Cell Transplantation

No results are available from prospective, randomized trials comparing alloSCT with either ASCT or conventional treatment. In contrast to ASCT, long-term disease control and potential cure after alloSCT for SLL/CLL was demonstrated more than 10 years ago.[113,123–125] The myeloablative conditioning regimens used in these early studies were quite toxic, however, leading to nonrelapse mortality at day 100 of up to 57%.[125] Consequently, nonrandomized comparisons of ASCT and alloSCT for patients who had CLL showed superior survival outcomes for ASCT.[126]

Unlike ASCT, the efficacy of alloSCT against SLL/CLL relies more on an immunologic "graft-versus-lymphoma" (GvL) effect than on the antitumor activity of the conditioning regimen itself. This effect is demonstrated by a decreased risk of relapse in patients who have chronic graft-versus-host disease (GvHD),[127] by increased risk of relapse with T-cell depletion of the graft, and by induction of response through donor lymphocyte infusion.[113] Thus, reduced-intensity conditioning (RIC) regimens were developed that are nonmyeloablative but are highly immunosuppressive, allowing engraftment of the allogeneic stem cells. Their reduced acute toxicity makes RIC protocols more suitable for the mostly elderly patients who have SLL/CLL, and RIC protocols now are the most commonly used type of conditioning regimens, resulting in markedly reduced TRM (13%–26%) at 1 year. The RIC protocols, however, were associated with considerable rates of grade 2 through grade 4 acute GvHD (34%–61%) and with extensive chronic GvHD (21%–58%) (**Table 3**).[128–133] No formal assessment of RIC compared with myeloablative alloSCT has been undertaken, but in an analysis of European Bone Marrow Transplant registry data the outcome of 73 patients who received a RIC alloSCT was compared with 82 matched patients who had had undergone myeloablative alloSCT for CLL. The analysis revealed significantly reduced TRM

Table 3
Outcome of RIC alloSCT in patients who had disseminated SLL or CLL

Study	N	Chemo-refractory (%)	TRM (%)	Acute Grade 2–4	Chronic Extensive	Survival Rate (%)
				GvHD (%)		
Khouri et al, 1994[116]	39	Not stated	22 overall	45	58	4 years: OS 48 PFS 44
Schetelig et al, 2003[128]	30	47	13 overall	56	21	2 years: OS 72 PFS 67
Dreger et al, 2003[129]	77	33	18 at 12 months	34	58	2 years: OS 72 PFS 56
Sorror et al, 2005[130]	64	53	22 overall	61	50	2 years: OS 60 PFS 52
Brown et al, 2006[132]	46	57	17 overall	34	43	2 years: OS 54 PFS 34
Delgado et al, 2006[133]	41	27	26 overall	10, grade 3–4	33	2 years: OS 51 PFS 45

but increased relapse rates with RIC and no differences between the two groups in PFS or OS.[134] One important question with RIC alloSCT for SLL/CLL is how much GvL effect can be expected and how much intensity of the conditioning regimen is needed to achieve disease control. The fact that donor lymphocyte infusions alone were able to induce a remission in only 20% of patients suggests that the GvL effect is limited and smaller than in other diseases such as AML.[128,130,133] On the other hand, DFS and OS after RIC alloSCT have been shown to be no different in patients who have poor-prognosis CLL (11q or 17p deletion or unmutated IgV_H) from those who have good-prognosis CLL.[135] Fludarabine-based RIC regimens currently are considered the most promising protocols for alloSCT in patients who have SLL/CLL and continue to be explored in ongoing trials.[136–138]

In a recent analysis of patients who had SLL or CLL undergoing alloSCT, the patients who had SLL had significantly better 5-year PFS and OS than those who had CLL. The authors attribute this finding to the greater incompetence of the immune system in the patients who had CLL.[139]

SUMMARY

The rarity of SLL and its similarity to the much more common CLL hamper the conduction of larger trials that would define further the particularities of SLL and its management. For clinical practice, it is important to identify patients who have early-stage SLL, because these patients should be treated with radiotherapy with curative intent. The differences in receptor expression between SLL and CLL are of only academic interest thus far and have not yet gained clinical relevance. Therefore, disseminated SLL is treated in the same way as CLL, and many studies include patients who have both disease subentities.

Although the data from the supporting study is not yet formally reported, the combination of FCR is the emerging standard for systemic treatment of SLL/CLL. Treatment with a lower intensity (eg, rituximab or chlorambucil alone) still can be an appropriate choice in elderly or frail patients with a view to sequential rather than combined administration of active agents.

The most promising new agents for SLL/CLL are immunologically active drugs, especially lenalidomide, which already has shown remarkable activity as single agent in the setting of relapsed/refractory disease.

ASCT generally has not proven beneficial compared with standard systemic treatment and therefore should be reserved for clinical trials and for specific clinical situations. In young patients and/or those who have high-risk SLL/CLL, alloSCT should be considered, especially if a matched sibling donor is available, and planned early enough in the course of the disease to avoid the development of chemoresistance or histologic transformation, because alloSCT still is the only treatment modality with curative potential.

In many clinical situations, there is no clear evidence as to the best treatment option for patients who have SLL/CLL. Therefore the inclusion of patients who have SLL/CLL in clinical trial remains highly desirable.

LYMPHOPLASMACYTIC LYMPHOMA/WALDENSTROM'S MACROGLOBULINEMIA

The terms "lymphoplasmacytic lymphoma" and "Waldenstrom's macroglobulinemia" were first described by the Swedish physician Jan Gösta Waldenström in the mid-1940s. LPL/WM has long been considered a clinical syndrome and only recently has been defined as a distinct clinicopathological entity.[140,141] The definition of LPL/WM continues to be revised and further refined, with the most widely accepted definition resulting from the Second International Workshop on Waldenstrom's Macroglobulinemia in 2002 (**Table 4**).[142] Differences in the diagnostic criteria used in different clinical trials hamper cross-trial comparisons and interpretation of outcomes, however. As in multiple myeloma, recent definitions of LPL/WM include a category of IgM monoclonal gammopathy of undetermined significance (IgM MGUS).

Epidemiologic data reveal that LPL/WM is a rare disease accounting for only 1% to 2% of all hematologic malignancies, that is, an incidence of approximately three per million people per year.[143,144] As with SLL/CLL, it is a disease of the elderly, with a median age at diagnosis of about 65 years and a male predominance of 55% to 70%.[145] A large retrospective analysis of 146,394 patients who had hepatitis C infection found an increased risk for WM of about threefold.[146] Otherwise, no specific etiologic factors are known, but familial clustering of LPL/WM and other B-cell malignancies suggests genetic predisposition as an important factor for the manifestation of LPL/WM.[147-152]

The risk of developing LPL/WM is 46 times higher in patients who have IgM MGUS than in the general population, but what what triggers the progression is unknown.[153]

Table 4	
Diagnostic criteria for the diagnosis of WM following the Second International Workshop on Waldenstrom's Macroglobulinemia in 2002	
Test	**Finding**
Serum protein electrophoresis	Monoclonal gammopathy IgM
Bone marrow cytology/histology	Diffuse, interstitial or nodular infiltrate of small lymphocytes, lymphoplasmacytoid cells, and plasma cells
Flow cytometry	Surface Ig+, CD5−, CD10−, CD19+, CD20+, CD23−

Data from Owen RG, Treon SP, Al-Katib A. Clinicopathological definition of Waldenstrom's macroglobulinemia: consensus panel recommendations from the Second International Workshop on Waldenstrom's Macroglobulinemia. Semin Oncol 2003;30(2):110–5.

PATHOLOGY/BIOLOGY

Unlike other malignancies, no pathognomonic morphologic, immunophenotypic, or genetic abnormalities are specific for LPL/WM. Thus, other lymphoid malignancies must be excluded, and pathologic as well as clinical characteristics must be taken into account to establish the diagnosis.

The most recent definition formulated at the second International Workshop on Waldenstrom's Macroglobulinemia requires a bone marrow infiltration of lymphoplasmacytic cells (LPCs) in association with a monoclonal IgM, with or without lymphadenopathy (**Table 4**).[142] The cells of LPL/WM show a small B-cell morphology with varying degrees of plasmacytoid features and sometimes a predominance of CD138-positive plasma cells, which also are of monoclonal origin.[142,154,155] The bone marrow infiltrate characteristically is intertrabecular.[142]

A typical morphologic feature is the presence of mast cells, which frequently are seen in the areas of the lymphoplasmacytic infiltrate. These cells are nonclonal but are thought to support survival and proliferation of the LPL cells and to stimulate immunoglobulin production by the expression of CD40 ligand, vascular endothelial growth factor, B-lymphocyte stimulator protein, and platelet-derived growth factor-α.[23,154,156,157]

Immunophenotypic analysis of the LPL cells shows expression of the B-cell markers CD19 and CD20, bright surface IgM, and light-chain restriction. The LPL cells are negative for CD3 and CD103.[158] According to the WHO classification, LPL cells also are negative for CD5, CD10, and CD23, but some groups have found a few cases to be positive for CD5 and/or CD10, and up to 61% of the cases were CD23 positive.[159,160] More refined analyses suggest a more indolent behavior of LPL among FMC7-positive and CD5-negative cases, whereas patients who had FMC7-negative and CD5-positive disease were characterized by high IgM levels and extensive bone marrow infiltration.[161] Recently, it was shown that the LPCs secrete soluble CD27, which seems to stimulate expression of CD40 ligand and other factors important for the pathogenesis of LPL.[162]

The cell of origin from which LPL/WM develops has not been defined, but currently LPCs are thought to resemble memory B cells most closely. Most LPC are of postgerminal center nature, preferentially using the V_H3 family.[163–165] In many cases, two different LPL clones seem to be present with distinct IgH VDJ sequences.[166]

Contrary to previous assumptions, recent studies have shown that LPCs also can undergo isotype class-switch recombination, although the fidelity seems to be impaired.[167,168]

Cytogenetics in Lymphoplasmacytic Lymphoma

Most cases of LPL/WM display a normal karyotype.[169–171] In the rare cases with an abnormal karyotype, a 6q deletion was the most common finding; with interphase FISH this deletion was detectable in about half the samples.[171–174] Some investigators have suggested that a 6q deletion is associated with an adverse prognosis,[175] but others could not confirm this suggestion.[176] Deletions of 13q14 and 17p13.1 are found rarely at the time of diagnosis but can be detected in about 15% of patients at the time of disease progression.[177]

As in multiple myeloma, LPCs express high levels of IL-6 consistent with the high serum levels of C-reactive protein frequently seen in patients who have WM and probably contributing to the disease-related anemia.[178,179]

DIFFERENTIAL DIAGNOSIS

The differential diagnosis of LPL/WM includes all other mature B-cell neoplasms (ie, SLL/CLL, multiple myeloma, marginal zone lymphoma, mantle cell lymphoma, follicular lymphoma). Because there are no pathognomonic features defining LPL/WM, other disease entities must be excluded, and doing so sometimes can be problematic, especially in the case of marginal zone lymphoma.

Given the prognostic implications, it also is important to distinguish between IgM MGUS (< 10% bone marrow infiltration, IgM < 30 g/L) and asymptomatic or symptomatic LPL/WM. Patients who have IgM MGUS have a risk of progression to LPL/WM of about 1.5% per year. The mortality rate of patients who have asymptomatic LPL/WM was found to be similar to that of the general population, whereas patients who have symptomatic disease have a more than five times higher risk of death.[180,181] Therefore, thorough staging at the time of diagnosis is very important.

Diagnostic Testing

For measurement of the paraprotein level, a serum protein electrophoresis usually is optimal. Additional immunofixation usually is required only to characterize the monoclonal protein at the time of diagnosis or in the rare case of a CR. For reasons of comparability, it is important to use the same laboratory method consistently for paraprotein quantification. It is useful to determine the whole blood viscosity at diagnosis because high IgM levels frequently lead to hyperviscosity and rheologic impairment. During further follow-up, however, it often is possible to determine the individual IgM level in a given patient that results in symptomatic hyperviscosity; this knowledge saves frequent viscosity measurements.[182]

In addition to standard routine biochemical assessments, β_2-microglobulin also should be measured because of its prognostic impact.[183,184] A 24-hour urine collection should be performed to assess creatinine clearance and to detect potential Bence-Jones-proteinuria, although Bence-Jones-proteinuria is not common in LPL/WM and rarely causes renal failure.[185] To assess lymphadenopathy and/or hepatosplenomegaly, a CT scan should be performed routinely. A bone scan is recommended only in the case of bone pain or purely plasmacytic morphology.[186–188]

Additional assessments of potential value are coagulation studies, test for amyloid (Congo red stain of the bone marrow, echocardiogram), cryoglobulins, nerve conduction studies, and lymph node biopsies in selected cases.

SYMPTOMS

The most common signs at diagnosis are nonspecific constitutional symptoms, particularly fatigue and malaise.[184,189] The anemia usually is of multifactorial origin resulting from bone marrow infiltration, increased plasma volume, elevated IL-6 levels, and hyperviscosity, which can lead to reduced erythropoietin production.[190] Thrombocytopenia is rare at the time of diagnosis and may be caused by heavy bone marrow infiltrate, splenomegaly, or immune thrombocytopenia.[184,189]

Hepatomegaly, splenomegaly, and lymphadenopathy caused by infiltration by LPCs are each present in about 15% to 20% of cases at diagnosis.[183,184,189,191]

Hyperviscosity

Although it is a classical symptom of LPL/WM, serum hyperviscosity is found only in about 15% of patients at diagnosis.[182,192,193] The physical properties of the pentameric IgM molecule are responsible for slower transit through capillaries. This slower transit can result in typical symptoms (eg, mucosal oronasal bleeding, retinal bleeding, headaches, or neurologic deficits). Often there are only subtle and nonspecific signs such as fatigue, confusion, or impaired cognition that should raise the suspicion of hyperviscosity.[194,195]

The clinical signs correlate with the IgM level, but the threshold for the development of symptoms shows great interpatient variability. At serum viscosity levels below 4 centipoises (cp), clinical signs of hyperviscosity are uncommon, at 5 to 8 cp most patients and above 8 cp virtually all patients are symptomatic. As stated earlier, the IgM threshold for the development of symptoms is fairly consistent for an individual patient.[182,192,193] It is important to note that additional factors such as transfusion of red blood cells can increase the viscosity further and precipitate symptomatic hyperviscosity syndrome.

If high levels of IgM are present, and a patient displays symptoms suggestive of hyperviscosity, plasmapheresis should be performed to reduce the serum paraprotein rapidly. An ophthalmoscopic examination, which can reveal venous engorgement, hemorrhage, or exudates as typical manifestations, is a sensitive method for identifying symptomatic hyperviscosity syndrome.[196]

Peripheral Neuropathy

Another relatively common symptom occurring in about 20% of patients is peripheral neuropathy that is caused mostly by the monoclonal IgM acting as an autoantibody against the myelin sheath.[197,198] Besides the typical chronic, symmetric sensory neuropathy, proprioception also can be affected, resulting in ataxia.[199,200] Other causes for neuropathy in patients who have LPL/WM include amyloid, vitamin B_{12} deficiency, and cryoglobulins.

Amyloidosis

LPL/WM can cause light-chain–associated amyloidosis that seems to carry a higher risk of cardiomyopathy and pleural or pulmonary manifestations than seen in amyloidosis of other causes.[201,202] The development of amyloidosis adversely affects the prognosis of patients who have LPL/WM, and more patients die from complications of cardiac amyloidosis than from the underlying disease itself.[203]

PROGNOSIS

The prognosis of LPL/WM shows great interpatient variability with an estimated median OS of 5 years.[204] Because of the mostly indolent course of the disease and the advanced age of the patients, other causes of death significantly affect the OS. Therefore, the disease-specific survival probably is much higher and was found in a recent analysis to be closer to 11 years.[205] In this study, age greater than 65 years and organomegaly were negative prognostic factors.

In a relatively large study of 232 patients treated with chemotherapy before the era of purine analogues, age greater than 65 years, albumin levels below 40 g/L, and cytopenias (hemoglobin < 120 g/L, platelet count < 150 × 10^9/L, white blood cell count < 4 × 10^9/L) were associated with shorter OS.[204] No difference was found between an initial strategy of watchful waiting and immediate initiation of treatment. The prognostic model based on these findings was validated in two subsequent studies.[206,207]

More recently, an International Prognostic Scoring System was proposed based on the analysis of 587 patients. In this study, age greater than 65 years, cytopenias (hemoglobin < 115 g/L, platelet count < 100 × 10^9/L), and a paraprotein level greater than 70 g/L and a β_2-microglobulin level greater than 3 mg/L were evaluated. A prognostic score was defined based on these parameters: low risk (one or no adverse characteristics other than age > 65 years), intermediate risk (two adverse characteristics or age > 65 years), and high risk (more than two adverse parameters). This score separated the patients into three different prognostic categories with 5-year-survival rates of 87%, 68%, and 36%, respectively.[208]

TREATMENT

Like patients who have other indolent lymphomas (ie, follicular lymphoma or SLL), patients who have LPL/WM often do not require immediate treatment at diagnosis but can be observed until they become symptomatic and/or until disease progression. There is no evidence of survival benefit from treatment of asymptomatic LPL/WM.[181,209] High but asymptomatic IgM levels in themselves are not an indication for treatment.

The accepted indications for treatment are signs of hyperviscosity, symptomatic adenopathy or organomegaly, neuropathy, constitutional symptoms, systemic amyloidosis, transformation to a high-grade lymphoma, cytopenias (typically hemoglobin less than 100 g/L, platelet count $< 100 \times 10^9$/L, or earlier if the patient is symptomatic), cryoglobulinemia, or any other end-organ damage thought to be related to the LPL/WM.[210]

Given the incurability of the disease and the generally advanced age of the patients, symptom relief and prevention of organ damage are the main therapeutic goals.

There usually are several therapeutic options for a patient, and no single treatment regimen has been proven superior. This paucity of evidence results from the relatively small numbers of participants even in phase III trials and the repeated changes in disease definition and response criteria that make interpretation of study results and especially cross-trial comparisons more difficult.

The most widely accepted treatment recommendations were published as a result of the Third International Workshop on Waldenstrom's Macroglobulinemia.[210] Four different acceptable first-line treatment options are listed, so the choice is determined by the characteristics of the individual patient and the preferences of the treating physician (**Box 1**).

Box 1
First-line and salvage treatment of LPL/WM: Consensus Panel recommendations following the Third International Workshop on Waldenstrom's Macroglobulinemia

First-line treatment

Alkylating agents (eg, chlorambucil, cyclophosphamide)

Purine nucleoside analogues (fludarabine, cladribine, pentostatin)

Monoclonal antibody (rituximab)

Combination therapy

Salvage treatment

Reuse of initial therapy if not refractory or alternative first-line agent

Combination therapy

Thalidomide ± steroids

Autologous stem cell transplantation

Alemtuzumab

Data from Treon SP, Gertz MA, Dimopoulos M, et al. Update on treatment recommendations from the Third International Workshop on Waldenstrom's macroglobulinemia. Blood 2006;107(9):3442–6.

One of the main outstanding questions is whether treatment with a purine analogue is superior to the long-standing standard treatment with an alkylating agent. It is hoped that the answer will come from the results of a randomized, phase III trial comparing chlorambucil versus fludarabine as first-line treatment. This trial has been completed, but the results are not yet available.[211]

For decades the standard treatment for LPL/WM has been oral alkylators such as chlorambucil, melphalan, or cyclophosphamide, which generally are well tolerated. Chlorambucil has been the most commonly used agent, resulting in a response rate of about 50% and a median OS of 5 years.[189] Continuous application of 0.1 mg/kg/d or pulsed doses of 0.3 mg/kg/d for 7 days every 28 days were found to be equivalent with regard to response rate (79% and 68%, respectively) and OS.[212] The optimal duration of treatment has not been established; a reasonable strategy is to treat until a response plateau is achieved and then stop treatment and monitor. Prolonged treatment increases the risk of therapy-related myelodysplasias and leukemias.[212–214] Prolonged treatment also carries the risk of impairing the collection of hematopoietic stem cells for a subsequent ASCT, which makes this class of agents less suitable for the first-line treatment of younger patients. Given their favorable safety profile, alkylators are still an attractive treatment option for elderly patients.

Rituximab

Another generally well-tolerated treatment option that can be administered as single agent or in combination with chemotherapy is rituximab. First studies in patients who had chemotherapy-refractory disease have shown symptomatic improvements and objective responses.[215–218] The overall response rate was 44% to 60%, including minor responses, and did not differ between pretreated and treatment-naïve patients.[218,219] When the standard regimen with four weekly infusions of rituximab (375 mg/m^2) was used, the median time to response was 3.3 months, and the median duration of response was 16 months.[219]

Further experience has shown that the best response to rituximab may be delayed until many months after treatment initiation. Therefore, a potential response may be missed in an early evaluation, and overall response rates may improve with prolonged rituximab treatment. In fact, in a study with two 4-week courses of rituximab (weeks 1–4 and 12–16), the median time to best response was 17 months, the overall response rate was 66%, and only two of 19 patients had experienced relapse at a median follow-up of 29 months.[220]

Rituximab is generally well tolerated; the most common side effects are infusion-related reactions. The B-cell depletion induced by rituximab rarely results in infectious complications.[221] Apart from slight enhancement of neutropenias, the side-effect profile of rituximab does not overlap with that of cytostatic agents, making rituximab an important partner in combination chemotherapy, as discussed later.

A characteristic of rituximab treatment in patients who have LPL/WM is the rituximab flare, a paradoxical rise in the IgM paraprotein level that sometimes is detected early after treatment initiation.[222,223] This flare can lead to the manifestation of hyperviscosity in a previously asymptomatic patient. Therefore, in a patient who has high IgM levels, plasmapheresis may be considered before initiation of rituximab treatment; when combined chemoimmunotherapy is planned, rituximab may be omitted in the first cycle to avoid this complication.[219]

Alemtuzumab

The anti-CD52 antibody alemtuzumab also is a promising treatment option for LPL/WM, although the clinical experience in this disease is still limited.[224] Possible limitations are the substantial toxicity of alemtuzumab (myelosuppression, infections) and the fact that CD52 is expressed on the malignant B lymphocytes but to a much lesser extent on the plasma cells.[225] At present, alemtuzumab should be considered an option in the relapsed setting in patients who have a good performance status.

Purine Nucleoside Analogues

Purine nucleoside analogues, mainly fludarabine and cladribine, have been shown to be highly effective against LPL/WM in both untreated and pretreated patients.

When fludarabine was used as first-line treatment, responses were achieved in 40% to 86% of patients and lasted for 40 to 50 months.[183,226,227] Cladribine has shown similar efficacy in previously untreated patients, resulting in response rates of 64% to 90%.[228-233]

In the salvage setting, there is more experience with fludarabine. In a randomized trial comparing fludarabine with the combination of cyclophosphamide, doxorubicin, and prednisone, the response rate with fludarabine was significantly higher (28% versus 11%). Fludarabine also was superior in time to treatment failure, but there was no difference in OS.[234]

The available data also indicate that cladribine is highly efficacious as salvage treatment, resulting in response rates of 38% to 63%.[235,236]

Generally, the success with nucleoside analogues as salvage treatment is higher, and toxicity is lower, in patients who are treated relatively early in the course of the disease and before they are alkylator refractory.[237] Usually, there is cross-resistance among the different nucleoside analogues.

The main side effects of nucleoside analogues are myelosuppression and immunosuppression from T-cell depletion, which predispose patients to developing opportunistic infections, especially if the nucleoside analogues are combined with corticosteroids.[238-240] High rates of acute neutropenia (up to 77%) have been reported, as has considerable thrombocytopenia.[232,241]

Fludarabine pretreatment adversely affects the ability to mobilize peripheral blood stem cells,[118-121] but a new combination of stem cell factor and high-dose granulocyte colony-stimulating factor has been shown to result in adequate peripheral blood stem cell collection in 75% of patients aged under 50 years, despite prior exposure to fludarabine.[122]

Combination Therapy

The question whether combination chemotherapy should be used in LPL/WM brings up conflicting arguments similar to those arising from the question about when treatment should be initiated. Because the disease usually is indolent, it may be hard to prove a survival advantage with combination therapy as opposed to the sequential administration of single agents. In favor of combinations are the higher chance of achieving a response and therefore symptom reduction and the longer duration of response. On the other hand, this strategy may affect the patient's quality of life and places this elderly patient population at increased risk of infections.

Purine nucleoside combinations

In an early study at the MD Anderson Cancer Center, cladribine (0.1 mg/kg/d) administered subcutaneously on days 1 through 3 was combined with intravenous cyclophosphamide (500 mg/m^2) on day 1 and oral prednisolone, resulting in a response rate of 88%. The rate of grade 4 neutropenia was 11%, and no treatment-related deaths were observed.[242] In a follow-up study a higher dose of cladribine (5.6 mg/m^2) was given in combination with cyclophosphamide (up to 300 mg/m^2), both on days 1 through 3, with a response rate of 58%. The main side effects were neutropenia and severe infections (in 4% of cycles), and thrombocytopenia. Thrombocytopenia led to early treatment termination in 31% of patients.[243]

Several studies have demonstrated the high efficacy of the combination of fludarabine and cyclophosphamide. In a trial including 49 patients who had LPL/WM, 14 of whom were previously untreated, fludarabine was administered at 30 mg/m^2 and cyclophosphamide 300 mg/m^2, both intraveneously, on days 1 through 3 of a 28-day cycle. The overall response rate was 78% (all PRs); 18% had stable disease, and disease progressed in only 4%. The median time to treatment failure was 27 months.[244] In a small study, 14 patients who had WM were treated with pentostatin (4 mg/m^2), cyclophosphamide (600 mg/m^2), and, in eight cases, also with rituximab (375 mg/m^2), all on day 1 of a 21-day cycle. The response rate was 65% overall and was 77% in the patients receiving rituximab; of note, two patients achieved a CR.[245] The authors' group studied the outcome of patients who had WM who were treated with different fludarabine-based combinations.[84,246] A recent updated analysis of 24 patients (25% pretreated) receiving FCR (n = 11), FC (n = 9), fludarabine and mitoxantrone (n = 3), or fludarabine and rituximab (n = 1) revealed an overall response rate of 78%. The median time to progression was 43 months, and the 5- and 10-year actuarial survival rates were 72% and 63%, respectively. The overall tolerability was very good, with only 3% of cycles being complicated by grade 3 or 4 infections; however, two heavily pretreated patients subsequently developed MDS/AML.[247] Similar results, but with a shorter follow-up, were found in an Italian and in a French study using FCR for pretreated as well as for therapy-naïve patients who had WM.[248,249]

Other chemotherapy combination therapies

Because the combination of rituximab and cyclophosphamide, hydroxydaunorubicin, vincristine, and prednisone chemotherapy has shown efficacy in other indolent lymphomas, this combination was tested in a small study of 13 patients who had WM, 10 of whom had been treated previously. Six cycles of combination therapy were followed by rituximab maintenance treatment. The results were very encouraging, with three unconfirmed CRs, eight PRs, and one minor response.[250] A further study with 16 patients confirmed the excellent response rate but was closed early because of poor accrual. At the time of presentation, the follow-up was still too short to assess response duration, PFS, and OS.[251]

Stem Cell Transplantation

Data on transplantation in patients who have LPL/WM are scarce. Because of the lack of prospective data, results from two retrospective analyses of patients who had LPL/WM and who received transplants have been published recently (**Table 5**). A French study reports on 54 patients who received transplantation between 1990 and 2006. Thirty-two of these patients had high-dose chemotherapy with or without total-body irradiation followed by ASCT. The median age in this group was 56 years. After a median follow-up of 45 months the 1-, 3-, and 5-year OS rates were 87%, 77%, and 58%, respectively; the event-free survival at 5 years was 25%.[252] The largest study yet published analyzed 201 patients (median age, 53 years) who had advanced WM and who were treated with ASCT between 1992 and 2005. Most patients received conditioning with high-dose bischloroethylnitrosourea, etoposide, cytarabine, and melphalan or a combination of an alkylator and total-body irradiation. With a relatively short median follow-up of 26 months, the estimated 5-year PFS was 33%. The actuarial OS rates at 1 year, 3 years, and 5 years were 86%, 75%, and 61%, respectively.[253]

Study	N	Type of Transplant	5-Year EFS/PFS	OS
Table 5				
Outcome of ASCT and alloSCT in patients who had LPL/WM				
Dhedin et al, 2007[252]	32	ASCT	EFS 25%	1/3/5-year OS 87/77/58%
Kyriakou et al, 2007[253]	201	ASCT	PFS 33%	1/3/5-year OS 86/75/61%
Dhedin et al, 2007[252]	22	alloSCT 11 MA 11 RIC	EFS 48% 68%	1/3/5-year OS 64/54/54% 82/68/68%
Kyriakou et al, 2007[254]	106	alloSCT 44 CT 62 RIC	PFS 54% 39%	1/3/5-year OS 65/59/59% 71/66/66%

Abbreviations: CT, conventional therapy conditioning; MA, myeloablative conditioning; RIC, reduced intensity conditioning.

These studies confirm that ASCT is feasible in selected patients who have LPL/WM and has the potential of prolonged remissions; however, the results are not definitively superior to those achieved with active combinations of conventional chemoimmuno-therapy,[247] and ASCT certainly does not have the potential for cure. This approach should be considered in younger patients who have relapsed disease after treatment with alkylating agents, nucleoside analogues, and rituximab.

AlloSCT may have curative potential in patients who have LPL/WM. In the French retrospective analysis mentioned earlier, 22 patients received an alloSCT, 11 with myeloablative conditioning and 11 with RIC. The OS rates at 1, 3, and 5 years were similar to the results with ASCT, but the event-free survival rate at 5 years seemed better in the myeloablative group (48%) and even more so in the patients treated with RIC (68%), suggesting superior disease control than with the autograft strategy.[252]

A retrospective European multicenter study analyzed 106 patients who had WM who underwent an alloSCT between 1989 and 2005. The median patient age was 49 years; 62 patients received a RIC regimen, and 44 patients were treated with conventional conditioning. In this study, also, the OS rates at 1, 3, and 5 years did not seem to differ significantly from those achieved with ASCT (65%, 59%, and 59%, respectively for the patients in the conventional treatment group; 71%, 66%, and 66%, respectively, for patients receiving RIC). Again, in a cross-trial comparison PFS seemed better after alloSCT than after ASCT; contrary to the French trial, how-ever, in this larger retrospective analysis conventional conditioning seemed to provide better tumor control than RIC. The PFS rates at 1, 3, and 5 years were 60%, 54%, and 54%, respectively, in the CT group as opposed to 61%, 44%, and 39%, respectively, for the patients who received RIC (see **Table 5**).[254] Given the often indolent disease course and the ability to induce remissions recurrently with chemotherapy with or without ASCT, 10- and 15-year PFS and OS data are needed to determine whether long-term disease control and potential cure can be achieved with an allogeneic strategy.

New Agents

Bortezomib is a proteasome inhibitor that is thought to exert its antitumor activity by the inhibition of nuclear factor kappa B, but the exact mechanism is not known.

Studies in pretreated patients who had WM with single-agent bortezomib in the standard schedule as it is used in multiple myeloma (1.3 mg/m^2 on days 1, 4, 8, and 11 of a 21-day cycle) showed impressive reductions in paraprotein, response rates of up to 85%, median PFS figures of 7.9 to more than 11 months, and overall good tolerability.[255,256] Some uncertainty remains about the drug's effectiveness in clearing marrow or organ infiltration. Another trial in 17 patients who had relapsed WM combined bortezomib (1.6 mg/m^2) on days 1, 8, and 15 of a 28-day cycle for six cycles with rituximab (375 mg/m^2) on days 1, 8, 15, and 22 of cycles 1 and 4. The overall response rate was 85%, and none of the patients had progressed at the time of analysis, which was too early to assess PFS or OS.[257]

An ongoing study for primary treatment of patients who have WM combines the standard bortezomib regimen with dexamethasone (40 mg) on the days of bortezomib administration and rituximab (375 mg/m^2) on day 11 of the 21-day cycles. An interim analysis revealed a 100% overall response rate while maintaining a favorable toxicity profile; data for PFS or OS were not available.[258]

Thalidomide has been used at a relatively high dosage of 200–600 mg daily as an immunomodulatory and antiangiogenic agent in a phase II trial with 10 untreated and 10 pretreated patients. The overall response rate was 25%, but the median time to progression was less than 3 months.[259] Therefore, at least as a single agent, thalidomide seems to be only moderately active in WM and may be suitable only for selected patients, (eg, those who have severe cytopenias).[260]

Several other agents for the treatment of LPL/WM are currently under investigation, but the results are too preliminary to have relevance outside clinical trials.

Other Therapeutic Interventions

As mentioned earlier, plasmapheresis is a very effective procedure in patients who have LPL/WM who present with symptomatic hyperviscosity or to prevent such symptoms in a patient who is about to start treatment with rituximab-containing chemotherapy. Plasmapheresis has no effect on the tumor burden, however. Usually, a volume of 1 to 1.5 of the total plasma volume is exchanged with a solution containing 5% albumin in normal saline, which reduces the plasma IgM levels by 60% to 75%.[261] Because the IgM level rises again quickly after plasmapheresis, cytoreductive treatment should be initiated soon thereafter, or recurrent plasma exchanges should be performed. Occasionally, this strategy has been pursued long-term to control the IgM levels in elderly or frail patients who have chemotherapy-refractory disease.[262]

There are case reports of patients who had dominant splenic disease who benefited considerably from a splenectomy. Given the difficulties in the differential diagnosis of LPL/WM, however, it is unclear whether some of these cases represented splenic marginal zone lymphomas rather than true WM.

Very rarely, the occurrence of a localized nodal or extranodal LPL has been described without involvement of other lymph nodes, liver, spleen, or bone marrow and without the presence of an IgM paraprotein. In these unusual situations local radiotherapy is the appropriate treatment and may result in a lasting remission.[263–265]

SUMMARY

As outlined in the previous sections, treatment for LPL/WM should be initiated only when the patient becomes symptomatic or the disease shows clear signs of progression and is likely to cause complications soon. The best treatment for LPL/WM is still undetermined, because intensive combination therapy has been shown to increase response rates and PFS, but no advantage in OS could be demonstrated. Therefore, this decision must be made individually for each patient. Sequential therapies with single agents such as alkylators, rituximab, or nucleoside analogues can be as appropriate as intensive combinations of all three. In younger patients who have few or no comorbidities and/or relatively aggressive disease, high-dose chemotherapy and ASCT can be an adequate means for achieving a long-term remission. Results of alloSCT suggest that there is a GvL effect in LPL that can result in prolonged remissions and possibly cure; however, the follow-up is not yet long enough to support this conclusion.

Research in LPL/WM is becoming increasingly active, and numerous new agents such as proteasome inhibitors and immunomodulatory agents are being explored as treatment options. As in multiple myeloma, these drugs soon may change the treatment paradigms in LPL/WM.

REFERENCES

1. Müller-Hermelink HKME, Catovsky D, Harris NL. Chronic lymphocytic leukemia/ small lymphocytic lymphoma. In: Jaffe ES, Harris NL, Stein H, et al, editors. World Health Organization classification of tumours pathology and genetics of tumours of haematopoietic and lymphoid tissues. Lyon (France): IARCPress; 2001. p. 127–30.
2. Morrison W, Hoppe R, Weiss L, et al. Small lymphocytic lymphoma. J Clin Oncol 1989;7(5):598–606.
3. Evans HLBJ, Youness EL. Malignant lymphoma, small lymphocytic type: a clinicopathologic study of 84 cases with suggested criteria for intermediate lymphocytic lymphoma. Cancer 1978;41(4):1440–55.
4. Ahmed S, Shahid RK, Sison CP, et al. Orbital lymphomas: a clinicopathologic study of a rare disease. Am J Med Sci 2006;331(2):79–83.
5. Medeiros LJ, Harris NL. Lymphoid infiltrates of the orbit and conjunctiva. A morphologic and immunophenotypic study of 99 cases. Am J Surg Pathol 1989; 13(6):459–71.
6. Marti GE, Rawstron AC, Ghia P, et al. Diagnostic criteria for monoclonal B-cell lymphocytosis. Br J Haematol 2005;130(3):325–32.
7. Hallek M, Cheson BD, Catovsky D, et al. Guidelines for the diagnosis and treatment of chronic lymphocytic leukemia: a report from the International Workshop on Chronic Lymphocytic Leukemia (IWCLL) updating the National Cancer Institute-Working Group (NCI-WG) 1996 guidelines. Blood 2008;111(12):5446–56.
8. Ben-Ezra J, Burke J, Swartz W, et al. Small lymphocytic lymphoma: a clinicopathologic analysis of 268 cases. Blood 1989;73(2):579–87.
9. Jemal A, Siegel R, Ward E, et al. Cancer statistics, 2007. CA Cancer J Clin 2007; 57(1):43–66.
10. Tsimberidou AM, Wen S, O'Brien S, et al. Assessment of chronic lymphocytic leukemia and small lymphocytic lymphoma by absolute lymphocyte counts in 2,126 patients: 20 years of experience at the University of Texas M.D. Anderson Cancer Center. J Clin Oncol 2007;25(29):4648–56.
11. Rawstron AC, Green MJ, Kuzmicki A, et al. Monoclonal B lymphocytes with the characteristics of "indolent" chronic lymphocytic leukemia are present in 3.5% of adults with normal blood counts. Blood 2002;100(2):635–9.
12. The Non-Hodgkin's Lymphoma Classification Project. A clinical evaluation of the International Lymphoma Study Group classification of non-Hodgkin's lymphoma. Blood 1997;89(11):3909–18.

13. National Cancer Institute sponsored study of classification of non-Hodgkin's lymphomas: summary and description of a working formulation for clinical usage. Non-Hodgkin's Lymphoma Classification Project. Cancer 1982;49: 2112–35.

14. Cheson B, Bennett J, Grever M, et al. National Cancer Institute-sponsored Working Group guidelines for chronic lymphocytic leukemia: revised guidelines for diagnosis and treatment. Blood 1996;87(12):4990–7.

15. Olejniczak SH, Stewart CC, Donohue K, et al. A quantitative exploration of surface antigen expression in common B-cell malignancies using flow cytometry. Immunol Invest 2006;35(1):93–114.

16. Trentin L, Cabrelle A, Facco M, et al. Homeostatic chemokines drive migration of malignant B cells in patients with non-Hodgkin lymphomas. Blood 2004;104(2): 502–8.

17. Wong S, Fulcher D. Chemokine receptor expression in B-cell lymphoproliferative disorders. Leuk Lymphoma 2004;45(12):2491–6.

18. Hamblin TJ, Orchard JA, Gardiner A, et al. Immunoglobulin V genes and CD38 expression in CLL. Blood 2000;95(7):2455–7.

19. Jaksic O, Kardum P, Mirjana M, et al. CD38 on B-cell chronic lymphocytic leukemia cells has higher expression in lymph nodes than in peripheral blood or bone marrow. Blood 2004;103(5):1968–9.

20. Nagy B, Ferrer A, Larramendy M, et al. Lymphotoxin beta expression is high in chronic lymphocytic leukemia but low in small lymphocytic lymphoma: a quantitative real-time reverse transcriptase polymerase chain reaction analysis. Haematologica 2003;88(6):654–8.

21. Horning SJ, Rosenberg SA. The natural history of initially untreated low-grade non-Hodgkin's lymphomas. N Engl J Med 1984;311(23):1471–5.

22. Carbone PP, Kaplan HS, Musshoff K, et al. Report of the Committee on Hodgkin's Disease Staging Classification. Cancer Res 1971;31(11):1860–1.

23. Pangalis GA, Angelopoulou MK, Vassilakopoulos TP, et al. B-chronic lymphocytic leukemia, small lymphocytic lymphoma, and lymphoplasmacytic lymphoma, including Waldenström's macroglobulinemia: a clinical, morphologic, and biologic spectrum of similar disorders. Semin Hematol 1999;36(2):104–14.

24. Binet JLAA, Dighiero G, Chastang C, et al. A new prognostic classification of chronic lymphocytic leukemia derived from a multivariate survival analysis. Cancer 1981;48(1):198–206.

25. Rai K, Sawitsky A, Cronkite E, et al. Clinical staging of chronic lymphocytic leukemia. Blood 1975;46(2):219–34.

26. Binet J-L, Caligaris-Cappio F, Catovsky D, et al. Perspectives on the use of new diagnostic tools in the treatment of chronic lymphocytic leukemia. Blood 2006; 107(3):859–61.

27. Dohner H, Stilgenbauer S, Benner A, et al. Genomic aberrations and survival in chronic lymphocytic leukemia. N Engl J Med 2000;343(26):1910–6.

28. Dohner H, Fischer K, Bentz M, et al. p53 gene deletion predicts for poor survival and non-response to therapy with purine analogs in chronic B-cell leukemias. Blood 1995;85(6):1580–9.

29. Grever MR, Lucas DM, Dewald GW, et al. Comprehensive assessment of genetic and molecular features predicting outcome in patients with chronic lymphocytic leukemia: results from the US Intergroup Phase III Trial E2997. J Clin Oncol 2007;25(7):799–804.

30. Byrd JC, Gribben JG, Peterson BL, et al. Select high-risk genetic features predict earlier progression following chemoimmunotherapy with fludarabine

and rituximab in chronic lymphocytic leukemia: justification for risk-adapted therapy. J Clin Oncol 2006;24(3):437–43.

31. Cuneo A, Rigolin GM, Bigoni R, et al. Chronic lymphocytic leukemia with 6q- shows distinct hematological features and intermediate prognosis. Leukemia 2004;18(3):476–83.

32. Damle RN, Wasil T, Fais F, et al. Ig V gene mutation status and CD38 expression as novel prognostic indicators in chronic lymphocytic leukemia. Blood 1999; 94(6):1840–7.

33. Hamblin TJ, Davis Z, Gardiner A, et al. Unmutated Ig VH genes are associated with a more aggressive form of chronic lymphocytic leukemia. Blood 1999;94(6): 1848–54.

34. Orchard JA, Ibbotson RE, Davis Z, et al. ZAP-70 expression and prognosis in chronic lymphocytic leukaemia. Lancet 2004;363(9403):105–11.

35. Crespo M, Bosch F, Villamor N, et al. ZAP-70 expression as a surrogate for immunoglobulin-variable-region mutations in chronic lymphocytic leukemia. N Engl J Med 2003;348(18):1764–75.

36. Ghia P, Guida G, Stella S, et al. The pattern of CD38 expression defines a distinct subset of chronic lymphocytic leukemia (CLL) patients at risk of disease progression. Blood 2003;101(4):1262–9.

37. Molica S, Brugiatelli M, Callea V, et al. Comparison of younger versus older B-cell chronic lymphocytic leukemia patients for clinical presentation and prognosis. A retrospective study of 53 cases. Eur J Haematol 1994;52(4):216–21.

38. Montserrat E, Gomis F, Vallespi T, et al. Presenting features and prognosis of chronic lymphocytic leukemia in younger adults [see comments]. Blood 1991; 78(6):1545–51.

39. Catovsky D, Fooks J, Richards S. Prognostic factors in chronic lymphocytic leukaemia: the importance of age, sex and response to treatment in survival. A report from the MRC CLL 1 trial. MRC Working Party on Leukaemia in Adults. Br J Haematol 1989;72(2):141–9.

40. Jaksic B, Vitale B, Hauptmann E, et al. The roles of age and sex in the prognosis of chronic leukaemias. A study of 373 cases. Br J Cancer 1991;64(2): 345–8.

41. Hallek M, Wanders L, Ostwald M, et al. Serum beta(2)-microglobulin and serum thymidine kinase are independent predictors of progression-free survival in chronic lymphocytic leukemia and immunocytoma. Leuk Lymphoma 1996; 22(5–6):439–47.

42. Keating MJ, Kantarjian H, Freireich EJ, et al. The serum β2-microglobulin (beta2m) level is more powerful than stage in predicting response and survival in chronic lymphocytic leukemia (CLL). Blood 1995;86:606.

43. Reinisch W, Willheim M, Hilgarth M, et al. Soluble CD23 reliably reflects disease activity in B-cell chronic lymphocytic leukemia. J Clin Oncol 1994;12(10): 2146–52.

44. Calin GA, Ferracin M, Cimmino A, et al. A microRNA signature associated with prognosis and progression in chronic lymphocytic leukemia. N Engl J Med 2005; 353(17):1793–801.

45. Del Poeta G, Del Principe MI, Luciano F, et al. High CD69 protein expression predicts a poor prognosis in B-cell chronic lymphocytic leukemia (B-CLL). ASH Annual Meeting Abstracts 2007;110(11):750.

46. Nowakowski GS, Hoyer JD, Shanafelt TD, et al. Percentage of smudge cells on blood smear predicts prognosis in chronic lymphocytic leukemia: a multicenter study. ASH Annual Meeting Abstracts 2007;110(11):745.

47. Weisenburger DD, Nathwani BN, Diamond LW, et al. Malignant lymphoma, intermediate lymphocytic type: a clinicopathologic study of 42 cases. Cancer 1981; 48(6):1415–25.
48. Dighiero G, Maloum K, Desablens B, et al. Chlorambucil in indolent chronic lymphocytic leukemia. N Engl J Med 1998;338(21):1506–14.
49. Shustik CMR, Silver R, Sawitsky A, et al. Treatment of early chronic lymphocytic leukemia: intermittent chlorambucil versus observation. Hematol Oncol 1988; 6(1):7–12.
50. CLL Trialists' Collaborative Group. Chemotherapeutic options in chronic lymphocytic leukemia: a meta-analysis of the randomized trials. J Natl Cancer Inst 1999; 91(10):861–8.
51. Keating MJ, O'Brien S, Lerner S, et al. Long-term follow-up of patients with chronic lymphocytic leukemia (CLL) receiving fludarabine regimens as initial therapy. Blood 1998;92(4):1165–71.
52. Bosch F, Ferrer A, Lopez-Guillermo A, et al. Fludarabine, cyclophosphamide and mitoxantrone in the treatment of resistant or relapsed chronic lymphocytic leukaemia. Br J Haematol 2002;119(4):976–84.
53. Keating MJ, O'Brien S, Albitar M, et al. Early results of a chemoimmunotherapy regimen of fludarabine, cyclophosphamide, and rituximab as initial therapy for chronic lymphocytic leukemia. J Clin Oncol 2005;23(18):4079–88.
54. Wierda W, O'Brien S, Wen S, et al. Chemoimmunotherapy with fludarabine, cyclophosphamide, and rituximab for relapsed and refractory chronic lymphocytic leukemia. J Clin Oncol 2005;23(18):4070–8.
55. Rawstron AC, Kennedy B, Evans PAS, et al. Quantitation of minimal disease levels in chronic lymphocytic leukemia using a sensitive flow cytometric assay improves the prediction of outcome and can be used to optimize therapy. Blood 2001;98(1):29–35.
56. Koehi U, Ying Yang L, Nowak B, et al. Effect of combined treatment with 4-hydroperoxycyclophosphamide and fludarabine on cytotoxicity and repair of damaged DNA. Acute leukemias VII: experimental approaches and novel therapies. Berlin: Springer-Verlag; 1998. p. 549–55.
57. Catovsky D, Richards S, Matutes E, et al. Assessment of fludarabine plus cyclophosphamide for patients with chronic lymphocytic leukaemia (the LRF CLL4 Trial): a randomised controlled trial. Lancet 2007;370(9583):230–9.
58. Eichhorst BF, Busch R, Hopfinger G, et al. Fludarabine plus cyclophosphamide versus fludarabine alone in first-line therapy of younger patients with chronic lymphocytic leukemia. Blood 2006;107(3):885–91.
59. Tsimberidou AM, Keating MJ, Giles FJ, et al. Fludarabine and mitoxantrone for patients with chronic lymphocytic leukemia. Cancer 2004;100(12):2583–91.
60. Seymour JF, Grigg AP, Szer J, et al. Fludarabine and mitoxantrone: effective and well-tolerated salvage therapy in relapsed indolent lymphoproliferative disorders. Ann Oncol 2001;12(10):1455–60.
61. Mauro F, Foa R, Meloni G, et al. Fludarabine, ara-C, novantrone and dexamethasone (FAND) in previously treated chronic lymphocytic leukemia patients. Haematologica 2002;87(9):926–33.
62. Robertson LE, O'Brien S, Kantarjian H, et al. Fludarabine plus doxorubicin in previously treated chronic lymphocytic leukemia. Leukemia 1995;9(6): 943–5.
63. Rummel MJ, Kafer G, Pfreundschuh M, et al. Fludarabine and epirubicin in the treatment of chronic lymphocytic leukaemia: a German multicenter phase II study. Ann Oncol 1999;10(2):183–8.

64. Weiss MA, Maslak PG, Jurcic JG, et al. Pentostatin and cyclophosphamide: an effective new regimen in previously treated patients with chronic lymphocytic leukemia. J Clin Oncol 2003;21(7):1278–84.
65. Robak T, Blonski JZ, Gora-Tybor J, et al. Cladribine alone and in combination with cyclophosphamide or cyclophosphamide plus mitoxantrone in the treatment of progressive chronic lymphocytic leukemia: report of a prospective, multicenter, randomized trial of the Polish Adult Leukemia Group (PALG CLL2). Blood 2006;108(2):473–9.
66. Zhou LJ, Tedder TF. CD20 Workshop Panel report. In: Schlossman SF, Boumsell L, Gilks W, et al, editors. Leucocyte typing v white cell differentiation antigens. Oxford (UK): Oxford University Press; 1995. p. 511–4.
67. McLaughlin P, Grillo-Lopez A, Link B, et al. Rituximab chimeric anti-CD20 monoclonal antibody therapy for relapsed indolent lymphoma: half of patients respond to a four-dose treatment program. J Clin Oncol 1998;16(8):2825–33.
68. O'Brien SM, Kantarjian H, Thomas DA, et al. Rituximab dose-escalation trial in chronic lymphocytic leukemia. J Clin Oncol 2001;19(8):2165–70.
69. Hainsworth JD, Litchy S, Barton JH, et al. Single-agent rituximab as first-line and maintenance treatment for patients with chronic lymphocytic leukemia or small lymphocytic lymphoma: a phase II trial of the Minnie Pearl Cancer Research Network. J Clin Oncol 2003;21(9):1746–51.
70. Gilleece M, Dexter T. Effect of Campath-1H antibody on human hematopoietic progenitors in vitro. Blood 1993;82(3):807–12.
71. Keating MJ, Flinn I, Jain V, et al. Therapeutic role of alemtuzumab (Campath-1H) in patients who have failed fludarabine: results of a large international study. Blood 2002;99(10):3554–61.
72. Rai KR, Freter CE, Mercier RJ, et al. Alemtuzumab in previously treated chronic lymphocytic leukemia patients who also had received fludarabine. J Clin Oncol 2002;20(18):3891–7.
73. Ferrajoli A, O'Brien SM, Cortes JE, et al. Phase II study of alemtuzumab in chronic lymphoproliferative disorders. Cancer 2003;98(4):773–8.
74. Stilgenbauer S, Döhner H. Campath-1H-induced complete remission of chronic lymphocytic leukemia despite p53 gene mutation and resistance to chemotherapy. N Engl J Med 2002;347(6):452–3.
75. Lozanski G, Heerema NA, Flinn IW, et al. Alemtuzumab is an effective therapy for chronic lymphocytic leukemia with p53 mutations and deletions. Blood 2004; 103(9):3278–81.
76. Lundin J, Kimby E, Bjorkholm M, et al. Phase II trial of subcutaneous anti-CD52 monoclonal antibody alemtuzumab (Campath-1H) as first-line treatment for patients with B-cell chronic lymphocytic leukemia (B-CLL). Blood 2002;100(3): 768–73.
77. Faderl S, Thomas DA, O'Brien S, et al. Experience with alemtuzumab plus rituximab in patients with relapsed and refractory lymphoid malignancies. Blood 2003;101(9):3413–5.
78. Cruz RI, Hernandez-Ilizaliturri FJ, Olejniczak S, et al. CD52 over-expression affects rituximab-associated complement-mediated cytotoxicity but not antibody-dependent cellular cytotoxicity: preclinical evidence that targeting CD52 with alemtuzumab may reverse acquired resistance to rituximab in non-Hodgkin lymphoma. Leuk Lymphoma 2008;48(12):2424–36.
79. Alas S, Emmanouilides C, Bonavida B. Inhibition of interleukin 10 by rituximab results in down-regulation of Bcl-2 and sensitization of B-cell non-Hodgkin's lymphoma to apoptosis. Clin Cancer Res 2001;7(3):709–23.

80. Chow K, Sommerlad W, Boehrer S, et al. Anti-CD20 antibody (IDEC-C2B8, rituximab) enhances efficacy of cytotoxic drugs on neoplastic lymphocytes in vitro: role of cytokines, complement, and caspases. Haematologica 2002;87(1):33–43.

81. Di Gaetano N, Xiao Y, Erba E, et al. Synergism between fludarabine and rituximab revealed in a follicular lymphoma cell line resistant to the cytotoxic activity of either drug alone. Br J Haematol 2001;114(4):800–9.

82. Tam CS, Keating MJ. Chemoimmunotherapy of chronic lymphocytic leukemia. Best Pract Res Clin Haematol 2007;20(3):479–98.

83. Roche Press Release (Basel, Switzerland). Available at: http://www.roche.com/med-cor-2008-01-25. 2007.

84. Tam CS, Wolf M, Prince HM, et al. Fludarabine, cyclophosphamide, and rituximab for the treatment of patients with chronic lymphocytic leukemia or indolent non-Hodgkin lymphoma. Cancer 2006;106(11):2412–20.

85. Keating MJ, O'Brien S, Lerner S, et al. Chemoimmunotherapy with fludarabine (F), cyclophosphamide (C), and rituximab (R) improves complete response (CR), remission duration and survival as initial therapy of chronic lymphocytic leukemia (CLL) [abstract 6565]. J Clin Oncol 2004;22. (14S:Proceedings of the ASCO Annual Meeting).

86. Byrd JC, Murphy T, Howard RS, et al. Rituximab using a thrice weekly dosing schedule in B-cell chronic lymphocytic leukemia and small lymphocytic lymphoma demonstrates clinical activity and acceptable toxicity. J Clin Oncol 2001;19(8):2153–64.

87. O'Brien S, Wierda WG, Faderl S, et al. FCR-3 as frontline therapy for patients with chronic lymphocytic leukemia (CLL). ASH Annual Meeting Abstracts 2005;106(11):2117.

88. Faderl S, Wierda W, O'Brien S, et al. A phase II study of fludarabine (F), cyclophosphamide (C), and mitoxantrone (M) plus rituximab (R) (FCM-R) in previously untreated patients (pts) with CLL < 70 years (yrs) [abstract 6607]. J Clin Oncol 2006;24. (18S: Proceedings of the ASCO Annual Meeting).

89. Faderl S, Wierda W, Ferrajoli A, et al. Update of experience with fludarabine, cyclophosphamide, mitoxantrone plus rituximab (FCM-R) in frontline therapy for chronic lymphocytic leukemia (CLL). ASH Annual Meeting Abstracts 2007;110(11):627.

90. Kay NE, Geyer SM, Call TG, et al. Combination chemoimmunotherapy with pentostatin, cyclophosphamide, and rituximab shows significant clinical activity with low accompanying toxicity in previously untreated B chronic lymphocytic leukemia. Blood 2007;109(2):405–11.

91. Lamanna N, Kalaycio M, Maslak P, et al. Pentostatin, cyclophosphamide, and rituximab is an active, well-tolerated regimen for patients with previously treated chronic lymphocytic leukemia. J Clin Oncol 2006;24(10):1575–81.

92. Yunus F, George S, Smith J, et al. Phase II multicenter trial of pentostatin and rituximab in patients with previously treated and untreated chronic lymphocytic leukemia [abstract 5168]. Blood 2003;102.

93. Kennedy B, Rawstron A, Carter C, et al. Campath-1H and fludarabine in combination are highly active in refractory chronic lymphocytic leukemia. Blood 2002;99(6):2245–7.

94. Sayala H, Moreton P, Richard JA, et al. Interim report of the UKCLL02 trial: a phase II study of subcutaneous alemtuzumab plus fludarabine in patients with fludarabine refractory CLL (on behalf of the NCRI CLL trials sub-group). ASH Annual Meeting Abstracts 2005;106(11):2120.

95. Elter T, Borchmann P, Schulz H, et al. Fludarabine in combination with alemtuzumab is effective and feasible in patients with relapsed or refractory b-cell chronic lymphocytic leukemia: results of a phase II trial. J Clin Oncol 2005;23(28): 7024–31.

96. Chanan-Khan A, Miller KC, Takeshita K, et al. Results of a phase 1 clinical trial of thalidomide in combination with fludarabine as initial therapy for patients with treatment-requiring chronic lymphocytic leukemia (CLL). Blood 2005;106(10): 3348–52.

97. Furman RR, Leonard JP, Allen SL, et al. Thalidomide alone or in combination with fludarabine are effective treatments for patients with fludarabine-relapsed and refractory CLL [abstract 6640]. J Clin Oncol 2005;23. (16S:Proceedings of the ASCO Annual Meeting).

98. Giannopoulos K, Dmoszynska A, Kowal M, et al. Thalidomide alone and in combination with fludarabine exerts distinct molecular and antileukemic effects in B-cell chronic lymphocytic leukemia. ASH Annual Meeting Abstracts 2007; 110(11):3124.

99. Chanan-Khan A, Miller KC, Musial L, et al. Clinical efficacy of lenalidomide in patients with relapsed or refractory chronic lymphocytic leukemia: results of a phase II study. J Clin Oncol 2006;24(34):5343–9.

100. Chanan-Khan A, Whitworth A, Lawrence D, et al. Clinical activity of lenalidomide in relapsed or refractory chronic lymphocytic leukemia (CLL) patients: updated results of a phase II clinical trial. Leuk Lymph 2007;48:S166.

101. Ferrajoli A, Lee B-N, Schlette EJ, et al. Lenalidomide induces complete and partial remissions in patients with relapsed and refractory chronic lymphocytic leukemia. Blood 2008;111(11):5291–7.

102. Ferrajoli A, O'Brien SM, Faderl SH, et al. Lenalidomide induces complete and partial responses in patients with relapsed and treatment-refractory chronic lymphocytic leukemia (CLL). ASH Annual Meeting Abstracts 2006; 108(11):305.

103. Ferrajoli A, Keating MJ, Wierda WG, et al. Lenalidomide is active in patients with relapsed/refractory chronic lymphocytic leukemia (CLL) carrying unfavorable chromosomal abnormalities. ASH Annual Meeting Abstracts 2007;110(11):754.

104. Chanan-Khan AA, Cheson BD. Lenalidomide for the treatment of B-cell malignancies. J Clin Oncol 2008;26(9):1544–52.

105. O'Brien S, Moore JO, Boyd TE, et al. Randomized phase III trial of fludarabine plus cyclophosphamide with or without oblimersen sodium (Bcl-2 antisense) in patients with relapsed or refractory chronic lymphocytic leukemia. J Clin Oncol 2007;25(9):1114–20.

106. Byrd JC, O'Brien S, Flinn I, et al. Safety and efficacy results from a phase i trial of single-agent lumiliximab (anti-CD23 antibody) for chronic lymphocytic leukemia. ASH Annual Meeting Abstracts 2004;104(11):2503.

107. Coiffier B, Tilly H, Pedersen LM, et al. Significant correlation between survival endpoints and exposure to ofatumumab (HuMax-CD20) in chronic lymphocytic leukemia. ASH Annual Meeting Abstracts 2006;108(11):2842.

108. Byrd JC, Lin TS, Dalton JT, et al. Flavopiridol administered using a pharmacologically derived schedule is associated with marked clinical efficacy in refractory, genetically high-risk chronic lymphocytic leukemia. Blood 2007;109(2):399–404.

109. Shanafelt TD, Geyer SM, Kay NE. Prognosis at diagnosis: integrating molecular biologic insights into clinical practice for patients with CLL. Blood 2004;103(4): 1202–10.

110. Seiler T, Döhner H, Stilgenbauer S. Risk stratification in chronic lymphocytic leukemia. Semin Oncol 2006;33(2):186–94.

111. Dreger P, Stilgenbauer S, Benner A, et al. The prognostic impact of autologous stem cell transplantation in patients with chronic lymphocytic leukemia: a risk-matched analysis based on the VH gene mutational status. Blood 2004;103(7):2850–8.

112. Pavletic ZS, Bierman PJ, Vose JM, et al. High incidence of relapse after autologous stem-cell transplantation for B-cell chronic lymphocytic leukemia or small lymphocytic lymphoma. Ann Oncol 1998;9(9):1023–6.

113. Gribben JG, Zahrieh D, Stephans K, et al. Autologous and allogeneic stem cell transplantations for poor-risk chronic lymphocytic leukemia. Blood 2005; 106(13):4389–96.

114. Milligan DW, Fernandes S, Dasgupta R, et al. Results of the MRC pilot study show autografting for younger patients with chronic lymphocytic leukemia is safe and achieves a high percentage of molecular responses. Blood 2005;105(1):397–404.

115. Rabinowe S, Soiffer R, Gribben J, et al. Autologous and allogeneic bone marrow transplantation for poor prognosis patients with B-cell chronic lymphocytic leukemia. Blood 1993;82(4):1366–76.

116. Khouri I, Keating M, Vriesendorp H, et al. Autologous and allogeneic bone marrow transplantation for chronic lymphocytic leukemia: preliminary results. J Clin Oncol 1994;12(4):748–58.

117. Jantunen E, Itälä M, Siitonen T, et al. Autologous stem cell transplantation in patients with chronic lymphocytic leukaemia: the Finnish experience. Bone Marrow Transplant 2006;37(12):1093–8.

118. Tournilhac O, Cazin B, Lepretre S, et al. Impact of frontline fludarabine and cyclophosphamide combined treatment on peripheral blood stem cell mobilization in B-cell chronic lymphocytic leukemia. Blood 2004;103(1):363–5.

119. Michallet M, Thiebaut A, Dreger P, et al. Peripheral blood stem cell (PBSC) mobilization and transplantation after fludarabine therapy in chronic lymphocytic leukaemia (CLL): a report of the European Blood and Marrow Transplantation (EBMT) CLL subcommittee on behalf of the EBMT Chronic Leukaemias Working Party (CLWP). Br J Haematol 2000;108(3):595–601.

120. Morgan SJ, Seymour JF, Grigg A, et al. Predictive factors for successful stem cell mobilization in patients with indolent lymphoproliferative disorders previously treated with fludarabine. Leukemia 2004;18(5):1034–8.

121. Micallef IN, Apostolidis J, Rohatiner AZ, et al. Factors which predict unsuccessful mobilisation of peripheral blood progenitor cells following G-CSF alone in patients with non-Hodgkin's lymphoma. Hematol J 2000;1(6):367–73.

122. Seymour JF, Morgan S, Prince M, et al. Ancestim (SCF) and high-dose twice-daily filgrastim (G-CSF) is superior to G-CSF alone or cyclophosphamide plus G-CSF for mobilization of peripheral blood stem cells (PBSC) in patients with indolent lymphoproliferative disorders previously treated with fludarabine; results of a historically-controlled phase-II study. ASH Annual Meeting Abstracts 2006; 108(11):3066.

123. Michallet M, Archimbaud E, Bandini G, et al. HLA-identical sibling bone marrow transplantation in younger patients with chronic lymphocytic leukemia. Ann Intern Med 1996;124(3):311–5.

124. Khouri I, Champlin R. Allogeneic bone marrow transplantation in chronic lymphocytic leukemia [abstract]. Ann Intern Med 1996;125(9):780-a-.

125. Doney KC, Chauncey T, Appelbaum FR. Seattle Bone Marrow Transplant Team. Allogeneic related donor hematopoietic stem cell transplantation for treatment of chronic lymphocytic leukemia. Bone Marrow Transplant 2002;29(10):817–23.

126. Horowitz M, Montserrat E, Sobocinski K, et al. Haemopoietic stem cell transplantation for chronic lymphocytic leukemia. Blood 2000;(Suppl I):96 [abstract 522].

127. Toze CL, Galal A, Barnett MJ, et al. Myeloablative allografting for chronic lymphocytic leukemia: evidence for a potent graft-versus-leukemia effect associated with graft-versus-host disease. Bone Marrow Transplant 2005;36(9): 825–30.

128. Schetelig J, Thiede C, Bornhauser M, et al. Evidence of a graft-versus-leukemia effect in chronic lymphocytic leukemia after reduced-intensity conditioning and allogeneic stem-cell transplantation: the Cooperative German Transplant Study Group. J Clin Oncol 2003;21(14):2747–53.

129. Dreger P, Brand R, Hansz J, et al. Treatment-related mortality and graft-versus-leukemia activity after allogeneic stem cell transplantation for chronic lymphocytic leukemia using intensity-reduced conditioning. Leukemia 2003;17(5): 841–8.

130. Sorror ML, Maris MB, Sandmaier BM, et al. Hematopoietic cell transplantation after nonmyeloablative conditioning for advanced chronic lymphocytic leukemia. J Clin Oncol 2005;23(16):3819–29.

131. Khouri IF. Reduced-intensity regimens in allogeneic stem-cell transplantation for non-Hodgkin lymphoma and chronic lymphocytic leukemia. Hematology/The Education Program of the American Society of Hematology 2006;390–7.

132. Brown JR, Kim HT, Li S, et al. Predictors of improved progression-free survival after nonmyeloablative allogeneic stem cell transplantation for advanced chronic lymphocytic leukemia. Biol Blood Marrow Transplant 2006;12(10):1056–64.

133. Delgado J, Thomson K, Russell N, et al. Results of alemtuzumab-based reduced-intensity allogeneic transplantation for chronic lymphocytic leukemia: a British Society of Blood and Marrow Transplantation Study. Blood 2006;107(4):1724–30.

134. Dreger P, Brand R, Milligan D, et al. Reduced-intensity conditioning lowers treatment-related mortality of allogeneic stem cell transplantation for chronic lymphocytic leukemia: a population-matched analysis. Leukemia 2005;19(6): 1029–33.

135. Caballero D, Garcia-Marco JA, Martino R, et al. Allogeneic transplant with reduced intensity conditioning regimens may overcome the poor prognosis of B-cell chronic lymphocytic leukemia with unmutated immunoglobulin variable heavy-chain gene and chromosomal abnormalities (11q- and 17p-). Clin Cancer Res 2005;11(21):7757–63.

136. Sorror ML, Storer B, Sandmaier BP, et al. Long-term follow up of patients (pts) with high-risk chronic lymphocytic leukemia (CLL) given nonmyeloablative allogeneic hematopoietic cell transplantation (HCT). ASH Annual Meeting Abstracts 2007;110(11):1662.

137. Schetelig J, van Biezen A, Caballero D, et al. Allogeneic hematopoietic cell transplantation for chronic lymphocytic leukemia (CLL) with 17p deletion: a retrospective EBMT analysis. ASH Annual Meeting Abstracts 2007;110(11):47.

138. Shea TC, Johnston J, Walsh W, et al. Reduced intensity allogeneic transplantation provides high disease-free and overall survival in patients (Pts) with advanced indolent NHL and CLL: CALGB 109901. ASH Annual Meeting Abstracts 2007;110(11):486.

139. Dickinson JD, Loberiza F, Whalen V, et al. Outcomes of hematopoietic stem cell transplantation for chronic lymphocytic leukemia (CLL)/small lymphocytic lymphoma (SLL). ASH Annual Meeting Abstracts 2007;110(11):3045.

140. Waldenstrom J. Incipient myelomatosis or 'essential' hyperglobulinemia with fibrinogenemia: a new syndrome? Acta Med Scand 1944;117:216–22.

141. Harris N, Jaffe E, Stein H, et al. A revised European-American classification of lymphoid neoplasms: a proposal from the International Lymphoma Study Group [see comments]. Blood 1994;84(5):1361–92.
142. Owen RG, Treon SP, Al-Katib A. Clinicopathological definition of Waldenstrom's macroglobulinemia: consensus panel recommendations from the Second International Workshop on Waldenstrom's Macroglobulinemia. Semin Oncol 2003; 30(2):110–5.
143. Herrinton L, Weiss N. Incidence of Waldenstrom's macroglobulinemia. Blood 1993;82(10):3148–50.
144. Groves FD, Lois BT, Devesa SS, et al. Waldenström's macroglobulinemia. Cancer 1998;82(6):1078–81.
145. Dimopoulos MA, Panayiotidis P, Moulopoulos LA, et al. Waldenstrom's macroglobulinemia: clinical features, complications, and management. J Clin Oncol 2000;18(1):214.
146. Giordano TP, Henderson L, Landgren O, et al. Risk of non-Hodgkin lymphoma and lymphoproliferative precursor diseases in US veterans with hepatitis C virus. JAMA 2007;297(18):2010–7.
147. Brown AK, Elves MW, Gunson HH, et al. Waldenströms macroglobulinaemia. A family study. Acta Haematol 1967;38(3):184–92.
148. McMaster ML, Giambarresi T, Vasquez L, et al. Cytogenetics of familial Waldenstrom's macroglobulinemia: in pursuit of an understanding of genetic predisposition. Clin Lymphoma 2005;5(4):230–4.
149. McMaster ML, Goldin LR, Bai Y, et al. Genomewide linkage screen for Waldenstrom macroglobulinemia susceptibility loci in high-risk families. Am J Hum Genet 2006;79(4):695–701.
150. Treon SP, Hunter ZR, Aggarwal A, et al. Characterization of familial Waldenstrom's macroglobulinemia. Ann Oncol 2006;17(3):488–94.
151. McMaster ML, Csako G, Giambarresi TR, et al. Long-term evaluation of three multiple-case Waldenstrom macroglobulinemia families. Clin Cancer Res 2007;13(17):5063–9.
152. Linet MS, Humphrey RL, Mehl ES, et al. A case-control and family study of Waldenstrom's macroglobulinemia. Leukemia 1993;7(9):1363–9.
153. Kyle RA, Therneau TM, Rajkumar SV, et al. A long-term study of prognosis in monoclonal gammopathy of undetermined significance. N Engl J Med 2002; 346(8):564–9.
154. Dutcher TF, Fahey JL. The histopathology of the macroglobulinemia of Waldenström. J Natl Cancer Inst 1959;22(5):887–917.
155. Kucharska-Pulczynska M, Ellegaard J, Hokland P. Analysis of leucocyte differentiation antigens in blood and bone marrow from patients with Waldenström's macroglobulinaemia. Br J Haematol 1987;65(4):395–9.
156. Tournilhac O, Santos DD, Xu L, et al. Mast cells in Waldenstrom's macroglobulinemia support lymphoplasmacytic cell growth through CD154/CD40 signaling. Ann Oncol 2006;17(8):1275–82.
157. Elsawa SF, Novak AJ, Grote DM, et al. B-lymphocyte stimulator (BLyS) stimulates immunoglobulin production and malignant B-cell growth in Waldenstrom macroglobulinemia. Blood 2006;107(7):2882–8.
158. Lin P, Medeiros LJ. Lymphoplasmacytic lymphoma/Waldenstrom macroglobulinemia: an evolving concept. Adv Anat Pathol 2005;12(5):246–55.
159. Konoplev S, Medeiros LJ, Bueso-Ramos CE, et al. Immunophenotypic profile of lymphoplasmacytic lymphoma/Waldenström macroglobulinemia. Am J Clin Pathol 2005;124(3):414–20.

160. Remstein ED, Hanson CA, Kyle RA. Despite apparent morphologic and immunophenotypic heterogeneity, Waldenstrom's macroglobulinemia is consistently composed of cells along a morphologic continuum of small lymphocytes, plasmacytoid lymphocytes, and plasma cells. Semin Oncol 2005;30(2): 182–6.

161. San Miguel JF, Vidriales MB, Ocio E, et al. Immunophenotypic analysis of Waldenstrom's macroglobulinemia. Semin Oncol 2003;30(2):187–95.

162. Ho AW, Hatjiharissi E, Ciccarelli BT, et al. CD27–CD70 interactions in the pathogenesis of Waldenstrom's macroglobulinemia. Blood 2008 [epub].

163. Wagner S, Martinelli V, Luzzatto L. Similar patterns of V kappa gene usage but different degrees of somatic mutation in hairy cell leukemia, prolymphocytic leukemia, Waldenstrom's macroglobulinemia, and myeloma. Blood 1994;83(12): 3647–53.

164. Sahota SS, Garand R, Bataille R, et al. VH gene analysis of clonally related IgM and IgG from human lymphoplasmacytoid B-cell tumors with chronic lymphocytic leukemia features and high serum monoclonal IgG. Blood 1998;91(1): 238–43.

165. Kriangkum J, Taylor BJ, Reiman T, et al. Origins of Waldenstrom's macroglobulinemia: does it arise from an unusual B-cell precursor? Clin Lymphoma 2005; 5(4):217–9.

166. Kriangkum J, Taylor BJ, Treon SP, et al. Molecular characterization of Waldenstrom's macroglobulinemia reveals frequent occurrence of two B-cell clones having distinct IgH VDJ sequences. Clin Cancer Res 2007;13(7):2005–13.

167. Kriangkum J, Taylor BJ, Strachan E, et al. Impaired class switch recombination (CSR) in Waldenstrom macroglobulinemia (WM) despite apparently normal CSR machinery. Blood 2006;107(7):2920–7.

168. Martin-Jimenez P, Garcia-Sanz R, Sarasquete ME, et al. Functional class switch recombination may occur 'in vivo' in Waldenström macroglobulinaemia. Br J Haematol 2007;136(1):114–6.

169. Contrafatto G. Marker chromosome of macroglobulinemia identified by G-banding. Cytogenet Cell Genet 1977;18(6):370–3.

170. Han T, Sadamori N, Takeuchi J, et al. Clonal chromosome abnormalities in patients with Waldenstrom's and CLL-associated macroglobulinemia: significance of trisomy 12. Blood 1983;62(3):525–31.

171. Schop RFJ, Kuehl WM, Van Wier SA, et al. Waldenstrom macroglobulinemia neoplastic cells lack immunoglobulin heavy chain locus translocations but have frequent 6q deletions. Blood 2002;100(8):2996–3001.

172. Mansoor A, Medeiros LJ, Weber DM, et al. Cytogenetic findings in lymphoplasmacytic lymphoma/Waldenström macroglobulinemia. Chromosomal abnormalities are associated with the polymorphous subtype and an aggressive clinical course. Am J Clin Pathol 2001;116(4):543–9.

173. Jankovic GM, Colovic MD, Wiernik PH, et al. Multiple karyotypic aberrations in a polymorphous variant of Waldenstrom macroglobulinemia. Cancer Genet Cytogenet 1999;111(1):77–80.

174. Wong KF, So CC. Waldenstrom macroglobulinemia with karyotypic aberrations involving both homologous 6q. Cancer Genet Cytogenet 2001;124(2):137–9.

175. Ocio EM, Schop RFJ, Gonzalez B, et al. 6q deletion in Waldenström macroglobulinemia is associated with features of adverse prognosis. Br J Haematol 2007; 136(1):80–6.

176. Chang H, Qi X, Xu W, et al. Analysis of 6q deletion in Waldenstrom macroglobulinemia. Eur J Haematol 2007;79(3):244–7.

177. Schop RFJ, Jalal SM, Van Wier SA, et al. Deletions of 17p13.1 and 13q14 are uncommon in Waldenstrom macroglobulinemia clonal cells and mostly seen at the time of disease progression. Cancer Genet Cytogenet 2002;132(1):55–60.
178. Hatzimichael EC, Christou L, Bai M, et al. Serum levels of IL-6 and its soluble receptor (sIL-6R) in Waldenström's macroglobulinemia. Eur J Haematol 2001; 66(1):1–6.
179. Gutierrez NC, Ocio EM, de las Rivas J, et al. Gene expression profiling of B lymphocytes and plasma cells from Waldenstrom's macroglobulinemia: comparison with expression patterns of the same cell counterparts from chronic lymphocytic leukemia, multiple myeloma and normal individuals. Leukemia 2007;21(3): 541–9.
180. Kyle RA, Therneau TM, Rajkumar SV, et al. Long-term follow-up of IgM monoclonal gammopathy of undetermined significance. Blood 2003;102(10):3759–64.
181. Gobbi PG, Baldini L, Broglia C, et al. Prognostic validation of the international classification of immunoglobulin M gammopathies: a survival advantage for patients with immunoglobulin M monoclonal gammopathy of undetermined significance? Clin Cancer Res 2005;11(5):1786–90.
182. Gertz MA, Kyle RA. Hyperviscosity syndrome. J Intensive Care Med 1995;10(3): 128–41.
183. Dhodapkar MV, Jacobson JL, Gertz MA, et al. Prognostic factors and response to fludarabine therapy in patients with Waldenstrom macroglobulinemia: results of United States intergroup trial (Southwest Oncology Group S9003). Blood 2001;98(1):41–8.
184. Garcia-Sanz R, Montoto S, Torrequebrada A, et al. Waldenström macroglobulinaemia: presenting features and outcome in a series with 217 cases. Br J Haematol 2001;115(3):575–82.
185. Kyle RA, Garton JP. The spectrum of IgM monoclonal gammopathy in 430 cases. Mayo Clin Proc 1987;62:719–31.
186. Zarrabi MH, Stark RS, Kane P. IgM myeloma, a distinct entity in the spectrum of B-cell neoplasia. Am J Clin Pathol 1981;75(1):1–10.
187. Takahashi K, Yamamura F, Motoyama H. IgM myeloma—its distinction from Waldenström's macroglobulinemia. Acta Pathol Jpn 1986;36(10):1553–63.
188. Kondo H, Yokoyama K. IgM myeloma: different features from multiple myeloma and macroglobulinaemia. Eur J Haematol 1999;63(5):366–8.
189. Facon T, Brouillard M, Duhamel A, et al. Prognostic factors in Waldenstrom's macroglobulinemia: a report of 167 cases. J Clin Oncol 1993;11(8):1553–8.
190. Singh A, Eckardt KU, Zimmermann A, et al. Increased plasma viscosity as a reason for inappropriate erythropoietin formation. J Clin Invest 1993;91(1): 251–6.
191. Leblond V, Tournilhac O, Morel P. Waldenström's macroglobulinemia: prognostic factors and recent therapeutic advances. Clin Exp Med 2004;3(4):187–98.
192. Alexanian R. Blood volume in monoclonal gammopathy. Blood 1977;49(2): 301–7.
193. MacKenzie M, Lee T. Blood viscosity in Waldenstrom macroglobulinemia. Blood 1977;49(4):507–10.
194. Pavy MD, Murphy PL, Virella G. Paraprotein-induced hyperviscosity. A reversible cause of stroke. Postgrad Med 1980;68(3):109–12.
195. Mueller J, Hotson JR, Langston JW. Hyperviscosity-induced dementia. Neurology 1983;33(1):101–3.
196. Barras JP, Graf C. Hyperviscosity in diabetic retinopathy treated with Doxium (calcium dobesilate). Vasa 1980;9(2):161–4.

197. Vital C, Deminière C, Bourgouin B, et al. Waldenström's macroglobulinemia and peripheral neuropathy: deposition of M-component and kappa light chain in the endoneurium. Neurology 1985;35(4):603–6.

198. Ropper AH, Gorson KC. Neuropathies associated with paraproteinemia. N Engl J Med 1998;338(22):1601–7.

199. Dellagi K, Dupouey P, Brouet J, et al. Waldenstrom's macroglobulinemia and peripheral neuropathy: a clinical and immunologic study of 25 patients. Blood 1983;62(2):280–5.

200. Nobile-Orazio E, Marmiroli P, Baldini L, et al. Peripheral neuropathy in macroglobulinemia: incidence and antigen-specificity of M proteins. Neurology 1987;37(9):1506–14.

201. Gertz M, Kyle R, Noel P. Primary systemic amyloidosis: a rare complication of immunoglobulin M monoclonal gammopathies and Waldenstrom's macroglobulinemia. J Clin Oncol 1993;11(5):914–20.

202. Gertz MA, Lacy MQ, Dispenzieri A, et al. Amyloidosis. Best Pract Res Clin Haematol 2005;18(4):709–27.

203. Gertz MA, Kyle RA. Amyloidosis with IgM monoclonal gammopathies. Semin Oncol 2003;30(2):325–8.

204. Morel P, Monconduit M, Jacomy D, et al. Prognostic factors in Waldenstrom macroglobulinemia: a report on 232 patients with the description of a new scoring system and its validation on 253 other patients. Blood 2000;96(3):852–8.

205. Ghobrial IM, Fonseca R, Gertz MA, et al. Prognostic model for disease-specific and overall mortality in newly diagnosed symptomatic patients with Waldenstrom macroglobulinaemia. Br J Haematol 2006;133(2):158–64.

206. Kyrtsonis MC, Vassilakopoulos TP, Angelopoulou MK, et al. Waldenström's macroglobulinemia: clinical course and prognostic factors in 60 patients. Experience from a single hematology unit. Ann Hematol 2001;80(12):722–7.

207. Levy V, Morel P, Porcher R, et al. Advanced Waldenstrom's macroglobulinemia: usefulness of Morel's scoring system in establishing prognosis. Haematologica 2005;90(2):279–81.

208. Morel P, Duhamel A, Gobbi P, et al. International prognostic scoring system (IPSS) for Waldenstrom's macroglobulinemia (WM). ASH Annual Meeting Abstracts 2006;108(11):127.

209. Alexanian R, Weber D, Delasalle K, et al. Asymptomatic Waldenstrom's macroglobulinemia. Semin Oncol 2003;30(2):206–10.

210. Treon SP, Gertz MA, Dimopoulos M, et al. Update on treatment recommendations from the Third International Workshop on Waldenstrom's macroglobulinemia. Blood 2006;107(9):3442–6.

211. Johnson SA, Owen RG, Oscier DG, et al. Phase III study of chlorambucil versus fludarabine as initial therapy for Waldenstrom's macroglobulinemia and related disorders. Clin Lymphoma 2005;5(4):294–7.

212. Kyle RA, Greipp PR, Gertz MA, et al. Waldenström's macroglobulinaemia: a prospective study comparing daily with intermittent oral chlorambucil. Br J Haematol 2000;108(4):737–42.

213. Petersen HS. Erythroleukaemia in a melphalan-treated patient with primary macroglobulinaemia. Scand J Haematol 1973;10(1):5–11.

214. Cardamone JM, Kimmerle RI, Marshall EY. Development of acute erythroleukemia in B-cell immunoproliferative disorders after prolonged therapy with alkylating drugs. Am J Med 1974;57(5):836–42.

215. Weide R, Heymanns J, Köppler H. Induction of complete haematological remission after monotherapy with anti-CD20 monoclonal antibody (RITUXIMAB)

in a patient with alkylating agent resistant Waldenström's macroglobulinaemia. Leuk Lymphoma 1999;36(1–2):203–6.

216. Weide R, Heymanns J, Koppler H. The polyneuropathy associated with Waldenström's macroglobulinaemia can be treated effectively with chemotherapy and the anti-CD20 monoclonal antibody rituximab. Br J Haematol 2000;109(4): 838–41.

217. Byrd JC, White CA, Link B, et al. Rituximab therapy in Waldenstrom's macroglobulinemia: preliminary evidence of clinical activity. Ann Oncol 1999;10(12): 1525–7.

218. Treon SP, Agus DB, Link B, et al. CD20-directed antibody-mediated immunotherapy induces responses and facilitates hematologic recovery in patients with Waldenstrom's macroglobulinemia. J Immunother 2001;24(3):272–9.

219. Dimopoulos MA, Zervas C, Zomas A, et al. Treatment of Waldenstrom's macroglobulinemia with rituximab. J Clin Oncol 2002;20(9):2327–33.

220. Treon SP, Emmanouilides C, Kimby E, et al. Extended rituximab therapy in Waldenstrom's macroglobulinemia. Ann Oncol 2005;16(1):132–8.

221. Kimby E. Tolerability and safety of rituximab (MabThera(R)). Cancer Treat Rev 2005;31(6):456–73.

222. Treon SP, Branagan AR, Hunter Z, et al. Paradoxical increases in serum IgM and viscosity levels following rituximab in Waldenstrom's macroglobulinemia. Ann Oncol 2004;15(10):1481–3.

223. Ghobrial IM, Fonseca R, Greipp PR, et al. Initial immunoglobulin M 'flare' after rituximab therapy in patients diagnosed with Waldenstrom macroglobulinemia. Cancer 2004;101(11):2593–8.

224. Hunter ZR, Boxer M, Kahl B, et al. Phase II study of alemtuzumab in lymphoplasmacytic lymphoma: results of WMCTG trial 02-079. J Clin Oncol 2006;24(18S): [abstract 7523].

225. Owen RG, Hillmen P, Rawstron AC. CD52 expression in Waldenstrom's macroglobulinemia: implications for alemtuzumab therapy and response assessment. Clin Lymphoma 2005;5(4):278–81.

226. Foran JM, Rohatiner AZ, Coiffier B, et al. Multicenter phase II study of fludarabine phosphate for patients with newly diagnosed lymphoplasmacytoid lymphoma, Waldenström's macroglobulinemia, and mantle-cell lymphoma. J Clin Oncol 1999;17(2):546–53.

227. Thalhammer-Scherrer R, Geissler K, Schwarzinger I, et al. Fludarabine therapy in Waldenström's macroglobulinemia. Ann Hematol 2000;79(10):556–9.

228. Dimopoulos MA, Kantarjian H, Estey E, et al. Treatment of Waldenstrom macroglobulinemia with 2-chlorodeoxyadenosine. Ann Intern Med 1993;118(3):195–8.

229. Dimopoulos MA, Kantarjian H, Weber D, et al. Primary therapy of Waldenström's macroglobulinemia with 2-chlorodeoxyadenosine. J Clin Oncol 1994;12(12): 2694–8.

230. Delannoy A, Ferrant A, Martiat P, et al. 2-Chlorodeoxyadenosine therapy in Waldenstrom's macroglobulinaemia. Nouv Rev Fr Hematol 1994;36(4):317–20.

231. Fridrik MA, Jäger G, Baldinger C, et al. First-line treatment of Waldenström's disease with cladribine. Arbeitsgemeinschaft Medikamentöse Tumortherapie. Ann Hematol 1997;74(1):7–10.

232. Hellmann A, Lewandowski K, Zaucha JM, et al. Effect of a 2-hour infusion of 2-chlorodeoxyadenosine in the treatment of refractory or previously untreated Waldenström's macroglobulinemia. Eur J Haematol 1999;63(1):35–41.

233. Weber D, Treon SP, Emmanouilides C, et al. Uniform response criteria in Waldenstrom's macroglobulinemia: Consensus Panel recommendations from

the Second International Workshop on Waldenstrom's Macroglobulinemia. Semin Oncol 2003;30(2):127–31.

234. Leblond V, Lévy V, Maloisel F, et al. Multicenter, randomized comparative trial of fludarabine and the combination of cyclophosphamide-doxorubicin-prednisone in 92 patients with Waldenström macroglobulinemia in first relapse or with primary refractory disease. Blood 2001;98(9):2640–4.

235. Dimopoulos MA, Weber D, Delasalle KB, et al. Treatment of Waldenstrom's macroglobulinemia resistant to standard therapy with 2-chlorodeoxyadenosine: identification of prognostic factors. Ann Oncol 1995;6(1):49–52.

236. Betticher DC, Hsu Schmitz SF, et al. Cladribine (2-CDA) given as subcutaneous bolus injections is active in pretreated Waldenström's macroglobulinaemia. Swiss Group for Clinical Cancer Research (SAKK). Br J Haematol 1997;99(2):358–63.

237. Dimopoulos MA, Kyle RA, Anagnostopoulos A, et al. Diagnosis and management of Waldenstrom's macroglobulinemia. J Clin Oncol 2005;23(7):1564–77.

238. Seymour J, Kurzrock R, Freireich E, et al. 2-chlorodeoxyadenosine induces durable remissions and prolonged suppression of CD4+ lymphocyte counts in patients with hairy cell leukemia. Blood 1994;83(10):2906–11.

239. Cheson B. Infectious and immunosuppressive complications of purine analog therapy. J Clin Oncol 1995;13(9):2431–48.

240. Fenchel K, Bergmann L, Wijermans P, et al. Clinical experience with fludarabine and its immunosuppressive effects in pretreated chronic lymphocytic leukemias and low-grade lymphomas. Leuk Lymphoma 1995;18(5-6):485–92.

241. Liu ES, Burian C, Miller WE, et al. Bolus administration of cladribine in the treatment of Waldenström macroglobulinaemia. Br J Haematol 1998;103(3):690–5.

242. Laurencet FM, Zulian GB, Guetty-Alberto M, et al. Cladribine with cyclophosphamide and prednisone in the management of low-grade lymphoproliferative malignancies. Br J Cancer 1999;79(7-8):1215–9.

243. Van Den Neste E, Louviaux I, Michaux JL, et al. Phase I/II study of 2-chloro-2'-deoxyadenosine with cyclophosphamide in patients with pretreated B cell chronic lymphocytic leukemia and indolent non-Hodgkin's lymphoma. Leukemia 2000;14(6):1136–42.

244. Tamburini J, Lévy V, Chaleteix C, et al. Fludarabine plus cyclophosphamide in Waldenström's macroglobulinemia: results in 49 patients. Leukemia 2005;19(10):1831–4.

245. Hensel M, Villalobos M, Kornacker M, et al. Pentostatin/cyclophosphamide with or without rituximab: an effective regimen for patients with Waldenstrom's macroglobulinemia/lymphoplasmacytic lymphoma. Clin Lymphoma Myeloma 2005;6(2):131–5.

246. Tam CS, Wolf MM, Westerman D, et al. Fludarabine combination therapy is highly effective in first-line and salvage treatment of patients with Waldenström's macroglobulinemia. Clin Lymphoma Myeloma 2005;6(2):136–9.

247. Peinert S, Tam CS, Prince HM, et al. Fludarabine based combinations are highly effective and safe as first-line or salvage treatment for patients with Waldenström's macroglobulinemia. Accepted for publication.

248. Tedeschi A, Miqueleiz S, Ricci F, et al. Fludarabine, cyclophosphamide and rituximab in Waldenstrom's macroglobulinemia: an effective regimen requiring a new category of response criteria and a delayed assessment of results. ASH Annual Meeting Abstracts 2007;110(11):1290.

249. Vargaftig J, Pegourie-Bandelier B, Mahe B, et al. Fludarabine plus cyclophosphamide and rituximab (RFC) in Waldenstrom's macroglobulinemia (WM): results in 21 patients (pts). ASH Annual Meeting Abstracts 2006;108(11):4727.

250. Treon SP, Hunter Z, Barnagan AR. CHOP plus rituximab therapy in Waldenstrom's macroglobulinemia. Clin Lymphoma 2005;5(4):273–7.
251. Abonour R, Zhang LA, Rajkumar V, et al. Phase II pilot study of rituximab + CHOP in patients with newly diagnosed Waldenstrom's macroglobulinemia, an Eastern Cooperative Oncology Group Trial (Study E1A02). ASH Annual Meeting Abstracts 2007;110(11):3616.
252. Dhedin N, Tabrizi R, Bulabois PE, et al. Hematopoietic stem cell transplantation (HSCT) in Waldenstrom macroglobulinemia (WM), update of the French experience in 54 cases. ASH Annual Meeting Abstracts 2007;110(11):3015.
253. Kyriakou C, Canals C, Sureda A, et al. The role of autologous stem cell transplantation (ASCT) in patients with advanced Waldenstrom's macroglobulinemia. ASH Annual Meeting Abstracts 2007;110(11):941.
254. Kyriakou C, Canals C, Sureda A, et al. Allogeneic stem cell transplantation (allo-SCT) in the management of advanced Waldenstrom's macroglobulinemia (WM). ASH Annual Meeting Abstracts 2007;110(11):619.
255. Dimopoulos M, Anagnostopoulos A, Kyrtsonis M, et al. Treatment of relapsed or refractory Waldenstrom's macroglobulinemia with bortezomib. Haematologica 2005;90(12):1655–8.
256. Treon SP, Hunter ZR, Matous J, et al. Multicenter clinical trial of bortezomib in relapsed/refractory Waldenstrom's macroglobulinemia: results of WMCTG Trial 03-248. Clin Cancer Res 2007;13(11):3320–5.
257. Ghobrial IM, Padmanabhan S, Badros A, et al. Phase II trial of combination of bortezomib and rituximab in relapsed and/or refractory Waldenstrom macroglobulinemia: preliminary results. ASH Annual Meeting Abstracts 2007; 110(11):4494.
258. Treon SP, Soumerai JD, Patterson CJ, et al. Bortezomib, dexamethasone and rituximab (BDR) is a highly active regimen in the primary therapy of Waldenstrom's macroglobulinemia: planned interim results of WMCTG clinical trial 05-180. ASH Annual Meeting Abstracts 2006;108(11):2765.
259. Dimopoulos MA, Zomas A, Viniou NA, et al. Treatment of Waldenstrom's macroglobulinemia with thalidomide. J Clin Oncol 2001;19(16):3596–601.
260. Dimopoulos MA, Tsatalas C, Zomas A, et al. Treatment of Waldenstrom's macroglobulinemia with single-agent thalidomide or with the combination of clarithromycin, thalidomide and dexamethasone. Semin Oncol 2003;30(2):265–9.
261. Kaplan AA. Therapeutic apheresis for the renal complications of multiple myeloma and the dysglobulinemias. Ther Apher 2001;5(3):171–5.
262. Buskard NA, Galton DA, Goldman JM, et al. Plasma exchange in the long-term management of Waldenström's macroglobulinemia. Can Med Assoc J 1977; 117(2):135–7.
263. Orengo IF, Kettler AH, Bruce S, et al. Cutaneous Waldenström's macroglobulinemia. A report of a case successfully treated with radiotherapy. Cancer 1987; 60(6):1341–5.
264. Allbritton JI, Horn TD. Cutaneous lymphoplasmacytic lymphoma. J Am Acad Dermatol 1998;38(5 Pt 2):820–4.
265. Malik KJ, Berntson DG, Harrison AR. Lymphoplasmacytic lymphoma isolated to an extraocular muscle. Ophthal Plast Reconstr Surg 2006;22(5):400–1.

Diffuse Large B-Cell Lymphoma

Jonathan W. Friedberg, MD*, Richard I. Fisher, MD

KEYWORDS

• Chemotherapy • Pathology • Treatment

EPIDEMIOLOGY

Diffuse large B-cell lymphoma (DLBCL) is the most common of the aggressive non-Hodgkin's lymphomas (NHLs) in the United States. The rates of NHL, including DLBCL, have increased steadily in the United States by 3% to 4% each year from 1973 to the mid-1990s.[1] These increases in lymphoma have been observed in males and females, in whites and nonwhites, and in all age groups except the very young. With the exception of skin malignancies, such temporal increases in cancer incidence are unprecedented. Improved cancer reporting, more sensitive diagnostic techniques (particularly for borderline lesions), changes in the classification of lymphoproliferative diseases, and, in particular, the increasing occurrence of AIDS-associated DLBCL have contributed to the startling escalation of disease incidence.[2] Extensive analyses, however, have led to the conclusion that these factors account for only about 50% of the additional cases of NHL.[3] The incidence of non–AIDS-related NHL has continued to increase, specifically among females, older males, and blacks.[4]

For most patients, the origin of DLBCL is unknown. Factors thought to confer increased risk include immunosuppression (including AIDS and iatrogenic causes in the setting of transplantation or autoimmune diseases), ultraviolet radiation, pesticides, hair dyes, and diet.[5] A subset of DLBCL, including immunoblastic and primary central nervous system (CNS) disease, is highly associated with the Epstein-Barr virus although, unlike certain indolent histologies, the concept of antigen-driven lymphomagenesis is less developed in DLBCL.[6]

PATHOLOGY

DLBCL is a neoplasm of large B cells. Eighty percent of the neoplasms are composed of cells resembling germinal center centroblasts. The immunoblastic type (10% of

Dr. Friedberg is partially funded by a Scholar in Clinical Research award from the Leukemia & Lymphoma Society.
James P. Wilmot Cancer Center, University of Rochester, 601 Elmwood Avenue, Box 704, Room 1-4118C, Rochester, NY 14642, USA
* Corresponding author.
E-mail address: jonathan_friedberg@urmc.rochester.edu (J.W. Friedberg).

Hematol Oncol Clin N Am 22 (2008) 941–952
doi:10.1016/j.hoc.2008.07.002
0889-8588/08/$ – see front matter © 2008 Elsevier Inc. All rights reserved.

cases) has more than 90% immunoblasts. Other morphologic variants include the T-cell–rich/histiocyte-rich variant, which has a prominent background of reactive T cells and histiocytes. In the anaplastic type, the cells are morphologically similar to those of T/null anaplastic large-cell lymphoma, with pleomorphic nuclei, abundant cytoplasm, a sinusoidal growth pattern, and CD30 expression. Plasmablastic DLBCL, a very uncommon subtype, often occurs in HIV-positive patients.

A variety of chromosomal alterations have been described in DLBCL. The most common abnormality involves alterations of the BCL-6 gene at the 3q27 locus, which is critical for germinal center formation.[7] A substantial number of DLBCL cases have complex karyotypes.

Despite this significant morphologic and cytogenetic heterogeneity, it has been challenging to define unique therapies for each subgroup. To understand further the heterogeneity of this disease, gene-expression profiling has been used to investigate the different possible cellular origins of DLBCL, with the goal of identifying rational therapeutic targets. In 2002, the Leukemia and Lymphoma Molecular Profiling Project used DNA microarrays to analyze biopsy samples of DLBCL from 240 patients.[8] Subgroups with distinct gene-expression profiles were defined on the basis of hierarchical clustering. This study identified at least two independent gene-expression subgroups: the germinal-center B-cell–like (GCB) subtype and the activated B-cell–like (ABC) subtype. Patients in the GCB subgroup had a higher 5-year survival rate, independent of clinical international prognosis index (IPI) risk (see the article by Salles elsewhere in this issue). The group concluded that DNA microarrays can be used to formulate a molecular predictor of survival after chemotherapy for DLBCL. Using different methodology, other investigators have identified three different subgroups—oxidative-phosphorylation, B-cell receptor/proliferation, and host response—which also were associated with differential outcomes.[9]

Subsequent to these publications, a panel of three immunohistochemical stains (CD10, BCL6, and MUM1) has been proposed to distinguish the GCB and ABC subtypes.[10] Lossos and colleagues[11] evaluated 36 genes whose expression had been reported to predict survival in DLBCL using quantitative real-time polymerase chain reaction. The genes that were the strongest predictors were LMO2, BCL6, FN1, CCND2, SCYA3, and BCL2. The investigators concluded that measurement of the expression of these six genes was sufficient to predict overall survival in DLBCL.

Therefore, the disease DLBCL is clearly heterogeneous at a clinical, pathologic, and molecular level, as detailed further in the articles by Gascoyne and Rosenwald elsewhere in this issue. At the present time, the clinical approach to the disease generally does not take into account the distinct biology of these subtypes. Currently accruing clinical trials are underway to validate these findings prospectively in the modern therapeutic era and to determine whether novel targeted agents may be useful adjuncts to therapy in a molecularly defined subgroup of patients. The authors anticipate that future optimal therapy of DLBCL will incorporate this molecular information for appropriate risk-adapted therapy.

THERAPY OF EARLY-STAGE DIFFUSE LARGE B-CELL LYMPHOMA

In NHL, the term "early-stage" usually refers to disease limited to a single side of the diaphragm, including at most one contiguous extranodal site (see the article by CHeson elsewhere in this issue). During the past decade, a combined-modality approach incorporating chemotherapy of brief duration with subsequent radiation of the involved field has evolved to become the reasonable standard of care for most patients who have early-stage DLBCL. For most patients, outstanding results have been reported using this approach. As outcome data mature in the rituximab era, however, the optimal induction chemotherapy regimen and the role of involved-field radiation for most patients has been questioned again.

History—Before Rituximab

In 1998, Miller and colleagues[12] published results from a Southwest Oncology Group (SWOG) study that randomly assigned 401 patients who had nonbulky stage I or II aggressive NHL (mainly DLBCL) to three cycles of cyclophosphamide, hydroxydaunorubicin, vincristine, and prednisone (CHOP) (without rituximab) followed by involved-field radiation (40–50 Gy) or to eight cycles of CHOP (without rituximab) alone. Both progression-free survival and overall survival at 5 years were significantly superior for the combined-modality arm, with less life-threatening toxicity. Ten-year follow-up of this trial, however, has revealed an increase in late recurrences in patients treated with the combined modality and a continuous rate of death over the first 10 years with no evidence of plateau in the survival curve in either arm.[13]

In an older study of a combined-modality approach, the Eastern Cooperative Oncology Group enrolled 210 patients who had stage I disease with mediastinal or retroperitoneal involvement, bulky disease greater than 10 cm in diameter, or stage IE, II, or IIE disease and randomly assigned 172 patients who had attained a complete response after eight cycles of CHOP (without rituximab) to no further therapy or to involved-field radiation.[14] Disease-free survival at 6 years was superior for the combined-treatment arm (73% versus 56%), but there was no difference in overall survival.

These long-term results emphasize the importance of follow-up in interpreting the results of therapy of early-stage DLBCL and suggest that overall survival remains a key end point in this disease. In addition, these results suggest that early-stage disease may represent a distinct molecular entity, because late relapses in advanced-stage DLBCL are much less common events. Indeed, preliminary results from a gene-expression analysis comparing early-stage and advanced-stage DLBCL have revealed unique genes active in patients who have early-stage disease.[15]

Two French studies from the Groupe d'Etude des Lymphomes de l'Adulte (GELA) group evaluated the outcome of patients who had early-stage DLBCL before rituximab was available. One trial enrolled previously untreated patients younger than age 61 years who had localized stage I or II aggressive lymphoma and no IPI risk factors and compared three cycles of CHOP plus involved-field radiotherapy (329 patients) with chemotherapy alone with dose-intensified doxorubicin, cyclophosphamide, vindesine, bleomycin, and prednisone (ACVBP) plus sequential consolidation with high-dose methotrexate, etoposide, ifosfamide, and cytosine arabinoside (318 patients).[16] Of note, this trial, unlike the trials in the United States, included patients who had bulky stage II disease. The 5-year estimates of event-free survival were 82% for patients receiving ACVBP chemotherapy alone and 74% for those receiving standard CHOP plus radiotherapy. The 5-year estimates of overall survival in this trial were 90% and 81%, respectively. The survival benefit of ACBVP was smaller but remained significant in the subgroup of patients who had nonbulky disease. Vindesine currently is not available for use in the United States, limiting the applicability of this approach.

The GELA also has conducted a study of patients older than 60 years who had localized stage I or II aggressive lymphoma and no other adverse IPI factors. Patients were assigned randomly to receive either four cycles of CHOP (without rituximab) plus involved-field radiotherapy (299 patients) or CHOP alone (277 patients).[17] The 5-year estimates of event-free survival were 61% for patients receiving chemotherapy alone and 64% for patients receiving CHOP plus radiotherapy; the 5-year estimates of overall survival were 72% and 68%, respectively; differences were not significant at a median follow-up of 7 years.

The Rituximab Era and Risk-Adapted Therapy

When any risk factor in the IPI (age > 60 years, high lactate dehydrogenase level, stage II disease, or performance status ≥ 2) is present, the outcome is inferior to that seen in patients who have no risk factors. For example, the 5-year overall survival rates in the SWOG study were 94%, 71%, and 50%, respectively, for patients who had no, two, or three or more adverse risk factors (**Fig. 1**).[12] These findings have been confirmed by a Canadian experience using combined-modality treatment in a similarly defined group of patients who had early-stage disease. The overall survival rates at 5 years were 97% for patients who had no adverse factors, 77% for patients who had one or two adverse factors, and 58% for patients who had three adverse factors, with similar decrements in progression-free survival. In interpreting the results of various trials in early-stage disease, the clinical heterogeneity of these patients must be considered carefully. Therefore, more recent studies have been designed to improve outcome in this subgroup of patients at clinically high risk.

Rituximab has changed the prognosis and treatment paradigm for all patients who have DLBCL. Relatively few prospective studies focusing on early-stage disease have been published. The SWOG performed a pilot trial adding the monoclonal anti-CD20 antibody rituximab to three cycles of CHOP chemotherapy followed by radiotherapy.[18] This trial required patients to have at least one risk factor in the early-stage modification of the IPI. With the median follow-up of 5.3 years, treatment resulted in a progression-free survival of 93% at 2 years and 88% at 4 years. The overall survival rate was 95% at 2 years and 92% at 4 years, dramatically better than in historical controls. A pattern of continuing relapse with modest survival gains suggests that longer-term follow-up is required to clarify the magnitude of benefit in this setting.

The MabThera International Trial (MinT) enrolled young patients who had favorable risk factors and treated them with six cycles of CHOP-like chemotherapy with or

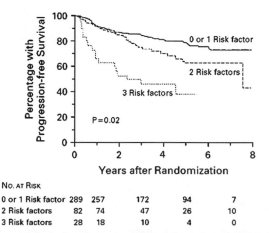

NO. AT RISK

0 or 1 Risk factor	289	257	172	94	7
2 Risk factors	82	74	47	26	10
3 Risk factors	28	18	10	4	0

Fig. 1. Progression-free survival of patients receiving eight cycles of CHOP alone and patients receiving three cycles of CHOP plus radiotherapy, according to the number of modified IPI risk factors. (*From* Miller TP, Dahlberg S, Cassady JR, et al. Chemotherapy alone compared with chemotherapy plus radiotherapy for localized intermediate- and high-grade non-Hodgkin's lymphoma. N Engl J Med 1998;339:24; with permission. Copyright © 1998, Massachusetts Medical Society.)

without rituximab.[19] Seventy-five percent of these patients had early-stage disease, and in early follow-up outstanding results were observed with six cycles of CHOP-like chemotherapy plus rituximab (R-CHOP) without radiation (except to bulk disease). Taken together, the MInT and SWOG studies suggest that the benefit of rituximab in early-stage DLBCL may be similar to that of radiation. Because of both short- and long-term toxicities of radiation, efforts again are underway to define a group of patients who do not require radiation therapy. In a preliminary report at the American Society of Hematology Meetings in 2007, Sehn and colleagues[20] reported on results from a single-arm, single-institution study suggesting that patients who have negative positron emission tomography scans after three cycles of R-CHOP therapy have excellent outcome without the addition of radiation therapy.

At present, the authors currently recommend three cycles of R-CHOP with involved-field radiation for most patients who have stage I and nonbulky stage II disease. This recommendation is extrapolated from the two previously mentioned SWOG studies. Based on the results of the MInT study, six cycles of R-CHOP chemotherapy without radiation seems to be another effective option for patients who do not have bulk disease. Patients who have bulky disease require more chemotherapy and possibly benefit from intensified regimens, as suggested by the GELA study. Current clinical trials in early-stage DLBCL use new agents such as radioimmunotherapy and continue the evaluation of fluorodeoxyglucose-positron emission tomography imaging to define which patients may not require external beam radiation. It is hoped that additional insights gained from gene-expression analyses concerning the possibly unique biology of early-stage disease may yield additional novel therapeutic approaches, particularly for the subset of patients at high risk.

THERAPY OF DISSEMINATED DIFFUSE LARGE B-CELL LYMPHOMA
In the Rituximab Era

Advanced-stage DLBCL is a curable disease when treated with systemic chemotherapy. The backbone of current therapy, CHOP, emerged as a standard following the United States Intergroup trial published in 1992, which compared CHOP, methotrexate, bleomycin, doxorubicin, cyclophosphamide, vincristine, and dexamethasone (m-BACOD) with prednisone, doxorubicin, cyclophosphamide, and etoposide plus cytarabine, bleomycin, and vincristine (ProMACE/CytaBOM) and methotrexate, doxorubicin, cyclophosphamide, vincristine, and bleomycin (MACOP-B).[21] The 6-year overall survival rate for the four regimens were 33% for CHOP; 36% for m-BACOD; 34% for ProMACE/CytaBOM; and 32% for MACOP-B. Because of its lower toxicity, the CHOP regimen emerged as a standard.

Rituximab has improved the outcome of advanced-stage DLBCL dramatically and when combined with CHOP chemotherapy has demonstrated benefit in overall survival in patients in all risk groups. The GELA group randomly assigned 399 previously untreated patients 60 to 80 years old who had DLBCL to receive either eight cycles of CHOP every 3 weeks or eight cycles of R-CHOP given on day 1 of each cycle.[22] Long-term follow-up has revealed significantly improved event-free survival, progression-free survival, disease-free survival, and overall survival in patients treated with R-CHOP (**Fig. 2**).[23] Moreover, no long-term toxicity seems to be associated with the R-CHOP combination, making this combination the standard of care in DLBCL.

A larger (n = 632) intergroup United States study randomly assigned a similar population of patients to CHOP versus R-CHOP in which rituximab was given on a slightly different schedule.[24] Responding patients then were assigned randomly to receive either rituximab maintenance therapy (four doses every 6 months for 2 years)

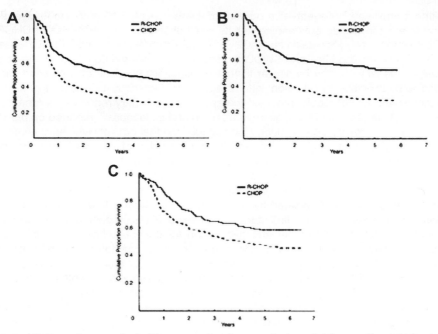

Fig. 2. (A) Event-free survival, (B) progression-free survival, and (C) overall survival with a median follow-up of 5 years in patients treated with CHOP and R-CHOP in the GELA study. (*From* Feugier P, Van Hoof A, Sebban C, et al. Long-term results of the R-CHOP study in the treatment of elderly patients with diffuse large B-cell lymphoma: a study by the Groupe d'Etude des Lymphomes de l'Adulte. J Clin Oncol 2005;23:4121; with permission.)

or no maintenance. There was no benefit to maintenance therapy after R-CHOP, and, in a secondary analysis that excluded patients receiving maintenance rituximab, R-CHOP alone reduced the risks of treatment failure and death compared with CHOP alone. Although rituximab maintenance provided a progression-free survival benefit in patients initially treated with CHOP alone, only R-CHOP induction seemed to increase the cure rate with longer follow-up of these patients.[25]

The German group has advocated greater dose intensity, with CHOP given every 14 days instead of every 21 days for elderly patients, and the addition of etoposide to CHOP chemotherapy for younger patients.[26,27] Rituximab adds benefit to these regimens, and a recent study has suggested that six cycles of intensified therapy (R-CHOP every 14 days) is adequate to provide maximal progression-free survival.[28] Ongoing studies are comparing these regimens with standard R-CHOP every 21 days.

Other attempts to improve the response to CHOP involve consolidation with high-dose therapy and autologous bone marrow transplantation (ASCT). Multiple studies have suggested that there is no clear indication for adding ASCT to the initial combination chemotherapy treatment for all patients who have aggressive lymphoma, but several studies evaluating ASCT as consolidation after CHOP-based therapy have suggested that ASCT is beneficial in patients who have high-intermediate or high IPI scores. For example, in a retrospective subset analysis of patients who had a high-intermediate risk of death, according to the age-adjusted IPI, a French study demonstrated the 5-year survival rate was significantly higher after high-dose therapy and ASCT consolidation than after CHOP (74% versus 44%).[29] These positive trials that included ASCT did not use rituximab in the induction chemotherapy. Because of the significant increase in cures observed with rituximab, a recently closed intergroup trial incorporated rituximab in the induction therapy followed by ASCT in patients who had high-intermediate or high-risk aggressive NHL; ultimately, the results of this trial should address this unresolved question. Until this study has matured, the authors do not advocate routine use of ASCT consolidation after R-CHOP induction therapy.

Primary Mediastinal Large B-Cell Lymphoma

Mediastinal (thymic) large B-cell lymphoma, originally considered a subtype of DLBCL arising in the mediastinum, is recognized now as a separate disease entity. The tumor is composed of large cells with variable nuclear features, often with abundant clear cytoplasm in a background compartmentalizing sclerosis. Expression of *FIG1*, amplification of the *REL* oncogene at chromosome 9p, and overexpression of the *MAL* gene at chromosome 2p13-15 are characteristic of primary mediastinal B-cell lymphoma but not of other DLBCLs.[30]

Gene-expression profiling shows that primary mediastinal B-cell lymphoma has an expression signature distinct from that of nodal DLBCL and with similarities to Hodgkin's lymphoma. In particular, loss of expression of B-cell receptor signaling genes and activation of both the Janus kinase-2 and nuclear factor-κB pathways were noticed, suggesting molecular mechanisms of transformation similar to those seen in a malignant clone.[31]

Primary DLBCL has a female predominance, and the median age of onset is in the fourth decade. Patients present with a locally invasive anterior mediastinal mass originating in the thymus, with frequent airway compromise and superior vena cava syndrome. Relapses tend to be extranodal, including liver, gastrointestinal tract, kidneys, ovaries, and the CNS.

In general, the treatment approach is similar to that for localized DLBCL. A recent series from Vancouver demonstrated favorable prognosis, with 5-year overall survival rates of 87%, 81% and 71% in patients younger than 65 years old treated with MACOP-B/etoposide, doxorubicin, cyclophosphamide, vincristine, prednisone, and bleomycin , CHOP-R, and CHOP-type chemotherapy, respectively.[32] The addition of radiation therapy did not improve survival in this series, and the role of radiation remains controversial in this histology. The prognosis of patients who have localized mediastinal large-cell NHL is similar to that of other patients who have poor-prognosis early-stage disease: approximately 50% of patients are alive and disease-free at 5 years.

In general, the authors' approach for patients who present with localized, bulky mediastinal diffuse large B-cell NHL is treatment with six cycles of R-CHOP followed by involved-field radiation therapy.

Testicular Lymphoma

DLBCL presenting in the testicle is approached like nodal DLBCL. CNS relapse has been reported with testicular lymphoma, however, and in some series the rate of relapse reaches 20%.[33] Most of these CNS relapses are parenchymal relapses not localized to the leptomeninges. For this reason, many advocate the use of CNS prophylaxis, with either intrathecal chemotherapy or high-dose systemic methotrexate with leucovorin rescue, in addition to standard R-CHOP therapy. The benefit of CNS prophylaxis never has been proven, and a recent analysis of SWOG data for all advanced-stage DLBCL suggested no benefit to the use of CNS prophylaxis in the setting of bone marrow involvement by lymphoma, another setting in which CNS relapses are common.

In addition to consideration of CNS prophylaxis, the authors recommend radiation to the contralateral testis after the completion of systemic therapy to avert relapses in that sanctuary site.

Lymphomatoid Granulomatosis

The entity described as "lymphomatoid granulomatosis" has been shown in most cases to be an Epstein-Barr virus–positive large B-cell lymphoma with a T-cell–rich background.[34] Patients typically present with extranodal disease, most commonly involving lung, CNS, and/or kidneys. Evidence of past or present immunosuppression may be found. Lymphomatoid granulomatosis is graded according to the number of large B cells. The prognosis for this entity is variable; for patients who have grade III disease the authors recommend an approach similar to that for disseminated DLBCL (ie, R-CHOP). For lower-grade disease, in addition to combination chemotherapy, responses have been reported with the use of interferon-α, rituximab, and high-dose therapy and autologous stem cell support.[35]

Future Therapy of Diffuse Large B-Cell lymphoma: Novel Agents

Despite the success of rituximab, a significant number of patients who have advanced-stage disease and clinical risk factors are not cured with R-CHOP–based therapy. Even if the findings of the intergroup trial of ASCT consolidation are positive, at least half of patients may not be eligible for this approach because of advanced age or medical comorbidities. Therefore, the authors believe that major improvements in the treatment of diffuse large B-cell NHL will include the incorporation of novel, rationally targeted agents into the standard treatment paradigm.

Bortezomib, a proteasome inhibitor that has demonstrated significant single-agent activity in mantle cell lymphoma,[36] is one example of such agents. Because of presumed effects targeting the nuclear factor-kB pathway, studies are underway evaluating bortezomib in combination with chemotherapy, particularly for patients who have mediastinal diffuse large B-cell NHL and patients who have the ABC genotype.

Enzastaurin, an inhibitor of protein kinase C-beta, is currently under investigation as a potential maintenance therapy following standard R-CHOP treatment in patients who have high-intermediate or high-risk DLBCL. This target was identified by gene-expression profiling studies suggesting that patients who have refractory disease overexpress protein kinase C-beta.[37] The agent has demonstrated modest single-agent activity, with the suggestion of an ability to stabilize disease.[38]

Lenalidomide, an analogue of thalidomide, is approved for myelodysplastic syndrome and myeloma. This agent has pleiotropic effects, including immunomodulatory activities and antiangiogenic effects. A study of lenalidomide in patients who have aggressive lymphomas, including DLBCL, suggests a response rate of 25% in patients who have refractory disease.[39] Efforts currently are underway to combine this agent with standard chemotherapy for this disease.

Radioimmunotherapy (discussed further in the article by Leonard and Elstrom elsewhere in this issue) is approved for treatment of indolent and transformed lymphoma. A phase II trial evaluating ibritumomab tiuxetan in patients who had relapsed or refractory DLBCL demonstrated responses of relatively short duration.[40] Studies of both ibritumomab tiuxetan and iodine-131 tositumomab consolidation after standard R-CHOP therapy for patients who have de novo DLBCL are underway.

Bevacizumab, an antibody directed against vascular endothelial growth factor, has demonstrated significant synergy with chemotherapy in multiple solid tumors. Although the agent has limited single-agent activity in DLBCL, studies combining bevacizumab with R-CHOP to treat DLBCL are ongoing.

Other agents under evaluation for DLBCL include inhibitors of *bcl-2*, inhibitors of *Syk* (a tyrosine kinase downstream of the B-cell receptor), inhibitors of the mammalian target of rapamycin pathway, and inhibitors of histone deacetylase.

THERAPY FOR RELAPSED OR REFRACTORY DISEASE

The authors strongly advocate obtaining a biopsy if disease progression is suspected. Both anatomic and functional imaging studies have limitations and may have false-positive results. Moreover, some patients who present with DLBCL are found to have a follicular lymphoma at the time of relapse, and this finding has profound implications for the further therapy of this disease.

The initial step in planning salvage chemotherapy is to determine the goal of treatment. Patients approached with curative intent (who can tolerate high-dose therapy and autologous stem cell transplantation) are treated with second-line combination chemotherapy regimens, usually including drugs such as cisplatin, ifosfamide, etoposide, and cytarabine, often in combination with rituximab.[41] The chances of achieving a complete remission with salvage therapy have varied widely in different studies, generally falling in the range of 20% to 40%, but responses occur in most patients.

The Parma study defined the role of autologous stem cell transplantation in relapsed DLBCL.[42] In this trial, 109 patients who had relapsed from complete remission and who responded to two cycles of dexamethasone, cytarabine, and cisplatin (DHAP) were allocated randomly to high-dose chemotherapy using the a regimen of carmustine, etoposide, cytarabine, and cyclophosphamide or to continued treatment with DHAP. Bone marrow transplantation was associated with a superior failure-free survival (51% versus 12% at 5 years) and overall survival (53% versus 32% at 5 years). Bone marrow transplantation remains the standard approach, although preliminary studies suggest an inferior outcome for ASCT in the rituximab era, as more patients are cured with initial therapy.

If patients are elderly or have comorbid conditions, the goal should be palliation. Radiotherapy frequently can be used to alleviate the symptoms at a particular site of involvement in patients who have relapsed DLBCL. Palliative chemotherapy approaches include single-agent treatment with vincristine, cytarabine, alkylating agents, or anthracyclines. Responses to single-agent rituximab occur in approximately 30% of these patients and generally are of brief duration.[43] The authors strongly believe that this setting is optimal for clinical trial enrollment, because many novel phase I and early phase II agents are investigated in this setting.

SUMMARY

The incorporation of rituximab into standard chemotherapeutic regimens has led to significant improvements in outcomes of patients who have early-stage or advanced-stage DLBCL. Insights into the biologic heterogeneity of DLBCL, particularly from gene-expression analyses, yield opportunities for rational targeted therapy, currently under investigation. Important clinical trials are underway that should define definitively the role of ASCT in first remission for patients who are at high clinical risk of relapse and should demonstrate the whether R-CHOP is given more effectively every 14 days or every 21 days. The authors anticipate that promising phase II results from ongoing studies evaluating novel agents eventually will improve outcomes for patients who have DLBCL.

REFERENCES

1. Fisher SG, Fisher RI. The epidemiology of non-Hodgkin's lymphoma. Oncogene 2004;23(38):6524–34.
2. Hartge P, Devesa SS. Quantification of the impact of known risk factors on time trends in non-Hodgkin's lymphoma incidence. Cancer Res 1992;52(19 Suppl): 5566s–9s.
3. Holford TR, Zheng T, Mayne ST, et al. Time trends of non-Hodgkin's lymphoma: are they real? What do they mean? Cancer Res 1992;52(19 Suppl):5443s–6s.
4. Eltom MA, Jemal A, Mbulaiteye SM, et al. Trends in Kaposi's sarcoma and non-Hodgkin's lymphoma incidence in the United States from 1973 through 1998. J Natl Cancer Inst 2002;94(16):1204–10.
5. Blinder V, Fisher SG. The role of environmental factors in the etiology of lymphoma. Cancer Invest 2008;26(3):306–16.
6. Fisher SG, Fisher RI. The emerging concept of antigen-driven lymphomas: epidemiology and treatment implications. Curr Opin Oncol 2006;18(5):417–24.
7. Spagnolo DV, Ellis DW, Juneja S, et al. The role of molecular studies in lymphoma diagnosis: a review. Pathology 2004;36(1):19–44.
8. Rosenwald A, Wright G, Chan WC, et al. The use of molecular profiling to predict survival after chemotherapy for diffuse large-B-cell lymphoma. N Engl J Med 2002;346(25):1937–47.
9. Monti S, Savage KJ, Kutok JL, et al. Molecular profiling of diffuse large B-cell lymphoma identifies robust subtypes including one characterized by host inflammatory response. Blood 2005;105(5):1851–61.
10. Hans CP, Weisenburger DD, Greiner TC, et al. Confirmation of the molecular classification of diffuse large B-cell lymphoma by immunohistochemistry using a tissue microarray. Blood 2004;103(1):275–82.
11. Lossos IS, Czerwinski DK, Alizadeh AA, et al. Prediction of survival in diffuse large-B-cell lymphoma based on the expression of six genes. N Engl J Med 2004;350(18):1828–37.
12. Miller TP, Dahlberg S, Cassady JR, et al. Chemotherapy alone compared with chemotherapy plus radiotherapy for localized intermediate- and high-grade non-Hodgkin's lymphoma. N Engl J Med 1998;339:21–6.
13. Miller TP, LeBlanc M, Spier C, et al. CHOP alone compared to CHOP plus radiotherapy for early stage aggressive non-Hodgkin's lymphomas: update of the Southwest Oncology Group (SWOG) randomized trial. Blood 2001;98: 724a–5a.
14. Horning SJ, Weller E, Kim K, et al. Chemotherapy with or without radiotherapy in limited-stage diffuse aggressive non-Hodgkin's lymphoma: Eastern Cooperative Oncology Group study 1484. J Clin Oncol 2004;22(15):3032–8.
15. Roberts R, Rimsza LM, Staudt L, et al. Gene expression differences between low and high stage diffuse large B cell lymphoma. Blood 2006;108(11):196a.
16. Reyes F, Lepage E, Ganem G, et al. ACVBP versus CHOP plus radiotherapy for localized aggressive lymphoma. N Engl J Med 2005;352(12):1197–205.
17. Bonnet C, Fillet G, Mounier N, et al. CHOP alone compared with CHOP plus radiotherapy for localized aggressive lymphoma in elderly patients: a study by the Groupe d'Etude des Lymphomes de l'Adulte. J Clin Oncol 2007;25(7): 787–92.
18. Persky DO, Unger JM, Spier CM, et al. Effect of adding rituximab to three cycles of CHOP plus involved-field radiotherapy for patients with limited stage aggressive B-cell lymphoma. J Clin Oncol, in press.

19. Pfreundschuh M, Trumper L, Osterborg A, et al. CHOP-like chemotherapy plus rituximab versus CHOP-like chemotherapy alone in young patients with good-prognosis diffuse large-B-cell lymphoma: a randomised controlled trial by the MabThera International Trial (MInT) Group. Lancet Oncol 2006;7(5):379–91.
20. Sehn L, Savage KJ, Hoskins P, et al. Limited-stage diffuse large B cell lymphoma patients with a negative PET scan following three cycles of R-CHOP can be effectively treated with abbreviated chemoimmunotherapy alone. Blood 2007;110:242a.
21. Fisher RI, Gaynor ER, Dahlberg S, et al. Comparison of a standard regimen (CHOP) with three intensive chemotherapy regimens for advanced non-Hodgkin's lymphoma. N Engl J Med 1993;328(14):1002–6.
22. Coiffier B, Lepage E, Briere J, et al. CHOP chemotherapy plus rituximab compared with CHOP alone in elderly patients with diffuse large-B-cell lymphoma. N Engl J Med 2002;346(4):235–42.
23. Feugier P, Van Hoof A, Sebban C, et al. Long-term results of the R-CHOP study in the treatment of elderly patients with diffuse large B-cell lymphoma: a study by the Groupe d'Etude des Lymphomes de l'Adulte. J Clin Oncol 2005;23(18):4117–26.
24. Habermann TM, Weller EA, Morrison VA, et al. Rituximab-CHOP versus CHOP alone or with maintenance rituximab in older patients with diffuse large B-cell lymphoma. J Clin Oncol 2006;24(19):3121–7.
25. Morrison VA, We EA, Erhardt W, et al. Maintenance rituximab compared to observation after R-CHOP or CHOP in older patients with diffuse large B-cell lymphoma. J Clin Oncol 2007;25:443s.
26. Pfreundschuh M, Truemper L, Kloess M, et al. 2-weekly or 3-weekly CHOP chemotherapy with or without etoposide for the treatment of young patients with good prognosis (normal LDH) aggressive lymphomas: results of the NHL-B1 trial of the DSHNHL. Blood Feb 24 2004.
27. Pfreundschuh M, Truemper L, Kloess M, et al. 2-weekly or 3-weekly CHOP chemotherapy with or without etoposide for the treatment of elderly patients with aggressive lymphomas: results of the NHL-B2 trial of the DSHNHL. Blood Mar 11 2004.
28. Pfreundschuh M, Schubert J, Ziepert M, et al. Six versus eight cycles of bi-weekly CHOP-14 with or without rituximab in elderly patients with aggressive CD20+ B-cell lymphomas: a randomised controlled trial (RICOVER-60). Lancet Oncol 2008;9(2):105–16.
29. Milpied N, Deconinck E, Gaillard F, et al. Initial treatment of aggressive lymphoma with high-dose chemotherapy and autologous stem-cell support. N Engl J Med 2004;350(13):1287–95.
30. Copie-Bergman C, Boulland ML, Dehoulle C, et al. Interleukin 4-induced gene 1 is activated in primary mediastinal large B-cell lymphoma. Blood 2003;101(7):2756–61.
31. Savage KJ, Monti S, Kutok JL, et al. The molecular signature of mediastinal large B-cell lymphoma differs from that of other diffuse large B-cell lymphomas and shares features with classical Hodgkin lymphoma. Blood 2003;102(12):3871–9.
32. Savage KJ, Al-Rajhi N, Voss N, et al. Favorable outcome of primary mediastinal large B-cell lymphoma in a single institution: the British Columbia experience. Ann Oncol 2006;17(1):123–30.
33. Zucca E, Conconi A, Mughal TI, et al. Patterns of outcome and prognostic factors in primary large-cell lymphoma of the testis in a survey by the International Extranodal Lymphoma Study Group. J Clin Oncol 2003;21(1):20–7.

34. Jaffe ES, Wilson WH. Lymphomatoid granulomatosis: pathogenesis, pathology and clinical implications. Cancer Surv 1997;30:233–48.
35. Wilson WH, Kingma DW, Raffeld M, et al. Association of lymphomatoid granulomatosis with Epstein-Barr viral infection of B lymphocytes and response to interferon-alpha 2b. Blood 1996;87(11):4531–7.
36. Fisher RI, Bernstein SH, Kahl BS, et al. Multicenter phase II study of bortezomib in patients with relapsed or refractory mantle cell lymphoma. J Clin Oncol 2006; 24(30):4867–74.
37. Shipp MA, Ross KN, Tamayo P, et al. Diffuse large B-cell lymphoma outcome prediction by gene-expression profiling and supervised machine learning. Nat Med 2002;8(1):68–74.
38. Robertson MJ, Kahl BS, Vose JM, et al. Phase II study of enzastaurin, a protein kinase C beta inhibitor, in patients with relapsed or refractory diffuse large B-cell lymphoma. J Clin Oncol 2007;25(13):1741–6.
39. Wiernik PH, Lossos I, Tuscano J, et al. Preliminary results from a phase II study of lenalidomide monotherapy in relapsed/refractory aggressive non-Hodgkin's lymphoma. Blood 2006;106:531.
40. Morschhauser F, Illidge T, Huglo D, et al. Efficacy and safety of yttrium-90 ibritumomab tiuxetan in patients with relapsed or refractory diffuse large B-cell lymphoma not appropriate for autologous stem-cell transplantation. Blood 2007;110(1):54–8.
41. Kewalramani T, Zelenetz AD, Nimer SD, et al. Rituximab and ICE as second-line therapy before autologous stem cell transplantation for relapsed or primary refractory diffuse large B-cell lymphoma. Blood 2004;103(10):3684–8.
42. Philip T, Guglielmi C, Hagenbeek A, et al. Autologous bone marrow transplantation as compared with salvage chemotherapy in relapses of chemotherapy-sensitive non-Hodgkin's lymphoma. N Engl J Med 1995;333(23):1540–5.
43. Coiffier B, Haioun C, Ketterer N, et al. Rituximab (anti-CD20 monoclonal antibody) for the treatment of patients with relapsing or refractory aggressive lymphoma: a multicenter phase II study. Blood 1998;92(6):1927–32.

Therapy of Mantle Cell Lymphoma: Current Standards and Future Strategies

Christian Schmidt, MD, Martin Dreyling, MD, PhD*

KEYWORDS

- Adult • Aged • Female • Humans • Rituximab
- Autologous transplant • Lymphoma • Male

Mantle cell lymphoma (MCL) represents a distinct histologic subtype of malignant B-cell neoplasia and accounts for 5% to 10% of all lymphoid malignancies corresponding to an incidence of two to three new cases per 100,000 inhabitants. In 1977, the Kiel classification described the disease as centrocytical lymphoma. In contrast, it was subsumed under different histologic entities. In the Working Formulation the term "mantle cell lymphoma" was first proposed by Banks and colleagues[1] 1992 and after introduction of the REAL and the current World Health Organization classification, MCL was established as an independent lymphoma entity.[2,3] MCL is cytomorphologically characterized by small- to medium-sized lymphoid cells with irregularly notched nuclei. Men are more often affected than women in a ratio of 4:1. The disease is usually clinically characterized by an aggressive course with only short-term remissions after conventional chemotherapy. The median survival in historical series is about 3 years, but this figure has recently improved.[4,5]

ETIOLOGY AND MOLECULAR PATHOGENESIS

The etiology and pathogenesis of MCL are not totally clarified and still an object of current research. Environmental toxins (eg, long-time exposure to herbicides) are discussed as risk factors, although population-based data so far are limited.

Nevertheless, increasing insights into the underlying molecular pathogenesis have been achieved within the last decade. On the genomic level, the chromosomal translocation (11; 14) represents the hallmark of MCL. Thereby, the cyclin-D1 gene on chromosome 11 is brought under the regulatory influence of the IgH gene promoter on chromosome 14, which results in inactivation of the retinoblastoma tumor suppression

Department of Medicine III, University of Munich, Hospital Grosshadern, Marchioninistrasse 15, D-81377 Munich, Germany
* Corresponding author.
E-mail address: martin.dreyling@med.uni-muenchen.de (M. Dreyling).

Hematol Oncol Clin N Am 22 (2008) 953–963
doi:10.1016/j.hoc.2008.07.001
0889-8588/08/$ – see front matter © 2008 Elsevier Inc. All rights reserved.

gene and finally a release of E2F-transcription factors and cell proliferation by various intracellular signal pathways.

Increased levels of cyclin-D1 form complexes with cyclin-dependent kinases 4 and 6, which lead to phosphorylation of the retinoblastoma protein. This process deregulates the cell cycle, promoting transition from G1 to S-phase. Another cell cycle regulator, p27, is secluded by cyclin E–cyclin-dependent kinase 2 complex disinhibition, which also results in an acceleration of cell cycle progression.

In a significant fraction of MCL reduced levels of cyclin-dependent kinase 4 and 6 inhibitors (eg, p16^{INK4a}) can be detected. About 20% of cases display homogenous deletions of chromosomal band 9p21 with the p16^{INK4a} gene being inactivated. Additionally p16^{ARF}, which is involved in DNA damage response by mdm2 and p53, is also encoded by the previously mentioned 9p21 gene locus and simultaneously deleted. These cases with 9p deletions often show the blastoid histology with a more aggressive clinical course. In as many as 75% of MCL the ataxia telangiectasia mutated gene on chromosomal band 11q22-23 is mutated, which causes impaired p53-mediated cell-cycle arrest, DNA repair, and apoptosis. Recent proteome analysis confirmed the central role of p53-triggered protein interactions in MCL.[6] Disruption of cell cycle regulation and concurrent DNA damage response are characteristics of MCL pathogenesis.[7,8]

HISTOLOGY

MCL is characterized by small- to medium-sized lymphoid cells with irregularly notched nuclei in a loose net of follicular, dendritic cells of reticulum. The growth pattern is often nodular but can also be diffuse. Cytomorphologically, it can be distinguished into a classical MCL and a blastoid variant.[3] Mixtures of cells (classical plus pleomorphic type) or transitions (classical-pleomorphic) are identified but more detailed classification is not of additional prognostic value.[9]

The lymphoma cells express IgM and often also IgD. The B-cell markers CD19, CD20, CD22, and CD79a are regularly expressed, and the T-cell antigen CD5; in contrast to chronic lymphocytic leukemia, cells typically do not express CD23. The typical translocation t[11;14][q13;q32] can be detected by classical cytogenetics or fluorescence in situ hybridization, with most of the breakpoints occurring in the major translocation cluster. Conventional genomic polymerase chain reaction is able to detect the translocation only in about 30% of cases, however, because of the wide genomic range of breakpoints. Resultant overexpression of this cell cycle regulator protein may be detected by cyclin-DI immunostaining in most patients, representing the hallmark of MCL diagnosis. Recently a few cyclin-D1–negative cases were identified.[10] Whether cases of atypical chronic lymphocytic leukemia with t[11;14] indicate a different disease entity is the subject of controversy.

CLINICAL PRESENTATION AND PROGNOSIS FACTORS

In general, MCL is characterized by a rapidly progressing clinical course. Most cases are diagnosed in an advanced stage (Ann Arbor III–IV) with generalized lymphadenopathy. B symptoms (fever, weight loss, and night sweats) additionally restrict the patient. In up to 50% of the cases, atypical lymphoma cells are detected in the differential blood count.

Extranodal manifestations emerge in up to 90% of all cases, with bone marrow involvement most frequent (60%–81%), followed by gastrointestinal tract and liver. In relapsed disease, central nervous system involvement is relatively frequent (4%–20%).[11]

MCL is characterized by a poor long-term prognosis. The median duration of survival has been reported to be in the range of 3 to 4 years with fewer than 15% long-term survivors,[4] whereas recent data suggest an improved outcome with a median overall survival (OS) of 5 years and longer.[5] The International Prognostic Index established in diffuse large cell lymphoma is only of minor relevance in MCL. In a multivariate analysis of more than 450 patients, age, performance status, lactate dehydrogenase, and leukocyte or lymphocyte count could be identified as independent prognostic factors, establishing a MCL-specific prognostic 12 score.[12]

Probably the most important prognostic parameter, however, is the rate of cell proliferation. A high rate of proliferation, identified either by RNA array or immunohistochemical staining (Ki67), is associated with a considerably worse prognosis.[10,13,14]

Minimal residual disease seems to be a strong prognostic factor in MCL patients after high-dose therapy and autologous hematopoietic stem cell transplantation. Data on combined immunochemotherapy, however, are contradictory.[15]

RECOMMENDATION FOR DIAGNOSTIC PROCEDURES

The histologic confirmation of diagnose is essential. A lymph node biopsy is strongly recommended. In the selected cases with retroperitoneal lymph nodes only, diagnosis can be confirmed by CT-guided core-needle biopsy. In contrast, fine-needle biopsy is not appropriate. Bone marrow aspiration alone is not sufficient but should be complemented by flow cytometry to identify the lymphoma-immune phenotype and bone marrow biopsy to quantify the percentage of infiltration. Because an accurate histologic diagnosis is essential, second opinion by an experienced hematopathologist is advisable.

The laboratory evaluation includes differential blood count and standard serum chemistry analysis including the determination of LDH as one of the major risk parameters. β_2-Microglobuline and thymidine kinase may also be determined.

Abdominal ultrasound and CT of the neck, chest, abdomen, and pelvis are obligatory. If there are hints of neurologic symptoms, cranial imaging with MRI and diagnostic lumbar puncture is recommended. PET scan is not included in the recent consensus recommendations based on scarce data and especially limited therapeutic consequences.[16]

Additional diagnostics depends on the clinical presentation and includes an ear-nose-throat consultation and gastroscopy and colonoscopy based on up to 60% asymptomatic infiltration of the bowel (lymphomatoid polyposis).[17]

THERAPY

The clinical course of MCL is especially aggressive with the worst long-time outcome of all B-cell lymphoma entities. A watch and wait strategy is rarely indicated, although conventional dosed chemotherapy is noncurative in advanced-stage disease.[18]

CONVENTIONAL CYTOTOXIC CHEMOTHERAPY

The superiority of anthracycline-containing regimens has not been confirmed in randomized trials. The CHOP-protocol (cyclophosphamide, doxorubicin, vincristine, and prednisone) achieved similar overall response rates (ORR) (89% versus 84%), median progression-free survival (PFS), and OS in comparison with an alkylator-based combination (COP).[18] Similarly ORRs after CHOP have only slightly improved in comparison with an anthrachinon-containing regimen (MCP) (87% versus 73%; $P = .080$) with a similar time to treatment failure (21 months versus 15 months; $P = .14$) and OS

(61 months versus 48 months; $P = .058$).[19] In contrast, retrospective analyses showed a longer survival after anthracycline-containing chemotherapy regimens in patients with low- or intermediate-risk disease.[20] CHOP remains the standard induction protocol for younger patients with MCL.

Fludarabine as a single agent displayed only moderate efficacy (30%–40% overall response) in MCL.[21] In contrast, combinations with either and idarubicin (FLU-ID) or cyclophosphamide achieved superior response rates (60% and 63%, respectively).[22,23] Hematologic toxicity and stem cell toxicity have to be considered, however, especially for patients who are potential candidates for autologous stem cell harvest.

Promising preliminary data have been recently presented for bendamustine.[24] A randomized phase III trial in patients with indolent non-Hodgkin's lymphoma and MCL demonstrated that bendamustine can efficaciously and safely replace cyclophosphamide in combination with vincristine and prednisone (BOP versus COP).[25] In a phase II trial, bendamustine in combination with rituximab showed an ORR of 75% with a complete response rate (CRR) of 50% in 16 patients with relapsed or refractory MCL.[26] Similarly, even in rituximab-pretreated patients with relapsed and refractory lymphoma including MCL, bendamustine in combination with mitoxantrone and rituximab was well-tolerated and highly effective with an ORR of 76% and a CRR of 38%[27] in another phase II trial.

INTENSIVE CHEMOTHERAPY

Recent studies confirmed the benefit of dose-intensified approaches in younger patients. Several studies show a high effectiveness of high-dose cytarabine in the therapy of MCLs. Lefrere and coworkers[28] analyzed the sequential administration of CHOP and DHAP (dexamethasone, high-dose cytarabine, cisplatin). After four cycles CHOP, only 7% of the patients reached complete remission. After four more cycles with DHAP the remission rate rose to over 80%. Another even more dose-intensified regimen of hyper-CVAD–MA (fractionated cyclophosphamide, doxorubicin, vincristine, dexamethasone; alternated with high-dose methotrexate and cytarabine) was introduced by the M.D. Anderson group and demonstrated a CRR of 38% and a partial response of 55.5% after four cycles in 45 patients with previously untreated and relapsed MCL.[29]

In the initial trials, both DHAP and hyper-CVAD protocols were applied as cytoreductive induction followed by consolidating myeloablative therapy and autologous hematopoietic stem cell transplantation. Meanwhile, even more impressive results have been reported when rituximab was combined with either the DHAP regimen[30] or the hyper-CVAD–MA regimen (**Table 1**).[31] Unfortunately, these excellent results could not be replicated in a multicenter study evaluating R-hyper-CVAD. ORR was 88% with only 2-year PFS of 63% (see **Table 1**).[32]

AUTOLOGOUS STEM CELL TRANSPLANTATION

Many studies suggested the efficacy of myeloablative high-dose therapy following autologous stem cell transfusion. In a randomized study high-dose consolidation achieved a significantly longer PFS in comparison with interferon maintenance (39 versus 17 months; $P = .0108$) with the tendency toward an improved OS, but longer follow-up times have to be awaited.[33]

In contrast to these results, the outcome in extensively pretreated patients is considerably worse. The myeloablative consolidation should be considered in the first remission for young patients. Unfortunately, even after such dose-intensified

Table 1
Clinical trials evaluating cytostatic chemotherapy combined with rituximab in mantle cell lymphoma

Author, Year	Phase and Disease Status	Regimen	N	Results	PFS/EFS	OS
Howard and colleagues, 2002[15]	Phase II, newly diagnosed MCL	CHOP + rituximab	40	CR/CRu: 4% PR: 48%	Median PFS: 16.6 mo	
Lenz and colleagues, 2005[39]	Phase III, newly diagnosed MCL	CHOP ± rituximab (followed by interferon maintenance versus ASCT)	122	CR: 34% versus 7% PR: 60% versus 68%	No significant difference in PFS Median TTF: 21 versus 14 mo	
Forstpointner and colleagues, 2004[40]	Phase III, relapsed or refractory MCL	FCM ± rituximab (followed by observation versus rituximab maintenance)	40	CR: 29% versus 0% PR: 29% versus 46%	Median PFS: 8 versus 4 mo	Median OS: NR versus 11 mo
Romaguera and colleagues, 2005[31]	Phase II, newly diagnosed MCL	Hyper-CVAD/MA + rituximab	97	CR/CRu: 87% PR: 10%	3-y EFS: 64%	3-y OS: 82%
de Guibert and colleagues, 2006[30]	Phase II, newly diagnosed MCL	DHAP + rituximab	24	CR/CRu: 92% PR: 4%	3-y EFS: 65%	3-y OS: 69%
Epner and colleagues, 2007[32]	Phase II, newly diagnosed MCL	Hyper-CVAD/MA + rituximab	97	CR/CRu: 58% PR: 30%	2-y PFS: 64%	2-y OS: 76%

Abbreviations: ASCT, autologous stem cell transplantation; CHOP, cyclophosphamide, doxorubicin, vincristine, and prednisone; CR, complete response rate; DHAP, dexamethasone, high dose Ara-C, cisplatium; EFS, event-free survival; FCM, fladarabine, cyclophosphamide, mitoxantrone; FFS, failure-free survival; hyper-CVAD/MA, fractionated cyclophosphamide, doxorubicin, vincristine, dexamethasone, alternated with high-dose methotrexate and cytarabine; MCL, mantle cell lymphoma; OS, overall survival; PFS, progression-free survival; PR, partial response rate; TTF, time to treatment failure.

approaches, most patients eventually relapse. A potential explanation for the high relapse rate is contamination of stem cell preparations by circulating MCL cells. Accordingly, recent series have reported an excellent outcome implementing in vitro purging before autologous stem cell transplantation.[34,35] It is not determined, however, which of the two published strategies, either sequential (CHOP induction followed by myeloablative consolidation) or upfront intensification (hyper-CVAD), is superior.[31,33]

A prospective trial evaluating the addition of high-dose cytarabine is currently accruing.[36] Interim analysis after inclusion of more than 300 patients did not detect a significant benefit so far. Response rates in the overall group have been 91% with 56% CRR-CRu after induction and 82% PFS after 12 months.

RITUXIMAB

Rituximab is a chimeric IgG_1 anti-CD20 monoclonal antibody that induces antibody-dependent cellular cytotoxicity and complement-dependent cytotoxicity. In addition, intracellular signaling may contribute to its efficacy; however, the exact in vivo function of CD20 is still unknown.[37] Rituximab is only moderately effective in treating MCL with response rates of 20% to 40%,[38] but based on an in vitro synergism the effectiveness of rituximab in combination with CHOP was analyzed in a phase III study. In the combination arm, 94% of the patients achieved a remission (CRR 34%) versus 75% (CRR 7%) in the control arm with only CHOP. In contrast, PFS differed only slightly.[39]

The combination of rituximab and FCM was also tested in relapsed MCL in comparison with only FCM chemotherapy. The combined study arm R-FCM achieved significantly superior ORR (ORR 58% versus 46%, CRR 29% versus 0%) and even OS.[40]

Rituximab maintenance therapy was initially investigated after antibody monotherapy induction, and no significant prolongation of PFS was observed.[37] In contrast, after a more effective initial tumor debulking (R-FCM) a significantly improved PFS was observed in relapsed MCL.[41]

Other monoclonal antibodies, either chimeric or fully humanized, targeting a variety of epitopes in addition to CD20,[42] such as CD22,[43,44] CD80,[45] or human leukocyte antigen (HLA)-DR,[46] are currently being investigated in preclinical and clinical trials; however, data in MCL are still scarce.

RADIOIMMUNOTHERAPY

Radioimmunotherapy has been explored in various studies of MCL because it is commonly considered to be inherently radiosensitive. Today there are two radioimmunoconjugates approved in either the United States or European Union: 90Y-ibritumomab tiuxetan and 131I-tositumomab. Both target CD20, which is expressed on virtually all B-cell lymphomas. Neither radioimmunoconjugate, however, is currently approved for the treatment of MCL. In two phase II trials the single agent activity of 90Y-ibritumomab tiuxetan in patients with relapsed or refractory MCL has been investigated.[47,48] ORR was 30% to 40% with only short durations of response. In contrast, data on radioimmunotherapy integrated into a multimodal therapeutic approach (ie, in segmental combination with chemotherapy either as induction or consolidation)[49] were more encouraging.[50] A promising option seems to be the application of radioimmunoconjugates in a combination with high-dose chemotherapy followed by autologous or even allogenic stem cell transplantation. In a phase II study 16 patients with relapsed or refracted MCL were enrolled to receive high-dose radioimmunotherapy with 131I-tositumomab followed by high-dose etoposide and cyclophosphamide as part of a myeloablative regimen before autologous hematopoietic stem cell transplantation.

ORR was remarkable (CRR 91%), with 3-year OS and PFS of 93% and 61%, respectively.[51]

ALLOGENIC BONE MARROW TRANSPLANTATION

The allogenic bone marrow transplantation remains the only therapeutic option with a curative potential in advanced-stage MCL. Several small studies document that, even on multiply pretreated patients, long-lasting remissions can be achieved.[52,53] In a phase II trial 33 patients with relapsed or refractory MCL were treated with non-myeloablative conditioning with fludarabine and 2-Gy total body irradiation followed by helical CT. The OS and disease-free survival at 2 years was 65% and 60%, respectively.[54] In another trial, patients with relapsed or refractory lymphoma including MCL received a conditioning therapy consisting of alemtuzumab, fludarabine, and melphalan before helical CT. OS at 3 years was 60% in the MCL subgroup.[55] Adverse effects associated with the transplantation, especially serious infections, appear often.

MOLECULAR TARGETED THERAPY

Bortezomib is a potent, selective, and reversible inhibitor of the 26S proteasome. Bortezomib as a single agent has proved to be effective in relapsed and refractory MCL in several phase II studies. In the largest trial of 141 patients a median response duration of 9.2 months and a median time to progression of 6.2 months were observed [56] with only minor toxicity; mild thrombocytopenia, neuropathy, and diarrhea was most common. Because preclinical data suggested a synergism of combination of bortezomib and cytarabine, preliminary clinical data confirmed the high efficacy of this combination.[57] Various ongoing trials are currently investigating different chemotherapy combinations.

Other promising small molecules are thalidomide and temsirolimus. Thalidomide is known to interfere with angiogenesis and the microenvironment. In a small phase II trial the combination with rituximab yielded an ORR of 81% and a CRR of 31%.[58] Recent data suggest an even higher efficacy of lenalidomide with a response rate of up to 50% in relapsed MCL. Temsirolimus inhibits the translation of cyclin-D1 messenger RNA by interfering with the mammalian target of rapamycin. In a phase II trial, single-agent treatment yielded an ORR of 38%, whereas the CRR was relatively low (3%) with a short median time to progression and duration of response short (6.5 and 6.9 months, respectively).[59] In future trials all of these approaches will be combined. Patients most like to respond to the different strategies should be identified.

REFERENCES

1. Banks PM, Chan J, Cleary ML, et al. Mantle cell lymphoma: a proposal for unification of morphologic, immunologic, and molecular data. Am J Surg Pathol 1992; 16:637–40.
2. Harris NL, Jaffe ES, Diebold J, et al. World Health Organization classification of neoplastic diseases of the hematopoietic and lymphoid tissues: report of the Clinical Advisory Committee meeting-Airlie House, Virginia, November 1997. J Clin Oncol 1999;17:3835–49.
3. Harris NL, Jaffe ES, Stein H, et al. A revised European-American classification of lymphoid neoplasms: a proposal from the International Lymphoma Study Group. Blood 1994;84:1361–92.
4. Dreyling M, Weigert O, Hiddemann W. Current treatment standards and future strategies in mantle cell lymphoma. Ann Oncl 2008;19(Suppl 4):iv41–4.

5. Herrmann A, Hoster E, Dreyling M, et al. Improvement of overall survival in mantle cell lymphoma during the last decades. Blood (ASH Annual Meeting Abstracts) 2006;108:2446.

6. Weinkauf M, Christopeit M, Hiddemann W, et al. Proteome- and microarray-based expression analysis of lymphoma cell lines identifies a p53-centered cluster of differentially expressed proteins in mantle cell and follicular lymphoma. Electrophoresis 2007;28:4416–26.

7. Fernandez V, Hartmann E, Ott G, et al. Pathogenesis of mantle-cell lymphoma: all oncogenic roads lead to dysregulation of cell cycle and DNA damage response pathways. J Clin Oncol 2005;23:6364–9.

8. Dreyling M, Bergsagel PL, Gordon LI, et al. The t(11;14) disorders: how biology can drive therapy. Alexandria (VA): ASCO Educational book; 2006. p. 476.

9. Tiemann M, Schrader C, Klapper W, et al. Histopathology, cell proliferation indices and clinical outcome in 304 patients with mantle cell lymphoma (MCL): a clinicopathological study from the European MCL Network. Br J Haematol 2005;131:29–38.

10. Rosenwald A, Wright G, Wiestner A, et al. The proliferation gene expression signature is a quantitative integrator of oncogenic events that predicts survival in mantle cell lymphoma. Cancer Cell 2003;3:185–97.

11. Ferrer A, Bosch F, Villamor N, et al. Central nervous system involvement in mantle cell lymphoma. Ann Oncol 2008;19:135–41.

12. Hoster E, Dreyling M, Klapper W, et al. A new prognostic index (MIPI) for patients with advanced-stage mantle cell lymphoma. Blood 2008;111:558–65.

13. Determann O, Hoster E, Ott G, et al. Ki-67 predicts outcome in advanced-stage mantle cell lymphoma patients treated with anti-CD20 immunochemotherapy: results from randomized trials of the European MCL Network and the German Low Grade Lymphoma Study Group. Blood 2008;111:2385–7.

14. Katzenberger T, Petzoldt C, Holler S, et al. The Ki67 proliferation index is a quantitative indicator of clinical risk in mantle cell lymphoma. Blood 2006;107:3407.

15. Howard OM, Gribben JG, Neuberg DS, et al. Rituximab and CHOP induction therapy for newly diagnosed mantle-cell lymphoma: molecular complete responses are not predictive of progression-free survival. J Clin Oncol 2002;20:1288–94.

16. Cheson BD, Pfistner B, Juweid ME, et al. Revised response criteria for malignant lymphoma. J Clin Oncol 2007;25:579–86.

17. Foss HD, Stein H. Pathology of intestinal lymphomas. Recent Results Cancer Res 2000;156:33–41.

18. Meusers P, Hense J, Brittinger G. Mantle cell lymphoma: diagnostic criteria, clinical aspects and therapeutic problems. Leukemia 1997;11(Suppl 2):S60–4.

19. Nickenig C, Dreyling M, Hoster E, et al. Combined cyclophosphamide, vincristine, doxorubicin, and prednisone (CHOP) improves response rates but not survival and has lower hematologic toxicity compared with combined mitoxantrone, chlorambucil, and prednisone (MCP) in follicular and mantle cell lymphomas: results of a prospective randomized trial of the German Low-Grade Lymphoma Study Group. Cancer 2006;107:1014–22.

20. Zucca E, Roggero E, Pinotti G, et al. Patterns of survival in mantle cell lymphoma. Ann Oncol 1995;6:257–62.

21. Foran JM, Rohatiner AZ, Coiffier B, et al. Multicenter phase II study of fludarabine phosphate for patients with newly diagnosed lymphoplasmacytoid lymphoma, Waldenstrom's macroglobulinemia, and mantle-cell lymphoma. J Clin Oncol 1999;17:546–53.

22. Zinzani PL, Magagnoli M, Moretti L, et al. Randomized trial of fludarabine versus fludarabine and idarubicin as frontline treatment in patients with indolent or mantle-cell lymphoma. J Clin Oncol 2000;18:773–9.
23. Cohen BJ, Moskowitz C, Straus D, et al. Cyclophosphamide/fludarabine (CF) is active in the treatment of mantle cell lymphoma. Leuk Lymphoma 2001;42: 1015–22.
24. Rummel MJ, von Gruenhagen U, Niederle N, et al. Bendamustine plus rituximab versus chop plus rituximab in the first-line treatment of patients with indolent and mantle cell lymphomas: first interim results of a randomized phase III study of the STIL (Study Group Indolent Lymphomas, Germany). Blood (ASH Annual Meeting Abstracts) 2007;110:385.
25. Herold M, Schulze A, Niederwieser D, et al. Bendamustine, vincristine and prednisone (BOP) versus cyclophosphamide, vincristine and prednisone (COP) in advanced indolent non-Hodgkin's lymphoma and mantle cell lymphoma: results of a randomised phase III trial (OSHO# 19). J Cancer Res Clin Oncol 2006;132: 105–12.
26. Rummel MJ, Al-Batran SE, Kim SZ, et al. Bendamustine plus rituximab is effective and has a favorable toxicity profile in the treatment of mantle cell and low-grade non-Hodgkin's lymphoma. J Clin Oncol 2005;23:3383–9.
27. Weide R, Hess G, Koppler H, et al. High anti-lymphoma activity of bendamustine/ mitoxantrone/rituximab in rituximab pretreated relapsed or refractory indolent lymphomas and mantle cell lymphomas. A multicenter phase II study of the German Low Grade Lymphoma Study Group (GLSG). Leuk Lymphoma 2007; 48:1299–306.
28. Lefrere F, Delmer A, Suzan F, et al. Sequential chemotherapy by CHOP and DHAP regimens followed by high-dose therapy with stem cell transplantation induces a high rate of complete response and improves event-free survival in mantle cell lymphoma: a prospective study. Leukemia 2002;16(4):587–93.
29. Khouri IF, Romaguera J, Kantarjian H, et al. Hyper-CVAD and high-dose methotrexate/cytarabine followed by stem-cell transplantation: an active regimen for aggressive mantle-cell lymphoma. J Clin Oncol 1998;16:3803–9.
30. de Guibert S, Jaccard A, Bernard M, et al. Rituximab and DHAP followed by intensive therapy with autologous stem-cell transplantation as first-line therapy for mantle cell lymphoma. Haematologica 2006;91:425–6.
31. Romaguera JE, Fayad L, Rodriguez MA, et al. High rate of durable remissions after treatment of newly diagnosed aggressive mantle-cell lymphoma with rituximab plus hyper-CVAD alternating with rituximab plus high-dose methotrexate and cytarabine. J Clin Oncol 2005;23:7013–23.
32. Epner EM, Unger J, Miller T, et al. A multi center trial of hyperCVAD + Rituxan in patients with newly diagnosed mantle cell lymphoma. Blood (ASH Annual Meeting Abstracts) 2007;110:387.
33. Dreyling M, Lenz G, Hoster E, et al. Early consolidation by myeloablative radiochemotherapy followed by autologous stem cell transplantation in first remission significantly prolongs progression-free survival in mantle-cell lymphoma: results of a prospective randomized trial of the European MCL Network. Blood 2005; 105:2677–84.
34. Geisler CH, Elonen E, Kolstad A, et al. Mantle cell lymphoma can be cured by intensive immunochemotherapy with in-vivo purged stem-cell support; final report of the Nordic Lymphoma Group MCL2 Study. Blood (ASH Annual Meeting Abstracts) 2007;110:Lb1.

35. Magni M, Di Nicola M, Devizzi L, et al. Successful in vivo purging of CD34-containing peripheral blood harvests in mantle cell and indolent lymphoma: evidence for a role of both chemotherapy and rituximab infusion. Blood 2000;96:864–9.

36. Dreyling MH, Hoster E, Hermine O, et al. European MCL Network: an update on current first line trials. Blood (ASH Annual Meeting Abstracts) 2007;110:388.

37. Cartron G, Watier H, Golay J,. et al. From the bench to the bedside: ways to improve rituximab efficacy. Blood 2004;104(9):2635–42.

38. Ghielmini M, Schmitz SF, Cogliatti S, et al. Effect of single-agent rituximab given at the standard schedule or as prolonged treatment in patients with mantle cell lymphoma: a study of the Swiss Group for Clinical Cancer Research (SAKK). J Clin Oncol 2005;23:705–11.

39. Lenz G, Dreyling M, Hoster E, et al. Immunochemotherapy with rituximab and cyclophosphamide, doxorubicin, vincristine, and prednisone significantly improves response and time to treatment failure, but not long-term outcome in patients with previously untreated mantle cell lymphoma: results of a prospective randomized trial of the German Low Grade Lymphoma Study Group (GLSG). J Clin Oncol 2005;23:1984–92.

40. Forstpointner R, Dreyling M, Repp R, et al. The addition of rituximab to a combination of fludarabine, cyclophosphamide, mitoxantrone (FCM) significantly increases the response rate and prolongs survival as compared with FCM alone in patients with relapsed and refractory follicular and mantle cell lymphomas: results of a prospective randomized study of the German Low-Grade Lymphoma Study Group. Blood 2004;104:3064.

41. Forstpointner R, Unterhalt M, Dreyling M, et al. Maintenance therapy with rituximab leads to a significant prolongation of response duration after salvage therapy with a combination of rituximab, fludarabine, cyclophosphamide, and mitoxantrone (R-FCM) in patients with recurring and refractory follicular and mantle cell lymphomas: results of a prospective randomized study of the German Low Grade Lymphoma Study Group (GLSG). Blood 2006;108:4003–8.

42. Morschhauser F, Leonard JP, Coiffier B, et al. Initial safety and efficacy results of a second-generation humanized anti-CD20 antibody, IMMU-106 (hA20), in non-Hodgkin's lymphoma. Blood (ASH Annual Meeting Abstracts) 2005;106:2428.

43. DiJoseph JF, Popplewell A, Tickle S, et al. Antibody-targeted chemotherapy of B-cell lymphoma using calicheamicin conjugated to murine or humanized antibody against CD22. Cancer Immunol Immunother 2005;54:11.

44. Leonard JP, Goldenberg DM. Preclinical and clinical evaluation of epratuzumab (anti-CD22 IgG) in B-cell malignancies. Oncogene 2007;26:3704–13.

45. Leonard JP, Friedberg JW, Younes A, et al. A phase I/II study of galiximab (an anti-CD80 monoclonal antibody) in combination with rituximab for relapsed or refractory, follicular lymphoma. Ann Oncol 2007;18:1216–23.

46. Rech J, Repp R, Rech D, et al. A humanized HLA-DR antibody (hu1D10, apolizumab) in combination with granulocyte colony-stimulating factor (filgrastim) for the treatment of non-Hodgkin's lymphoma: a pilot study. Leuk Lymphoma 2006;47:2147–54.

47. Weigert O, von Schilling C, Rummel MJ, et al. Efficacy and safety of a single-course of yttrium-90 (90Y) ibritumomab tiuxetan (Zevalin) in patients with relapsed or refractory mantle cell lymphoma (MCL) after/not appropriate for Autologous Stem Cell Transplantation (ASCT): a phase II trial of the European MCL network. Blood (ASH Annual Meeting Abstracts) 2005;106:4786.

48. Younes A, Pro B, Rodriguez MA, et al. Activity of yttrium 90 (90Y) ibritumomab tiuxetan (Zevalin) in 22 patients with relapsed and refractory mantle cell lymphoma (MCL). Blood (ASH Annual Meeting Abstracts) 2005;106:2452.
49. Weigert O, Jurczak W, Von Schilling C, et al. Efficacy of radioimmunotherapy with (90Y) ibritumomab tiuxetan is superior as consolidation in relapsed or refractory mantle cell lymphoma: results of two phase II trials of the European MCL network and the PLRG. ASCO Meeting Abstracts 2006;24:7533.
50. Smith MR, Zhang L, Gordon LI, et al. Phase II Study of R-CHOP followed by 90Y-ibritumomab tiuxetan in untreated mantle cell lymphoma: Eastern Cooperative Oncology Group Study E1499. Blood (ASH Annual Meeting Abstracts) 2007; 110:389.
51. Gopal AK, Rajendran JG, Petersdorf SH, et al. High-dose chemo-radioimmuno-therapy with autologous stem cell support for relapsed mantle cell lymphoma. Blood 2002;99:3158–62.
52. Khouri IF, Lee MS, Saliba RM, et al. Nonablative allogeneic stem-cell transplantation for advanced/recurrent mantle-cell lymphoma. J Clin Oncol 2003;21: 4407–12.
53. Robinson SP, Goldstone AH, Mackinnon S, et al. Chemoresistant or aggressive lymphoma predicts for a poor outcome following reduced-intensity allogeneic progenitor cell transplantation: an analysis from the Lymphoma Working Party of the European Group for Blood and Bone Marrow Transplantation. Blood 2002;100:4310–6.
54. Maris MB, Sandmaier BM, Storer BE, et al. Allogeneic hematopoietic cell transplantation after fludarabine and 2 Gy total body irradiation for relapsed and refractory mantle cell lymphoma. Blood 2004;104:3535–42.
55. Morris E, Thomson K, Craddock C, et al. Outcomes after alemtuzumab-containing reduced-intensity allogeneic transplantation regimen for relapsed and refractory non-Hodgkin lymphoma. Blood 2004;104:3865–71.
56. Fisher RI, Bernstein SH, Kahl BS, et al. Multicenter phase II study of bortezomib in patients with relapsed or refractory mantle cell lymphoma. J Clin Oncol 2006;24: 4867–74.
57. Weigert O, Weidmann E, Mueck R, et al. High dose cytarabine salvage regimen combined with bortezomib is feasible and highly effective in relapsed mantle cell lymphoma. Blood (ASH Annual Meeting Abstracts) 2006;108:2449.
58. Kaufmann H, Raderer M, Wohrer S, et al. Antitumor activity of rituximab plus thalidomide in patients with relapsed/refractory mantle cell lymphoma. Blood 2004; 104:2269–71.
59. Witzig TE, Geyer SM, Ghobrial I, et al. Phase II trial of single-agent temsirolimus (CCI-779) for relapsed mantle cell lymphoma. J Clin Oncol 2005;23:5347–56.

Highly Aggressive Lymphomas in Adults

John W. Sweetenham, MD

KEYWORDS

- Burkitt • Burkitt-like • Lymphoblastic

Highly aggressive lymphomas are relatively uncommon in adults, comprising approximately 4% to 5% of all non-Hodgkin lymphomas (NHLs) in the United States and Western Europe. The designation of "highly aggressive" is generally restricted to precursor T-cell and B-cell lymphoblastic lymphoma/leukemia (LBL) and Burkitt's lymphoma/leukemia (BL). Additionally, Burkitt-like lymphoma, a variant of BL with some morphologic and molecular features that overlap with diffuse large B-cell lymphoma (DLBCL) is included in this category. Although LBL and BL are both characterized by highly aggressive clinical behavior, they are biologically and clinically distinct entities. Treatment strategies for both include complex, highly intensive combination chemotherapy regimens, which may be curative. As with other subtypes of NHL, emerging data from gene-expression profiling and related techniques are helping to define these entities more precisely and identify potential new rational therapeutic targets.

LYMPHOBLASTIC LYMPHOMA (PRECURSOR T-CELL AND B-CELL LYMPHOBLASTIC LYMPHOMA/LEUKEMIA)

Lymphoblastic lymphomas are rare diseases accounting for approximately 2% of all NHL in the United States and Western Europe.[1] They are neoplasm of lymphoblasts that, in older lymphoma classifications, have been designated as LBL versus acute lymphoblastic leukemia (ALL) based on their predominant involvement of lymph nodes rather then bone marrow or peripheral blood. However, the clinical distinction between LBL and ALL in the published literature has been very variable. Based on the morphologic, immunophenotypic and cytogenetic similarities between LBL and ALL, they are now regarded as part of a spectrum of the same disease, recognized in the World Health Organization (WHO) Classification as precursor T-cell and B-cell LBL.[2] Despite this, treatment approaches to LBL and ALL have evolved separately and in many centers are still distinct. Additionally, recent gene-expression profiling studies in precursor T-cell disease suggest that there are biologic differences between predominantly nodal-based compared with leukemic presentations, which may be related to

Cleveland Clinic Taussig Cancer Institute, 9500 Euclid Avenue, Cleveland, OH 44195, USA
E-mail address: sweetej@ccf.org

Hematol Oncol Clin N Am 22 (2008) 965–978
doi:10.1016/j.hoc.2008.07.009
0889-8588/08/$ – see front matter © 2008 Elsevier Inc. All rights reserved.

hemonc.theclinics.com

differences in interactions between malignant cells and the microenvironment.[3] For these reasons, LBL is still recognized as a distinct entity.

Clinical Features

Approximately 85% to 90% of cases of LBL are of precursor T-cell phenotype. The disease occurs most commonly in adolescent and young adult males, with a median age around 20 years.[4,5] Mediastinal masses predominate in 65% to 70% of patients, almost exclusively in those with T-cell phenotype, and are commonly associated with pleural or pericardial effusions. Cardiac tamponade or superior vena caval obstruction may also be presenting features. Around 70% of patients have peripheral lymph node involvement, which is usually supradiaphragmatic. The frequency of involvement of the bone marrow at presentation is difficult to determine from published series because the degree of marrow infiltration is used variably to distinguish between LBL and ALL in reports from different groups. Recent prospective studies identify marrow involvement in approximately 20% of patients, with leukemic involvement reported in some.[6] The presence of leukemic overspill is used in some centers to distinguish LBL and ALL and its incidence is therefore uncertain.

Although central nervous system (CNS) involvement at presentation is uncommon (5%–15%), it is a common site of relapse (up to 30% of patients) in the absence of adequate CNS prophylaxis.[7] The typical pattern of CNS involvement is leptomeningeal disease with associated cerebrospinal fluid pleocytosis or cranial nerve involvement.

Rare sites of involvement include subdiaphragmatic lymph nodes, liver, spleen, testes, and skin.

Prognostic Factors and Risk Stratification

Clinical factors

The rarity of LBL and the overlap with ALL have limited the emergence of well-defined clinical prognostic factors for LBL. Adverse prognostic factors identified in older series have included advanced age, presence of B symptoms, elevated lactate dehydrogenase (LDH), CNS or bone marrow involvement, and leukemic involvement.[8–10] Some reports have suggested a poorer outcome for B-cell compared with T-cell immunophenotype, although this has not been reproducible. The predictive value of the International Prognostic Index has also been variably described in this disease,[6,11,12] but no reliable clinical model for risk stratification exists.

Biologic factors

Few specific studies have been performed in patients with LBL, but for those with precursor T-cell lymphoblastic disease in general (including ALL), expression of T-cell antigens has been associated with more favorable outcome in adults.[13] About one third of all patents with precursor T-cell disease have genetic abnormalities, including deletion of 9p, but mainly involving the α and δ and less commonly the β T-cell receptor (TCR) loci. These translocations produce high levels of expression of TCR genes as well as transcription factors, including *HOX11/TLX, TAL1/SCL* and *LYL1*. Gene signatures have been identified in precursor T-cell disease that are characteristic of certain stages of thymocyte maturation.[14] For example, a *HOX11* signature has been described that is characteristic of early cortical thymocytes and that is associated with low *bcl-2* expression and a favorable prognosis. By contrast, expression of *TAL1 or LYL1* signatures was associated with higher levels of *bcl-2*, a drug resistant phenotype, and poorer prognosis. In a more recent study restricted to patients with LBL, Baleydier and colleagues[15] have described a TCR-based immunogenetic classification allowing the identification of three subcategories of LBL with different outcomes.

They described a favorable subgroup expressing *HOXA9* or *TLX1* transcripts characteristic of thymocytes with intermediate maturation. Although based on a small number of patients treated in multiple protocols, these patients had a more favorable prognosis compared with those with features of either mature or immature thymocyte maturation. Further prospective studies on larger number of patients treated on uniform protocols will be required to confirm these observations.

At present, no clinically reproducible prognostic factors have been described for LBL, and risk-stratified approaches are therefore not justified.

Treatment

In view of the high proliferative rate of LBL and the chemosensitive nature of this disease, there is a high risk of acute tumor lysis syndrome. Prophylaxis for tumor lysis syndrome is an essential component of all treatment regimens.

Standard induction therapy

As summarized in **Table 1**, early treatment approaches based on standard cyclical chemotherapy regimens developed for use in NHLs have proven inadequate for patients with LBL. This has remained true in more recent series of standard-dose induction chemotherapy, even if patients undergo high-dose therapy and stem cell transplantation (SCT) at the time of first remission. Jost and colleagues[16] reported 3-year overall survival (OS) and event-free survival (EFS) rates of only 48% and 31%, respectively, for 20 adult patients undergoing high-dose therapy and autologous SCT after MACOP-B (methotrexate, doxorubicin, cyclophosphamide, vincristine, prednisone, bleomycin) or VACOP-B (etoposide, doxorubicin, cyclophosphamide, vincristine, prednisone, bleomycin) induction. The Groupe d'Etudes des Lymphomes de L'Adulte reported results for the subset of patients with LBL treated on their successive LNH 87 and LNH 93 studies, both of which used standard-dose NHL induction protocols with a randomization to consolidation with high-dose therapy and autologous SCT.[17] A total of 92 patients with LBL were included on these two studies and, despite a high initial complete response (CR) rate of 71%, the 5-year OS and EFS were disappointing, at 32% and 22%, respectively. A report from the Dutch-Belgian Hemato-Oncology Cooperative Group describes a prospective evaluation of short induction therapy followed by high-dose therapy and autologous SCT.[18] Only 15 patients with LBL were included but, despite an initial CR rate of 73% to brief induction therapy, the 5-year actuarial OS and EFS were only 46% and 40%, respectively.

Table 1				
Results from recent series of "standard" NHL induction therapy with or without SCT in adult LBL				
Reference	Therapy	No. of Patients	DFS	OS
Anderson et al[19]	COMP	40 (pediatric)	34% (5 yr)	45% (5 yr)
Colgan[20]	CHOP-like	39	49% (6 yr)	51% (6 yr)
Jost[16]	MACOP-B + Autologous SCT	20	31% (3 yr)	48% (3 yr)
Kaiser[21]	CHOP-like	29	38% (3.5 yr)	41% (3.5 yr)
Le Gouill[17]	ACVBP type	92	22% (34 mo)	32% (34 mo)
van Imhoff[18]	CHOP-like	15	40% (5yr EFS)	46% (5yr)

Abbreviations: ACVBP, doxorubicinm cyclophosphamide, vindesine, bleomycin, prednisone; CHOP, cyclophosphamide-hydroxydaunomycin oncovin prednisone; COMP, cyclophosphamide, vincristine, methotrexate, prednisone; DFS, disease-free survival; EFS, event free survival; MACOP-B, methotrexate, doxorubicin, cyclophosphamide, vincristine, prednisone, bleomycin; OS, overall survival; SCT, stem cell transplantation.

These are small studies and, in some cases, subset analyses of much larger trials; it is therefore difficult to draw firm conclusions, although the results suggest that nonintensive induction regimens are probably inadequate, and that the use of consolidative high-dose therapy and autologous SCT does not compensate for a nonintensive induction approach.

Intensive induction therapy

The poor results reported for standard NHL induction regimens in this disease prompted several groups to explore the use of regimens initially used for the treatment of ALL in adults with LBL, based partly on experience in the pediatric population. The results of reports of these regimens are summarized in **Table 2**.

Common components of these regimens include intensive, multi-agent induction therapy, a phase of CNS prophylaxis, remission consolidation therapy that in some cases includes SCT, and maintenance therapy in many. Most of the reported series are small, single-center studies and are subject to potential selection bias. Direct comparison of these reports with those from standard induction regimens are therefore difficult, but in general the reported results from these studies have been superior to those of lower intensity regimens. For example, the use of the HyperCVAD (cyclophosphamide, vincristine, doxorubicin, dexamethasone) regimen, alternating with methotrexate and cytarabine in 33 adult patients with LBL has been reported from the MD Anderson Cancer Center.[23] This protocol included intrathecal prophylaxis with cytarabine and methotrexate (or more intensive intrathecal prophylaxis with or without CNS radiation for patients with CNS disease at presentation), and mediastinal irradiation, followed by cyclical intravenous maintenance therapy for 24 months. The CR rate in this study was 91%, with 3-year actuarial OS and progression free survival (PFS) rates of 70% and 66%, respectively. Similar results have recently been reported from Vancouver in an intent to treat analysis for patients receiving an intensive ALL type regimen, in this case consolidated with high-dose therapy and autologous or allogeneic SCT.[25] For this small series of 34 patients, the 4-year OS and EFS were 72% and 68%, respectively.

The results summarized above suggest that intensive induction therapy is essential to achieve long-term disease free survival (DFS), irrespective of the subsequent

Table 2
Results from recent series of intensive induction therapy with or without SCT in adult LBL

Reference	Therapy	No. of Patients	DFS	OS
Anderson[19]	LSA2L2	124 (pediatric)	64% (5 yr)	67% (5 yr)
Coleman[20]	ALL-type protocols, intensified CNS prophylaxis in the second	44	56% (3-yr FFS)	56% (3 yr)
Slater[8]	Various ALL protocols	51	N/A	45% (5 yr)
Bernasconi[9]	Various ALL protocols	31	45% (3-yr RFS)	59% (3 yr)
Morel[10]	ALL-type	80	46% (30 mo)	51% (30 mo)
Hoelzer[22]	ALL-type	45	62% (7 yr)	51% (7 yr)
Thomas[23]	HyperCVAD	33	66% (3 yr)	70% (3 yr)
Jabbour[24]	LMT-98	27	44% (5-yr FFP)	63% (5 yr)
Song[25]	Hybrid ALL/NHL	34	68% (4-yr EFS)	72% (4 yr)

Abbreviations: CVAD, cyclophosphamide, vincristine, adriamycin, and dexamethasone; FFP, freedom from progression; FFS, failure-free survival; RFS, recurrence-free survival.

consolidation or maintenance strategy. Regimens that include consolidation with SCT only appear to result in superior EFS and OS rates if the initial induction therapy is a relatively intensive ALL-type regimen. Studies of the exact role of post-induction SCT after intensive induction are discussed below.

Central nervous system prophylaxis

The reported incidence of CNS relapse in patients who do not receive prophylaxis is approximately 30%. Although prospective randomized studies have not been performed, historical cohort comparisons and experience in pediatric ALL/LBL suggested a benefit for CNS prophylaxis. In a study of sequential regimens from Stanford University, the incidence of CNS relapse in adult patients with LBL was 3%, using a regimen with early intrathecal chemotherapy and CNS irradiation, compared with 31% in the previous protocol, which included relatively late use of intrathecal chemotherapy only.[7] Although the benefit of CNS prophylaxis is therefore widely accepted, the optimal regimen is unclear. Cranial irradiation has been used widely in the past, but concerns for long-term neuropsychologic effects have limited its use more recently. Regimens incorporating high-dose systemic methotrexate and cytarabine plus intrathecal chemotherapy result in very low rates of CNS relapse and have largely replaced cranial irradiation. Pediatric studies from Europe have compared sequential trials using cranial irradiation or intrathecal prophylaxis and have shown no apparent difference in DFS or CNS relapse.[26] Published data therefore favors the use of chemotherapy regimens incorporating systemic methotrexate or cytarabine, with additional intrathecal prophylaxis but without the requirement for cranial irradiation.

Mediastinal radiation

Because bulky mediastinal disease is a frequent presenting feature of LBL, some groups have included mediastinal irradiation as a component of first-line therapy. No systematic evaluation of its role has been performed, and it has been used variably for patients in partial remission or CR after initial induction therapy. A retrospective study from the MD Anderson Cancer Center reported 43 adult patients with LBL who achieved a CR to induction therapy, 19 of whom had consolidative mediastinal radiation.[27] None of these patients relapsed in the mediastinum, in contrast to 24 patients who did not receive mediastinal radiation, 8 of whom relapsed at this site. However, the use of mediastinal irradiation was not associated with improved OS and the analysis was confounded by the fact that most of the patients receiving mediastinal irradiation had been treated with HyperCVAD induction, whereas those not receiving radiation had received other induction regimens. The German Multicenter Study Group for ALL has reported favorable results in a study of 43 adult patients with LBL treated with a regimen incorporating mediastinal radiation in the induction phase.[25] However, of the 15 patients who relapsed in this study, 7 relapsed in the mediastinum, of whom 6 had received mediastinal radiation.

There is no clear evidence for a benefit from mediastinal irradiation in this population and insufficient evidence to recommend this approach.

Stem Cell Transplantation

The use of high-dose therapy with autologous or allogeneic SCT to consolidate first remission in adults with LBL has been reported in small retrospective series in several single center and registry studies, and in a single small, randomized prospective trial. Results from the reports are summarized in **Table 3**. Interpretation and comparison of these series is difficult because most are small, retrospective studies with variable selection criteria. Additionally, most report survival from the time of transplant and

Table 3				
Results from recent series of SCT in first remission in adult LBL				
References	Therapy	No. of Patients	DFS	OS
Jost[16]	MACOP-B + Auto SCT	20	31% (3 yr)	48% (3 yr)
Sweetenham[28]	Multiple induction regimens + Auto SCT	105	63% (6 yr)	64% (6 yr)
Bouabdallah[11]	ALL type induction + auto or allo SCT	62 (30 in first CR)	58% (5-yr EFS)	60% (5 yr)
Song[25]	Hybrid ALL/NHL + auto or allo SCT	34	68% (4-yr EFS)	72% (4 yr)

do not account for the substantial bias inherent in retrospective transplant studies. Few of these series include intent to treat analysis.

Despite these limitations, the existing data do not provide clear evidence of a survival benefit from the use of SCT in first remission. Studies using less intensive induction therapy before transplant report results that are generally inferior to those using ALL-type remission induction therapy. This suggests that the intensity of the initial therapy is more important in achieving long-term disease control than the use of early SCT. The single small, randomized trial comparing SCT with standard consolidation and maintenance therapy after remission induction in adults with LBL showed no difference in OS between the two arms (3-year actuarial OS = 45% for conventional versus 55% for high-dose consolidation).[6] A trend for improved RFS was observed in the SCT arm but this did not achieve statistical significance. A recent study from Vancouver reported outcomes for 34 adults with LBL who received a hybrid induction regimen followed by SCT in first remission in 29.[27] Using an intent-to-treat analysis, the 4-year OS and EFS in this report were 72% and 68%, respectively. These results are comparable to many nontransplant series, and current evidence suggests that post-remission therapy using SCT or conventional-dose consolidation and maintenance therapy are probably equivalent in terms of long-term DFS.

In the setting of relapsed or refractory disease, retrospective data suggest that SCT may be superior to conventional dose salvage therapy alone, although this is based mostly on comparison with historical controls. In the largest published series from the European Blood and Marrow Transplant Group (EBMT), the 3-year OS and PFS after SCT in this patient group were 31% and 30%, respectively.[28] Corresponding OS and PFS rates in historical series of patients treated with conventional dose salvage are on the rage of 5% to 10%.

Autologous versus allogeneic stem cell transplantation
There is no clear evidence for a graft-versus-lymphoma effect in adult LBL. Most studies of SCT have used autologous stem cells as the source of rescue. Comparative registry-based studies of allogeneic and autologous SCT have been reported from the EBMT [29] and the International Blood and Marrow Transplant Registry.[30] Both studies showed a lower relapse rate in patients undergoing allogeneic SCT, which was offset by a higher treatment-related mortality. The overall survival was the same in both groups. Current evidence therefore does not support the use of allogeneic cells as the preferred stem cell source.

Novel Approaches

Recent molecular studies have identified different subtypes of LBL, based upon TCR genotyping and *HOXA/TLX1* expression that appear to have prognostic significance.[15] If confirmed, these observations may lead to the development of risk-stratified approaches to therapy, and may uncover new rational therapeutic targets. Gene-expression profiling has also identified differences between ALL and LBL that could be exploited therapeutically.[3] For example, *CARD 10,* a recently recognized caspase recruitment domain family member has been shown to be highly expressed in LBL. This family of molecules are involved in apoptotic signaling leading to activation of nuclear factor (NF)κB. This pathway may therefore be an appropriate one to target specifically in LBL.

Although relatively few agents have been developed with apparent specificity for T-cells, Nelarabine, a prodrug which is demethylated by adenosine deaminase in T-cells to 9-β-D-arabinofuranosyl-guanine (Ara-G) has been shown to be toxic to T-cells and has now been investigated in a phase II study in subjects with T-ALL and LBL.[31] Complete and overall response rates of 31% and 41%, respectively, were observed with a median DFS of 20 weeks and a 1-year OS of 20%. This represents remarkable activity in a group of patients with relapsed and refractory disease. This agent is now being incorporated into protocols investigating its use as a component of first-line therapy.

BURKITT AND BURKITT-LIKE LYMPHOMA

BL is a rare tumor of mature B-cells derived from the germinal center. It is a clinically aggressive disease in which extranodal presentation is common, classically involving the ileocecal region in the sporadic type most common in the United States and Western Europe. It may present as an acute leukemia, designated as either Burkitt leukemia, or L3-ALL in the French-American-British Classification. Patients with Burkitt leukemia have sometimes been included in studies for the treatment of B-ALL, and sometimes in studies for BL. They appear to have an inferior prognosis compared with other patients with BL, but there are no data to indicate whether outcome in this group is improved using protocols directed at BL compared with B-ALL. The pathology of this disease is discussed elsewhere in this issue. The three clinical forms of BL (see below) are all characterized by the presence of chromosomal translocations involving 8q24/*MYC*, resulting in deregulation of *MYC* by juxtaposition to regulatory genes encoding immunoglobulins. The most frequent translocation partner (85%) is the immunoglobulin heavy-chain gene locus on chromosome 14. In the remaining 15% of cases, the translocation partner is the κ or λ light-chain locus on chromosomes 2 and 22, respectively. Variant cases of BL, designated as atypical BL, Burkitt-like lymphoma, and BL with plasmacytoid differentiation, have also been recognized and are described in the WHO classification. Additionally, cases of DLBCL with *c-myc* over-expression are well described. The distinction between BL, atypical BL, or Burkitt-like lymphoma and DLBCL has therefore been variable. Recent gene-expression profiling studies have helped to distinguish between these entities, because BL is characterized by high expression of *c-myc* target genes, as well as germinal center-associated genes, and low expression of major histocompatibility class I and NF-κB target genes.[32,33] The next revision of the WHO classification is likely to classify all cases with evidence of *c-myc* deregulation and acceptable morphology as BL, and the "Burkitt-like" and "atypical Burkitt" categories will be abandoned. In reviewing the existing clinical literature on BL, it is important to recognize the evolution of diagnostic criteria because the patient populations treated in earlier studies may differ from those now recognized as "true" BL.

Clinical Features

Three clinical variants of BL are recognized, with distinct epidemiologic and features.

Endemic Burkitt's lymphoma

Endemic BL occurs most commonly in equatorial Africa, where it is the most common childhood tumor. It shows male predominance and a peak incidence at 4 to 7 years. The jaw and facial bones are involved in 50% to 70% of patients. The areas of peak incidence appear to coincide with the distribution of endemic malaria and almost 100% of cases have evidence of Epstein-Barr virus (EBV) infection.

Sporadic Burkitt's lymphoma

The sporadic BL variant comprises between 1% and 2% of all NHLs in the United States and Western Europe.[1] The peak incidence is in children and young adults, with male predominance and a median age of about 30 years. Abdominal presentation (most commonly ileo-cecal) is characteristic. Common presenting symptoms therefore include abdominal pain and distension, nausea and vomiting, gastrointestinal bleeding or perforation, and abdominal obstruction secondary to intussusception. Extradural extension of retroperitoneal disease with resulting spinal cord compression is well recognized. Other common sites of involvement are bone marrow (20%), pleural effusions (20%), and CNS disease (15%), most commonly presenting with cranial nerve abnormalities or cerebrospinal fluid pleocytosis. Breast involvement is characteristically seen in association with the onset of the disease at puberty or during pregnancy and lactation, and is typically bilateral and often bulky. Evidence of EBV infection is seen in 20% to 30% of cases.

BL in association with immunodeficiency

This variant is primarily seen in patients with AIDS and may also occur in other immune compromised patients, including those who receive immunosuppressive therapy following solid organ or bone marrow transplantation. The clinical presentation is most commonly nodal, with relatively frequent marrow involvement and an increased risk of CNS disease. Approximately 40% have evidence of EBV.

Prognostic Factors and Risk Stratification

Table 4 describes some of the previously published risk-stratification models developed for the treatment of BL. In general, these reflect disease bulk, surgical respectability for patients with abdominal presentations and LDH. The risk factors described for patients entered into the NCI-89-C-41 protocol have been most widely applied in adult trials.[34] A European trial of a modified version of this protocol used slightly modified risk factors, with low-risk patients defined as having a normal LDH level, WHO performance status of 0 or 1, Ann Arbor stage I or II, and no residual tumor masses greater than 10 cm.[35] As with LBL, the rarity of the disease and relatively small patient populations in the published studies has limited the definition of widely accepted prognostic factors.

Treatment

In common with LBL, predominant features of current treatment regimens for BL include the use of multi-agent, dose-intensive chemotherapy, including high-dose systemic methotrexate and cytosine arabinoside for control of potential CNS disease.

Patients with BL are also at high risk of tumor lysis syndrome. Prophylaxis is essential before therapy in all patients.

As with LBL, many of the regimens now used in adults have been adapted from pediatric protocols. Results from these regimens are summarized in **Table 5**. Common

Table 4
Risk factors for adult Burkitt's lymphoma

(BFM)[36]		LMB[37]		National Cancer Institute[34]	
Risk Group	**Features**	**Risk Group**	**Features**	**Risk Group**	**Features**
1	Complete resection	A	Complete resection stage I or abdominal stage II	Low risk	Stage I or II and LDH <150% of normal
2	Incomplete resection: Stage I and II Stage III with LDH <500 IU/L	B	All patients not in A or C	High risk	All other patients
3	Incomplete resection: Stage III with LDH 500 IU/L–999 IU/L Stage V or B-cell leukemia with LDH <1,000IU/L; CNS negative	C	Central nervous system involvement or bone marrow involvement with ≥ 25% blasts	—	—
4	Incomplete I resection: Stage III and LDH >999IU/L Stage IV or B-cell leukemia and LDH >999IU/L ±CNS	—	—	—	—

Abbreviation: BFM, Berlin-Frankfurt-Munich.

elements of these regimens include intensive induction chemotherapy, relatively short treatment duration, and hematopoietic growth factor support to allow rapid initiation of successive cycles of chemotherapy as soon as hematologic recovery from the prior cycle is achieved. This is thought to be particularly important in view of the high proliferation rate of these tumors. There is no clear evidence to support the use of prolonged maintenance therapy. In adult patients, most single-center studies have reported CR rates from 75% to 97%, and 5-year survival rates between 70% and 92%. Rates of OS and EFS for patients with BL (L3-ALL) have generally been inferior.

The NCI 89-C-41 protocol is now widely used in adult patients with BL.[34] In the initial report of this regimen, patients with low-risk disease, treated with 3 cycles of the CODOX-M regimen, achieved longterm DFS of 100%, although patient numbers in this series were small.

A multicenter European study of a modified NCI 89-C-41 protocol reported 2-year actuarial EFS of 83% in a population with higher median age and lower performance status than those in the original NCI study.[35]

The regimens summarized in **Table 5** report roughly comparable data. Most are small, single-center studies, subject to selection bias, particularly with respect to median age and performance status, which are typically low in these studies. Studies that have included older patients have modified chemotherapy intensity, particularly of drugs such as methotrexate and cytarabine. In the study of HyperCVAD reported from

Table 5
Results of recent reports of intensive combination chemotherapy regimens in adults with BL

Reference	Therapy	No. of Patients	FFS/RFS	OS
Soussain[38]	Various LMB protocols	65	N/A	74% (3 yr)
McMaster[39]	Novel intensive chemotherapy-only regimen	20	60% (5 yr)	60% (5 yr)
Magrath[34]	NCI 89-C-41	39	92% (2 yr)	92% (2 yr)
Mead[35]	Modified NCI 89-C-41	52	65% (2 yr)	73% (2 yr)
Thomas[40]	Hyper-CVAD	26	N/A	49% (3 yr)
Thomas[41]	Rituximab/HyperCVAD	31	89% (3-yr EFS)	88% (3 yr)

the MD Anderson Cancer Center, the median age of the patient population was 58 years.[40] The CR rate was 81% but the 3-year DFS and OS were 61% and 49%, respectively. The poorer outcome was attributed in part to the toxicities of this therapy in the older patient population. In a subsequent study, the same group added rituximab to the HyperCVAD regimen. In a small study of 28 subjects treated with this regimen, the 3-year EFS and OS rates were 89% and 88%, respectively.[41] Although these sequential studies cannot be compared directly, they suggest a potential role for rituximab in this disease that is now being prospectively evaluated in several phase II studies in which rituximab is added to dose-intensive regimens, such as NCI-89-C-41.

Central nervous system prophylaxis and therapy

The propensity for CNS involvement at presentation and relapse has resulted in inclusion of CNS prophylaxis or therapy into most current regimens for BL. Typically, this involves the use of high-dose systemic methotrexate and cytarabine, supplemented by intrathecal chemotherapy. In some regimens, the schedule of intrathecal therapy is intensified for patients with CNS disease at presentation compared with those in whom it is used as prophylaxis. The impact of CNS prophylaxis on the subsequent rate of relapse at this site is unclear, although its use is widely accepted and several recent studies report no cases of CNS relapse using a combined systemic and intrathecal chemotherapy approach.

There is no proven role for CNS irradiation as prophylaxis in those regimens that incorporate high-dose systemic methotrexate or cytarabine, or intrathecal prophylaxis. Although there are no prospective data to confirm this, sequential cohorts of patients treated in the CALGB 9251 study with and without CNS radiation had equivalent rates of OS and EFS, as well as equivalent rates of CNS recurrence.[42] Its use has therefore largely been abandoned, particularly in view of the risks of neuropsychologic toxicity in adult patients.

Stem Cell Transplantation

The role of high-dose therapy and SCT in BL is limited. There are limited published data on the use of SCT as a component of first-line therapy, partly because of the rarity of BL and partly because the high response and survival rates reported for BL using intensive regimens without SCT.

The EBMT have reported a retrospective, registry-based study which included 70 patients receiving autologous SCT in first CR after various induction chemotherapy regimens.[43] The actuarial 3-year progression free and overall survival rates were

72% and 73%, respectively. The selection bias inherent in retrospective registry-based studies limits interpretation of these data, but they do not appear to be superior to those reported for nontransplant-based regimens. Few studies with intent-to-treat analysis have been reported. Jost and colleagues[16] reported a study in which patients with LBL and BL received a brief-duration induction chemotherapy regimen followed by high-dose therapy and autologous SCT for responding patients. The estimated 3-year event-free and overall survival were 31% and 48%, respectively. More recently, Song and colleagues[44] have described experience in British Columbia in 43 adult patients with BL and L3 ALL treated with a local intensive induction therapy (79%) or CHOP-like regimens in the remainder, with intent to proceed to high-dose therapy and autologous SCT. Of the 43 patients included, only 27 proceeded to SCT. The most common reason for failure to proceed to SCT was refractoriness to first-line therapy. For the entire population, the 3-year EFS was approximately 30%.

At present there are therefore no data to suggest a benefit for early SCT in this disease.

Very few series have investigated the role of SCT in the context of relapsed or refractory disease. The outcome in this situation is known to be very poor, with reported median OS rates of only 6 months after conventional-dose salvage therapy. The EBMT study reported 32 subjects with relapsed and refractory disease.[43] A long-term PFS rate of 37% was reported for those with chemosensitive relapse. Patients with resistant relapses or primary refractory disease progressed rapidly after SCT, most relapsing within 6 months. For the minority of relapsing patients who respond to second-line therapy, there is therefore a role for SCT, although for those with disease that is refractory to first- or second-line therapy, no data support the use of this modality.

Autologous versus allogeneic SCT

There are anecdotal reports that suggest a possible graft-versus-lymphoma effect on this disease, but few comparative data with autologous SCT. A matched analysis from the EBMT included 71 patients with BL undergoing allogeneic transplantation who were matched with 416 patients receiving autologous transplants.[45] No differences in either relapse rates were reported and the OS was superior in those receiving autologous cells because of the high treatment-related mortality in the allogeneic group. There are therefore no data that suggest that allogeneic transplantation is associated with superior outcome.

Novel Approaches

The relatively favorable results of modern therapy for BL have limited studies of novel agents in this disease, partly because of its rarity and the difficulty of designing studies of sufficient statistical power to demonstrate improvements in outcome. Several studies are in progress to determine the benefit of addition of rituximab to existing chemotherapy protocols. In parallel with these studies, the improved identification of low-risk patients who can be treated with less-intensive regimens remains a goal of current studies. It remains to be seen whether data from gene-expression profiling and other molecular studies will have utility in identifying different prognostic groups in this disease.

Emerging data from molecular studies has identified NFκB, and other molecules involved in regulation of apoptosis as having a central function in BL, in addition to *MYC* target genes. Agents directed at these pathways represent potential new therapies.

REFERENCES

1. The non-Hodgkin's Lymphoma Classification Project: A clinical evaluation of the International Lymphoma Study Group classification of non-Hodgkin's lymphomas. Blood 1997;89:3909–18.
2. Jaffe ES, Harris NL, Stein H, et al. Tumors of the haematopoietic and lymphoid tissues. World Health Organization. Lyon (France): IARC Press; 2001.
3. Raetz EA, Perkins SL, Bhojwani D, et al. Gene expression profiling reveals intrinsic differences between T-cell acute lymphoblastic leukemia and T-cell lymphoblastic lymphoma. Pediatr Blood Cancer 2006;47:130–40.
4. Rosen PJ, Feinstein DI, Pattengale PK, et al. Convoluted lymphocytic lymphoma in adults: a clinicopathological entity. Ann Intern Med 1978;89:319–24.
5. Nathwani BN, Diamond LW, Winberg CD, et al. Lymphoblastic lymphoma: a clinicopathologic study of 95 patients. Cancer 1978;48:2347–57.
6. Sweetenham JW, Santini G, Qian W, et al. High-dose therapy and autologous stem-cell transplantation versus conventional dose consolidation/maintenance therapy as post-remission therapy for adult patients with lymphoblastic lymphoma: results of a randomized trial of the European Group for Blood and Marrow Transplantation and the United Kingdom Lymphoma Group. J Clin Oncol 2001; 19:2927–36.
7. Coleman NC, Picozzi VJ, Cox RS, et al. Treatment of lymphoblastic lymphoma in adults. J Clin Oncol 1986;4:1626–37.
8. Slater DE, Mertelsmann R, Koriner B, et al. Lymphoblastic lymphoma in adults. J Clin Oncol 1986;4:57–67.
9. Bernasconi C, Brusamolino E, Lazzarino M, et al. Lymphoblastic lymphoma in adult patients; clinicopathological features and response to intensive multi-agent chemotherapy analogous to that used in acute lymphoblastic leukemia. Ann Oncol 1990;1:141–60.
10. Morel P, Lepage E, Brice P, et al. Prognosis and treatment of lymphoblastic lymphoma in adults: a report on 80 patients. J Clin Oncol 1992;10:1078–85.
11. Bouabdallah R, Xerri L, Bardou V-J, et al. Role of induction chemotherapy and bone marrow transplantation in adult lymphoblastic lymphoma: a report on 62 patients from a single center. Ann Oncol 1998;9:619–25.
12. Voakes JB, Jones SE, McKelvey EM. The chemotherapy of lymphoblastic lymphoma. Blood 1981;57:186–8.
13. Czuczman MS, Dodge RK, Stewart CC, et al. Value of immunophenotype in intensively treated adult acute lymphoblastic leukemia: Cancer and Leukemia Group B study 8364. Blood 1999;93:3931–9.
14. Xia Y, Brown L, Yang CY, et al. TAL2, a helix-loop-helix gene activated by the t(7;9)(q34;q32) translocation in human T-cell leukemia. Proc Natl Acad Sci USA 1989;88:11416–20.
15. Baleydier F, Decouvelaere A-V, Bergeron J, et al. T cell receptor genotyping and *HOXA/TLX1* expression define three T lymphoblastic lymphoma subsets which might affect clinical outcome. Clin Cancer Res 2008;14:692–700.
16. Jost LM, Jacky E, Dommann-Scherrer C, et al. Short-term weekly chemotherapy followed by high dose therapy with autologous bone marrow transplantation for lymphoblastic and Burkitt's lymphomas in adult patients. Ann Oncol 1995;6: 445–51.
17. LeGouill S, Lepretre S, Briere J, et al. Adult lymphoblastic lymphoma: a retrospective analysis of 92 patients under 61 years included in the LNH87/93 trials. Leukemia 2003;17:2220–4.

18. van Imhoff GW, van der Holt B, MacKenzie MA, et al. Short intensive sequential therapy followed by autologous stem cell transplantation in adult Burkitt, Burkitt-like and lymphoblastic lymphoma. Leukemia 2005;19:945–52.
19. Anderson JR, Wilson JF, Jenkin DT, et al. Childhood non-Hodgkin's lymphoma. The results of a randomized therapeutic trial comparing a 4-drug regimen (COMP) with a 10-drug regimen (LSA_2L_2). N Engl J Med 1983;308: 559–65.
20. Colgan JP, Andersen J, Habermann TM, et al. Long-term follow up of a XCHOP-based regimen with maintenance therapy and central nervous system prophylaxis in lymphoblastic non-Hodgkin's lymphoma. Leuk Lymphoma 1994;15: 291–6.
21. Kaiser U, Uebelacker I, Havemann K. Non-Hodgkin's lymphoma protocols in the treatment of patients with Burkitt's lymphoma and lymphoblastic lymphoma: a report on 58 patients. Leuk Lymphoma 1999;36:101–8.
22. Hoelzer D, Gokbuget N, Digel W, et al. Outcome of adult patients with T-lymphoblastic lymphoma treated according to protocols for acute lymphoblastic leukemia. Blood 2002;99:4379–85.
23. Thomas DA, O'Brien S, Cortes J, et al. Outcome with the hyper-CVAD regimens in lymphoblastic lymphoma. Blood 2004;104:1624–30.
24. Jabbour E, Koscielny S, Sebban C, et al. High survival rate with the LMT-89 regimen in lymphoblastic lymphoma (LL), but not in T-cell acute lymphoblastic leukemia (T-ALL). Leukemia 2006;20:814–9.
25. Song KW, Barnett MJ, Gascoyne RD, et al. Primary therapy for adults with T-cell lymphoblastic lymphoma with hematopoietic stem-cell transplantation results in favorable outcomes. Ann Oncol 2007;18:535–40.
26. Burkhardt B, Woessmann W, Zimmermann M, et al. Impact of cranial radiotherapy on central nervous system prophylaxis in children and adolescents with central nervous system-negative stage III or IV lymphoblastic lymphoma. J Clin Oncol 2006;24:491–9.
27. Dabaja BS, Ha CS, Thomas DA, et al. The role of local radiation therapy for mediastinal disease for adults with T-cell lymphoblastic lymphoma. Cancer 2002;94:2738–44.
28. Sweetenham JW, Santini G, Pearce R, et al. High-dose therapy and autologous bone marrow transplantation for adult patients with lymphoblastic lymphoma: results from the European Group for Bone Marrow Transplantation. J Clin Oncol 1994;12:1358–65.
29. Peniket AJ, Ruiz de Elvira MC, Taghipour G, et al. An EBMT registry matched study of allogeneic stem cell transplants for lymphoma: allogeneic transplantation is associated with a lower relapse rate but a higher procedure-related mortality rate than autologous transplantation. Bone Marrow Transplant 2003;8: 667–78.
30. Levine JE, Harris RE, Loberiza FR, et al. A comparison of allogeneic and autologous bone marrow transplantation for lymphoblastic lymphoma. Blood 2003;101: 2476–82.
31. DeAngelo DJ, Yu D, Johnson JL, et al. Nelarabine induces complete remissions in adults with relapsed or refractory T-lineage acute lymphoblastic leukemia or lymphoblastic lymphoma: Cancer and Leukemia Group B Study 19801. Blood 2007;109:5136–42.
32. Dace S, Fu K, Wright GW, et al. Molecular diagnosis of Burkitt's lymphoma. N Engl J Med 2006;354:2431–42.

33. Hummel M, Bentinck S, Berger H, et al. A biologic definition of Burkitt's lymphoma from transcriptional and genomic profiling. N Engl J Med 2006;354:2419–30.
34. Magrath IM, Shad A, et al. Children and adults with small non-cleaved cell lymphoma have a similar excellent outcome when treated with the same chemotherapy regimen. J Clin Oncol 1996;14:925–34.
35. Mead GM, Sydes MR, Walewski J, et al. An international evaluation of CODOX-M and CODOX-M alternating with IVAC in adult Burkitt's lymphoma: results of United Kingdom Lymphoma Group LY06 study. Ann Oncol 2002;13:1264–74.
36. Reiter A, Schrappe M, Tiemann M, et al. Improved treatment results in childhood B-cell neoplasms with tailored intensification of therapy: a report of the Berlin-Frankfurt-Munich NHL-BFM 90. Blood 1999;94:3294–306.
37. Patte C, Michon J, Frappaz D, et al. Therapy of Burkitt and other B-cell acute lymphoblastic leukemia and lymphoma: experience with the LMB protocols of the SFOP (French Paediatric Oncology Society) in children and adults. Baillieres Clin Haematol 1994;2:339–48.
38. Soussain C, Patte C, Ostronoff M, et al. Small non-cleaved cell lymphoma and leukemia in adults. A retrospective study of 65 adults treated with the LMB pediatric protocols. Blood 1995;85:664–74.
39. McMaster M, Greer JP, Greco A, et al. Effective treatment of small-noncleaved cell lymphoma with high-intensity, brief duration chemotherapy. J Clin Oncol 1991;9:941–6.
40. Thomas DA, Cortes J, O'Brien S, et al. Hyper-CVAD program in Burkitt's type adult acute lymphoblastic leukemia. J Clin Oncol 1999;17:2461–70.
41. Thomas DA, Faderl S, O'Brien S, et al. Chemoimmunotherapy with Hyper-CVAD plus rituximab for the treatment of adult Burkitt and Burkitt-type lymphoma or acute lymphoblastic leukemia. Cancer 2006;106:1569–80.
42. Rizzieri DA, Johnson JL, Niedzwiecki D, et al. Intensive chemotherapy with and without cranial radiation for Burkitt leukemia and lymphoma. Cancer 2004;100:1438–48.
43. Sweetenham JW, Pearce R, Taghipour G, et al. Adult Burkitt's and Burkitt-like non-Hodgkin's lymphoma—outcome for patients treated with high-dose therapy and autologous stem cell transplantation in first remission or at relapse: results from the European Group for Blood and Marrow Transplantation. J Clin Oncol 1996;14:2465–72.
44. Song KW, Barnett MJ, Gascoyne RD, et al. Haematopoietic stem cell transplantation as primary therapy of sporadic adult Burkitt lymphoma. Br J Haematol 2006;133:634–7.
45. Chopra R, Goldstone AH, Pearce R, et al. Autologous versus allogeneic bone marrow transplantation for non-Hodgkin's lymphoma: a case controlled analysis of the European Bone Marrow Transplant Group registry data. J Clin Oncol 1992;10:1690–5.

Cutaneous T-cell Lymphoma

Frederick Lansigan, MD[a], Jaehyuk Choi, MD, PhD[b], Francine M. Foss, MD[c],*

KEYWORDS

• Cutaneous T-cell lymphoma • Mycosis fungoides
• Sézary syndrome

Cutaneous T-cell lymphoma (CTCL) comprises a heterogeneous group of lymphoproliferative disorders characterized by clonal expansions of mature, post-thymic T cells that infiltrate the skin.[1] The most recent Surveillance, Epidemiology, and End Results database shows that the incidence of CTLC rose dramatically between 1973 and 2002[2] and that CTLC now comprises 3.4% of all non-Hodgkin's lymphomas.

The World Health Organization-European Organization for Research and Treatment of Cancer (WHO-EORTC) classification of primary cutaneous lymphomas (**Table 1**) defines distinct categories of cutaneous lymphomas based on histopathologic, clinical, and molecular features.[3] Mycosis fungoides (MF) is the most common form of CTCL and accounts for approximately 44% of all cutaneous lymphomas, but it comprises only 1% to 2% of non-Hodgkin's lymphomas.[4] MF derived its name from the mushroom-like tumors seen in the skin in advanced stages of the disease. The median age at diagnosis is 55 to 60 years, and the disease affects males more commonly than females (2:1).[3] MF is a chronic, slowly progressing disease but may evolve into patches, more infiltrated plaques, and eventually to tumors and dissemination to lymph nodes, blood, bone marrow, and other organs.

The term "Sézary syndrome" (SS) refers to a more aggressive form of CTCL in which there are skin manifestations in the form of erythroderma as well as circulating malignant T cells with highly infolded cerebriform nuclei, first characterized as "cellules monstrueuses" by Albert Sézary in 1938.[5] SS accounts for 0~3% of cutaneous lymphoma and may arise de novo or as a progression of pre-existing MF. The minimal criterion for diagnosing SS is the identification of a T-cell clone in the peripheral blood, preferably the same clone as found in the skin. The International Society for Cutaneous Lymphomas (ISCL), however, has proposed new criteria for the diagnosis of SS.[6] Under this system, the diagnosis of SS would consist of one or more of the

[a] Yale University School of Medicine, 333 Cedar Street, New Haven, CT, USA
[b] Department of Dermatology, Yale University School of Medicine, 333 Cedar Street, LCI 501, PO Box 208032, New Haven, CT 06510, USA
[c] Department of Medical Oncology, Yale University School of Medicine, 333 Cedar Street, FMP 112, PO Box 208032, New Haven, CT 06510, USA
* Corresponding author.
E-mail address: francine.foss@yale.edu (F.M. Foss).

Hematol Oncol Clin N Am 22 (2008) 979–996
doi:10.1016/j.hoc.2008.07.014
0889-8588/08/$ – see front matter © 2008 Elsevier Inc. All rights reserved.
hemonc.theclinics.com

Table 1
Relative frequency and disease-specific 5-year survival of primary cutaneous T-cell lymphomas classified according to the WHO-EORTC classification

WHO-EORTC Classification	No	Frequency (%)	Disease-Specific 5-Year Survival (%)
Indolent clinical behavior			
Mycosis fungoides	800	44	88
Folliculotropic mycosis fungoides	86	4	80
Pagetoid reticulosis	14	< 1	100
Granulomatous slack skin	4	< 1	100
Primary cutaneous anaplastic large-cell lymphoma	146	8	95
Lymphomatoid papulosis	236	12	100
Subcutaneous panniculitis-like T-cell lymphoma	18	1	82
Primary cutaneous CD4+ small/ medium pleomorphic T-cell lymphoma	39	2	75
Aggressive clinical behavior			
Sézary syndrome	52	3	24
Primary cutaneous natural killer/ T-cell lymphoma, nasal-type	7	< 1	NR
Primary cutaneous aggressive CD8+ T-cell lymphoma	14	< 1	18
Primary cutaneous γ/δ T-cell lymphoma	13	< 1	NR
Primary cutaneous peripheral T-cell lymphoma, unspecified	47	2	16

Adapted from Willemze R, Jaffe ES, Burg G, et al. WHO-EORTC classification for cutaneous lymphomas. Blood 2005;105:3769; with permission. © 2005 American Society of Hematology.

following: (1) an absolute Sézary count of at least 1000 cells/mm^3 in the peripheral blood; (2) immunophenotypic abnormalities such as an expanded CD4+ T-cell population with a CD4/CD8 ratio greater than 10:1; (3) an aberrant loss or expression of pan–T-cell markers (CD2, CD3, CD4, CD5, CD7) by flow cytometry; (4) increased lymphocyte counts with evidence of a T-cell clone in the blood by the Southern blot or polymerase chain reaction technique; and (5) a chromosomally abnormal T-cell clone. This new classification, which needs to be validated, would have implications in staging and prognosis.

Although the etiology of MF/SS is unknown, one proposed hypothesis is that it may represent the emergence of a clonal proliferation resulting from a chronic antigenic stimulus. Associations with exposure to chemicals or pesticides have been proposed but not demonstrated definitely in case-controlled epidemiologic studies.[7,8] In other studies, an association with chlamydia infection of keratinocytes has been proposed, but data demonstrating chlamydia proteins in affected skin lesions are equivocal.[9,10] An association with retroviruses has been suggested, because there are reports that HTLV-like viral particles in affected skin lesions and antibodies to HTLV-1 tax protein have been detected in some patients who have MF/SS.[11–14] Although there is no known geographic clustering and no evidence of maternal transmission of the disease, there are reports of multiple cases of MF/SS in a small number of families.

STAGING AND PROGNOSIS OF MYCOSIS FUNGOIDES/SÉZARY SYNDROME

Staging systems for MF have been developed based on clinical features of skin involvement as well as infiltration of lymph nodes and viscera. The most commonly used staging system for MF/SS is based on a tumor (T)-node (N)-metastasis (M)-blood (B) classification (**Table 2**).[15] Skin involvement is defined by the type and extent of lesion. T1 and T2 disease are patches or plaques involving less than or more than 10% of the skin surface, respectively. T3 disease is the presence of at least one cutaneous tumor. T4 disease is erythroderma, which may be flat and patchlike or diffusely infiltrated and associated with a leathery skin appearance or with thickening and fissuring of the skin, particularly on the palms or soles of the feet (**Fig. 1**). Lymph node involvement has been classified by the degree of infiltration with malignant cells. The dermatopathologic node demonstrates small (LN2) or large (LN3) clusters of atypical T cells with preserved nodal architecture and often with expansion of the parafollicular zones. LN4 nodes are effaced by atypical T cells.[16] Rearrangements of the T-cell receptor are found in half the patients who have LN3 nodes and, rarely, in those who have LN2 histology.[17] Bone marrow involvement has been shown to have prognostic significance based on the degree of involvement; cytologically atypical lymphoid aggregates and infiltrative disease are associated with inferior survival.[18] In retrospective studies, bone marrow involvement was associated with blood involvement and advanced lymph node disease.[19–22]

Overall outcome in MF/SS is correlated with clinical stage, and retrospective studies have identified skin involvement and visceral disease as the most important prognostic factors.[19,20,22] Patients who have limited patch/plaque disease covering less than 10% of the skin surface have a prognosis indistinguishable from that of age-, sex-, and race- matched controls.[23] The 10-year disease-specific survival rate for patients who have more extensive skin involvement with patches or plaques is 83%; patients who

Table 2
Tumor-node-metastasis-blood classification and clinical staging system for mycosis fungoides

N	M	T1: Limited Patch/ Plaque (< 10% BSA)	T2: Generalized Patch/Plaque (≥ 10% BSA)	T3 Tumor	T4 Erythroderma
N0: Nodes clinically uninvolved	M0	IA	IB	IIB	IIIA
N1: Nodes enlarged, histologically uninvolved	M0	IIA			
N2–3: Nodes clinically normal (N2) or enlarged (N3), histologically involved	M0	IVA			
N0–3: Visceral involvement	M1	IVB			
B classification is not incorporated in the clinical stage					
B0 Absence of significant peripheral blood Sézary cells					
B1 Presence of significant peripheral blood Sézary cells					

Abbreviation: BSA, body surface area.
Adapted from Demierre MF, Kim YH, Zackheim HS. Prognosis, clinical outcomes and quality of life issues in cutaneous T-cell lymphoma. Hematol Oncol Clin N Am 2003;17(6):1487; with permission.

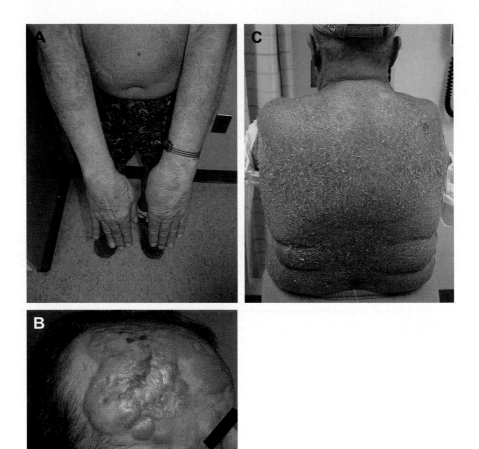

Fig. 1. Cutaneous manifestations of MF/SS. (*A*). Patch/plaque-stage disease. (*B*) Tumor-stage disease with ulceration. (*C*) Erythroderma with exfoliation.

have tumors or histopathologically documented lymph node involvement (LN3) have disease-specific 10-year survival rates of 42% and 20%, respectively. Effaced lymph nodes and the presence of large-cell transformation carry a uniformly poor prognosis.[24,25]

Previous staging systems have not accounted for blood involvement. In the proposed ISCL classification, blood involvement would be defined by the number of circulating Sézary cells. The B0 classification would signify no Sézary cells, B2 would signify more than 1000 Sézary cells/mm^3, and B1 would signify intermediate values between the B0 and B2 classifications. The new blood rating in the staging system of MF/SS may help differentiate patients who have SS (and therefore a worse prognosis) from their erythrodermic counterparts who have MF and is being applied prospectively in clinical trials.

TREATMENT

The diagnosis and initial treatment of CTCL usually takes place in the dermatologist's office. Because of the panoply of therapies available and the chronic progressive clinical course in most patients, management of the disease ideally involves a multidisciplinary team incorporating expertise in skin-directed therapy, radiation therapy, photopheresis, infusional and oral anti-neoplastic therapies, and combined-modality treatment. The therapeutic decision should incorporate the disease stage, overall prognosis, and quality-of-life issues, given the long duration of disease and therapy for most patients. In treating patients who have early-stage disease, for whom remission and possibly cure are likely, the goal should be to avoid long-term treatment-related toxicities. For patients who have advanced-stage disease, more aggressive combination strategies are warranted, and allogeneic stem cell transplantation should be considered as a potentially curative modality. Although the National Comprehensive Cancer Network recently has published guidelines for the treatment of MF and SS, the sequence of treatments frequently depends on the experience of the treating physicians and institution and on patient preference (**Table 3**).

Skin-Directed Therapies

The clinical manifestations of MF in its early and intermediate stages often are limited to the skin, without systemic involvement detectable by imaging studies. Skin-directed therapies can produce effective long-term responses in roughly 60% of

Table 3
Treatment algorithms according to disease stage

Stage	Initial Therapy	Relapsed/Refractory Disease
IA	Skin-directed therapy[a]	Additional skin-directed therapy or skin-directed therapy with biologic or single-agent therapy
IB/2A	Skin-directed therapy ± biologic therapy[b]	Skin-directed therapy + biologic or single-agent therapy
IIB	Skin-directed therapy (PUVA, electron beam radiation therapy) + biologic or single-agent therapy[c]	Multimodality combinations: skin-directed therapy + single-agent chemotherapy or biologic therapyMultiagent therapy Allogeneic stem cell transplantation
IIIA/B	ECP ± or skin-directed therapyMultimodality combinations with systemic or biologic therapies	Multimodality combinations with single-agent or multiagent therapyAllogeneic stem cell transplantation
IVA/B	Single-agent chemotherapy, combination biologic therapyMultiagent therapy[d]	Salvage chemotherapyAllogeneic stem cell transplantation

[a] Skin-directed therapy: topical steroids (intermediate and high potency), topical nitrogen mustard or bischloroethylnitrosourea ointment or aqueous solution, topical retinoids (bexarotene gel, tazarotene gel), phototherapy (UVB for patch or thin plaque, PUVA for thick plaque), electron beam irradiation (localized for limited disease, total skin for extensive skin involvement).
[b] Biologic therapies: interferon-α, retinoids (bexarotene, 13-*cis* retinoic acid, all-*trans*-retinoic acid), ECP, alemtuzumab.
[c] Single-agent therapy: methotrexate (low-dose oral or intravenous), denileukin diftitox, HDAC inhibitor (vorinostat), liposomal doxorubicin, gemcitabine, pentostatin, etoposide, cyclophosphamide, bortezomib, temozolomide.
[d] Multiagent combination therapies: biologic combinations (PUVA, UVB, or ECP + retinoids or interferon; PUVA UVB, ECP + retinoids + interferon; denileukin diftitox + bexarotene; retinoids + interferon; PUVA, UVB, or ECP with HDAC inhibitor [under investigation]); cytotoxic multiagent regimens (gemcitabine, venorelbine; liposomal doxorubicin; etoposide, vincristine, doxorubicin, cyclophosphamide, and oral prednisone; hyperfractionated cyclophosphamide, doxorubicin, vincristine, dexamethasone, alternating with methotrexate and cytarabine; etoposide, methylprednisolone, cytarabine, cisplatin; ifosfamide, carboplatin, etoposide).

patients who have limited patch or plaque disease. Patients who have early-stage disease usually have a relatively intact cellular immune response compared with patients who have SS or advanced MF, so treatment with non-immunosuppressive modalities is preferred.

Topical corticosteroids as monotherapy can induce clinical remission in 25% to 63% of patients, but the duration of benefit may be short.[26] Corticosteroids inhibit lymphocyte binding to endothelium and intercellular adhesion and can induce cell death of neoplastic lymphoid cells by up-regulating proapoptotic genes.[26] Long-term use of topical steroids can induce adrenal axis suppression in approximately 15% of patients and can lead to cutaneous atrophy. Oral corticosteroids also are effective, but they can cause the unwanted side effects of osteoporosis, adrenal suppression, altered glucose metabolism, and steroid-induced myopathies.

Mechlorethamine (nitrogen mustard) and carmustine are alkylating agents that have shown efficacy when applied to the involved skin. Nitrogen mustard liquid can be applied to the skin as an aqueous solution of 10 mg/dL or applied in an ointment base. Topical mechlorethamine has been shown to produce complete response (CR) rates of 26% to 76% in patch/plaque disease and CR rates of 22% to 49% in stage III disease. Relapses are frequent, however, even when therapy is continued after remission.[27–30] The time to response is stage dependent, and the duration of response is variable. Some patients who have stage IA disease may be cured, however. Mechlorethamine may cause an irritant reaction, and up to 40% of patients develop contact hypersensitivity. Mechlorethamine may be carcinogenic, and secondary cutaneous malignancies have been attributed to long-term use (8.6-fold and 1.8-fold increased risk for squamous and basal cell carcinoma, respectively).[29] Nonetheless, topical mechlorethamine in an ointment (Aquaphor) or water-based solution can be very effective in palliating involved skin lesions in patients at all disease stages, even when systemic treatment for CTCL is being administered. Carmustine is used less frequently because of the side effects of myelosuppression.

Topical retinoids, including 13-*cis* retinoic acid and tazarotene, have shown activity in patch and plaque lesions of CTCL. Recently, bexarotene (Targretin) was introduced in both an oral and topical formulation. Bexarotene is a novel, highly selective retinoid X receptor (RXR) retinoid that exerts its action by binding to RXR-γ and RXR-α receptors and altering gene transcription.[31] In phase I/II and III trials of bexarotene 1% gel, responses were seen in 44% to 64% of the patients who had stage I disease.[32,33] The time to response was 4.5 months,[32,33] and the median duration of response was 23 months.[33] Topical irritation and pruritus were the most common adverse events in these trials. The discomfort resulting from irritant dermatitis generally limits the use of the gel to patients who have involvement of less than 15% of the body surface area. Typically, bexarotene gel is applied to lesions once or twice a day with the frequency of application dictated by the irritant response. Regression of lesions may occur only after use of the gel is discontinued and the irritant response has subsided.

Psoralen plus UVA (PUVA) is a skin-directed therapy that penetrates into the deep dermis and induces apoptosis of both infiltrating tumor cells and mononuclear cells, including Langerhans cells that support the growth of the tumor cells in the skin microenvironment.[34,35] A retrospective study of PUVA monotherapy demonstrated a 63% response rate with 50% of responders showing sustained remissions,[35] although most of the responders had stage I disease. UVB, which is penetrates only through the epidermis, has been widely used in CTCL and in one study was associated with clinical CRs in 71% of patients who had early-stage CTCL with a reported response duration of 22 months.[36] Fewer durable responses were observed with infiltrated plaque-stage disease, however. Narrowband UVB can penetrate deeper in the dermis and in a small series of reports has demonstrated greater response than seen with broad-band UVB,[37–39] although a head-to-head comparison has not been done. Phototherapy can lead to irritation and skin erythema, however, and PUVA has been associated with increased risk of squamous and basal cell carcinomas and melanoma.

Electron beam radiation therapy is a therapeutic modality that uses electrons with limited skin penetration. Electrons ranging in energy between 4 and 7 MeV are used to treat the epidermis and dermis homogeneously. Structures below the deep dermis are relatively spared, because typically 80% of the dose is administered within the first 10 mm of depth, and less than 5% reaches a depth beyond 20 mm. Total-skin electron beam therapy (TSEBT) often is used in patients who have extensive patches or thin plaques refractory to PUVA or other skin-directed therapies. In patients who have limited involvement (stage IA disease), electron beam radiation may be curative. For patients at high risk for more generalized relapse in skin subsequent to TSEBT, adjuvant therapies, including interferons, retinoids, PUVA, or topical therapies, often are used.[40,41]

Clinical CR rates for patients who have T1 or T2 (patch or plaque) disease range from 71% to 98% and are higher in patients who have less extensive disease. Patients who have T1 and T2 disease treated with TSEBT have 5-year disease-free and overall survival rates of 50% to 65% and 80% to 90%, respectively, although patients who have antecedent or coexisting lymphomatoid papulosis or alopecia mucinosa (also known as "follicular mucinosis") seem to have shorter disease-free survival after TSEBT than those who do not. Patients who have more advanced T3 and T4 disease, however, have 5-year disease-free and overall survival rates of approximately 20% and 50%, respectively. For patients who have erythrodermic MF (T4 disease) who are managed with TSEBT alone (32–40 Gy), the CR rate may be as high as 70%, with a 5-year progression-free survival rate of 26%.[42] Long-term toxicities of electron beam radiation therapy include anhydrosis, telangiectasia, and secondary skin cancers.

Systemic Therapies

Patients are candidates for systemic therapy if they present with stage IIB disease or higher, have become refractory to skin-directed therapies, or have developed dose-limiting toxicities to UV or ionizing radiation. For these patients many systemic treatments, including novel therapies, are widely acceptable.

Extracorporeal photopheresis

One treatment modality that can be used in early- as well as advanced-stage disease and has a very low toxicity profile is extracorporeal photopheresis (ECP). ECP takes advantage of the principles derived from PUVA therapy and involves the extracorporeal exposure of peripheral blood mononuclear cells to photoactivated 8-methoxypsoralen with subsequent reinfusion of the treated cells. Activated 8-methoxypsoralen binds to thymidine and cross-links sister strands of DNA, leading to apoptosis of lymphocytes, whereas monocytoid cells are relatively resistant to this effect. Additionally, the process of leukapheresis and the subsequent passage of the blood through the narrow photoactivation plate induce differentiation of circulating monocytoid cells into immature dendritic cells.[43] By enriching the number of functional immature dendritic cells and inducing apoptosis in circulating tumor cells, the treatment is believed to induce an immune effector response against the tumor clone. It has been demonstrated that CD8+ T cells from patients who have SS and who have undergone ECP have the ability to kill autologous tumor cells in an major histocompatibility complex (MHC) class I–dependent manner ex vivo.[44]

Edelson and colleagues[45] treated patients who had refractory MF/SS with photopheresis in 1987 and reported a response rate of 73%. Other studies have shown similar responses to ECP monotherapy, but the best responders seem to be patients who have a short duration of disease, absence of bulky lymphadenopathy, leukocytosis less than 20,000/mm,[3] Sézary count of 10% to 20% of mononuclear cells, intact number of CD8+ cells, and lack of prior systemic chemotherapy.[46] ECP is administered either for 2 consecutive days one time per month or every 2 weeks, with therapy continued until maximal clearing is established. Although patients may show clinical improvement as early as the second month of therapy, most do not clear or achieve their maximal response until at least 4 to 6 months after starting therapy. After the patient's disease has stabilized, the interval between ECP treatments is prolonged gradually by 1 week per cycle every three cycles.

Combinations of ECP with other biologic agents such as interferon-α, interferon-γ, or retinoids have demonstrated efficacy. In one study, the combination of ECP administered during and after TSEBT seemed to improve survival ($P < .06$) for patients who had T3 or T4 disease who had achieved a CR to TSEBT. The group of treated patients was small, however, and the data are retrospective.[47]

Cytokines

Because the host immune response plays a pivotal role in the immune surveillance and clearing of CTCL tumor cells, biologic agents such as cytokines can be used to augment the immune response. CTCL tumor cells are thought to be CD4+ helper T (Th) cells that belong to the type 2 (Th2) subset and produce interleukin (IL)-4, IL-6, and IL-10. These cytokines enhance the differentiation of eosinophils and inhibit the production of interferon-γ, thus inhibiting cytotoxic T-cell responses. This Th2 skewing can predispose patients to infections, commonly the cause of serious morbidity and mortality in patients who have CTCL and other malignancies, and can lead to tumor cell evasion. It has been demonstrated that early MF lesions express a Th1 profile, whereas SS lesions exhibit a Th2 profile,[48] further characterizing the immune dysregulation in advanced disease. Additionally, in patients who have SS, Th2 cytokine production can be detected by flow cytometry in the serum and from the circulating and skin-infiltrating T cells.[49]

Interferon-alpha has been shown to suppress Th2 cytokine production and to increase MHC class I expression on lymphocytes.[50] Interferon-α also can enhance cell-mediated cytotoxicity directly by augmenting activation of CD8+ T cells and natural killer cells partly through the induction of IL-15.[51] Interferon-α was first shown to have activity in CTCL in 1984 by Bunn and coworkers.[52] Heavily treated patients who had advanced disease were treated with interferon-α and showed a 45% objective response rate. Subsequent studies confirmed activity in patients who had early- and late-stage disease, with 73% response in stage IA–IIA, and 60% response in stage IIB–IVA disease.[53]

In the practical management of early-stage CTCL, interferon-α can be added as an adjunct to topical therapy or after failure of skin-directed agents. For example, one study suggested synergistic effects obtained with ECP and interferon-α. Among the 10 patients treated with ECP alone in this two-arm study,[54] there was 1 CR and 1 minor response, whereas there were 4 CRs and 1 minor response among 9 patients treated with ECP and interferon-α. Combination therapies with interferon-α and PUVA, oral retinoids, and cytotoxic chemotherapy also have shown encouraging results.[50]

Bexarotene

Systemic retinoids often are the first systemic agents used in patients who have advanced or refractory MF/SS. Bexarotene, a highly selective RXR-binding retinoid, is an oral agent that has pleiotropic biologic activity including proapoptotic and immune-activating effects. Oral bexarotene administered at an initial dose of 300 mg/m^2/d in patients who had relapsed or refractory CTCL was associated with response rates of 54% in early-stage and 45% in advanced-stage CTCL.[55] The median response duration was 299 days with continuous dosing at a dose of 300 mg/m^2/d, and responses occurred in all groups of patients (57% at stage IIB, 32% at stage III, 44% at stage IVA, and 40% at IVB), including those who had large-cell transformation. A significant decrease in pruritus led to overall improvement in the quality-of-life indices of treated patients.

The major toxicities of bexarotene include elevations in serum lipids and cholesterol and suppression of thyroid function. Elevations in the lipids occurred rapidly, within 2 to 4 weeks, requiring the use of lipid-lowering agents in most patients. Patients taking bexarotene also developed a dose-dependent central hypothyroidism with low thyroid-stimulating hormone and free thyroxine levels within weeks of starting the medication. Symptoms of hypothyroidism may be subtle, because they include fatigue/asthenia, depression, cold intolerance, constipation, and other findings that may be attributed to malignancy. Supplementation with levothyroxine while patients were taking bexarotene was found to alleviate the symptoms and improve tolerance to treatment. The condition was reversible within 1 to 2 weeks after discontinuation of the drug.

Bexarotene has been used widely as a first systemic oral therapy for patients who have both early and advanced MF/SS. Therapy often is initiated at a low dose (two to four capsules per day) and titrated to achieve a therapeutic effect. Laboratory studies should be performed weekly until lipid and thyroid functions are stable and then performed intermittently during therapy.

The Development of Rationally Designed Targeted Therapy for Cutaneous T-Cell Lymphoma

The interleukin-2 receptor and denileukin diftitox

The IL-2 receptor (IL-2R) is a complex consisting of three parts: the α chain (CD25), which is required for high-affinity binding, the β chain (CD122), which participates in IL-2 and IL-15 signal transduction, and the common γ chain (CD132), which participates in downstream signal transduction of IL-2 and other cytokines.[56–58] IL-2R is expressed on less than 5% of normal circulating peripheral blood mononuclear cells but has been shown by immunohistochemistry to be overexpressed in most patients who have adult T-cell leukemia[59] and in about 50% of patients who have CTCL.[60]

Denileukin diftitox (Ontak) is a fusion protein toxin, which combines the IL-2R targeting ligand with a cytocidal moiety, such as a plant or bacterial toxin. Denileukin diftitox uses a truncated diphtheria toxin (DAB389) as the toxophore, which is fused to the full-length sequence of the IL-2 protein. The IL-2 moiety of the molecule directs the fusion toxin to cells bearing IL-2R. Upon internalization by receptor-mediated endocytosis, the fragment of diphtheria toxin is cleaved and translocates across the endosomal membrane into the cytosol where it inhibits protein synthesis via ADP-ribosylation of elongation factor-2, ultimately resulting in cell death.[61,62]

In the pivotal trial of denileukin diftitox in patients who had relapsed and refractory CTCL, a dose of 9 or 18 μg/kg/d was administered on 5 consecutive days every 3 weeks for up to eight cycles.[63] Overall, 30% of the 71 patients had an objective response, 20% had a partial response, and 10% had a CR. Reponses were rapid within the first three cycles in most patients, and the median duration of response was 6.9 months. Although the overall response rate was only 30%, 60% of patients had an improvement in overall disease burden, pruritus score, and quality-of-life index. Subsequent studies using denileukin diftitox in a population of less heavily pretreated patients who had CTCL have demonstrated a 50% overall response rate.[64] Not surprisingly, the degree of CD25 expression correlates with response to denileukin diftitox.[65] Overall, the most commonly reported adverse events included elevations of hepatic transaminases, flulike symptoms, hypoalbuminemia, acute hypersensitivity-type reactions, asthenia, nausea and vomiting, infections, and vascular leak syndrome.

Combination therapy with denileukin diftitox and retinoid therapy has been studied, because it has been demonstrated that both retinoid acid receptor A and RXR-binding retinoids are capable of up-regulating the CD25 subunit as well as the CD122 subunit of the IL-2R and thus sensitizing cell lines to the effects of denileukin diftitox.[66] In a phase I/II trial of bexarotene followed by denileukin diftitox,[67] up-regulation of the CD25 subunit of the IL-2R was demonstrated at bexarotene doses of at least 150 mg/d, and no overlapping toxicities were associated with these two agents. The response rate was 70%, and responders included patients who had stable disease or no response on denileukin diftitox alone.

Epigenetic Modification in Mycosis Fungoides/Sézary Syndrome

Genomic probing of cells in SS and MF has revealed general patterns of genetic and epigenetic changes and has led to the design of novel therapies. At varying frequencies, CTCL tumors have been found to have chromosomal deletions in 1p, 17p, 10q, and 19 with gains on chromosomes 4q, 18, and 17q, and these changes are associated with more advanced disease.[68] Each of these genetic regions contains known tumor suppressors or oncogenes. Point mutations in p53, found in chromosome 17p, were found in one third of the patients who had more advanced, tumor-stage MF but in no patients who had plaque-stage disease.[69] Further underscoring the relevance of specific genetic changes to the pathophysiology of the disease, Kari and colleagues[70] demonstrated gene signatures in patients who had SS that predicted a poor outcome and survival of less than 6 months, and recently Shin and colleagues[71] used lesional gene-expression profiling to identify clusters associated with disease outcome.

In an attempt to discover pathognomonic epigenetic changes, investigators performed a genome-wide screen for hypermethylation islands. DNA isolated from biopsy specimens from 28 patients who had CTCL revealed 35 CpG hypermethylated islands in at least 4 of the 28 CTCL samples.[72] It also has been shown that hypermethylation leading to gene silencing occurred in promoters of genes of cell-cycle regulation such as p16 and p15, DNA repair enzymes (eg, MGMT and hMLH1), proapoptotic pathways (eg, TMS1 and p73), and genes associated with chromosomal stability (eg, CHFR).[72–74]

Epigenetic modulation has emerged as an effective strategy in patients who have CTCL. Histone deacetylase (HDAC) inhibitors prevent the removal of the acetyl modification to lysine residues, leading to a more open chromatin structure and to global alterations in gene expression.[75] Depsipeptide (Romidepsin) was the first HDAC inhibitor tested in clinical trials at the National Cancer Institute, and responses were seen in patients who had T-cell lymphomas who received 14 mg/m^2 given intravenously on days 1, 8, and 15 of a 21-day cycle.[76] Among the 27 patients who had CTCL treated with depsipeptide, there were three CRs (all in patients who had SS) and five partial responses, including three in patients who had tumor-stage MF. The response durations ranged from 8 to 14 months. Toxicities included nausea, thrombocytopenia, leucopenia, and reversible ST-T segment changes and QT prolongation on electrocardiograms. In a recent study of 68 evaluable patients who had advanced CTCL treated with depsipeptide, the response rate was 35% with a median time to response of 8 weeks. More than 50% of patients reported improvement in pruritus.

Vorinostat (Zolinza), an oral HDAC inhibitor, was approved by the Food and Drug Administration in 2006 for the treatment of the skin manifestations of MF and SS. In preclinical studies, vorinostat was shown to induce apoptosis of Sézary cells in vitro.[77] In a phase II trial of vorinostat given at differing doses and schedules,[78] responses were seen in 30% of patients, and 42% experienced pruritus relief. A multicenter phase IIB trial[79] using vorinostat, 400 mg daily, also showed an overall response rate of 30% with one CR. The median time to response was 2 months, and the response duration was 9.8 months or longer. The most common side effects were diarrhea, nausea, fatigue, and anorexia. Pulmonary embolism occurred in 5% of patients. Asymptomatic QTc prolongation was observed on serial EKGs in 4% of patients. Other novel HDAC inhibitors such as belinostat and LBH589 are showing promising activity with good tolerability.

Purine Nucleoside Phosphorylase and Forodesine

A unique metabolic pathway important in normal T cells is the purine nucleoside phosphorylase (PNP) pathway. Patients who have genetic deletions in this gene have selective defects in T-cell function and numbers but not in B cell function and number.[80] PNP is responsible for catalyzing the cleavage of inosine, deoxyinosine, guanosine, and deoxyguanosine to their component base and sugar-1-phosphate. In the absence of this enzyme, PNP substrates accumulate. In T cells, where certain deoxynucleotide kinases are abundant, deoxyguanosine is converted to deoxyguanosine monophosphate and ultimately to deoxyguanosine triphosphate.[81] High levels of deoxyguanosine triphosphate, in turn, inhibit the enzymes that mediate the turnover of other DNA base components such as deoxycytidine triphosphate. In essence, PNP inhibition may activate a signaling cascade in T cells that ultimately leads to the accumulation of a toxic metabolite, inhibition of DNA synthesis, growth arrest, and finally apoptosis.[80] Two PNP inhibitors, arabinosylguanine and forodesine, have demonstrated efficacy in the clinic. Studies with intravenous and oral forodesine have shown encouraging results in patients who have MF and SS. In the phase I/II study of oral forodesine, the optimum biologic dose showed a 40% response rate, including in patients who had SS.[82]

Other Potential T-Cell Targets

Like their skin-homing T-cell counterparts, the malignant cells in MF and SS express a number of markers shared by most Th cells, including T-cell antigen receptor, CD4+, CCR4, and CD45RO+.[83] A number of humanized monoclonal antibodies have demonstrated efficacy in the treatment of MF and SS, but their use may be limited by T-cell depletion and immunosuppression. Alemtuzumab (Campath) targets cells that express the CD52 antigen, including lymphocytes and monocytes.[84] Despite reports of durable responses, treatment has been limited by the incidence of severe infections related to the immune-depleting effects of alemtuzumab. Recent studies with lower doses of alemtuzumab (10 mg three times per week) have reported responses in 6 of 10 patients (two CRs and four partial responses) with minimal immunosuppression.[85,86] Zanolimumab (HuMax-CD4), a high-affinity, fully humanized monoclonal antibody that targets the CD4 receptor, has shown promising results in 49 patients who had biopsy-proven CD4+ CTCL, including 23 patients who had advanced-stage disease.[87] Patients initially were treated with intravenous zanolimumab at a dose of 280 mg/week, which was increased to 560 mg/week in patients who had early-stage disease and to 980 mg/week in patients who had advanced disease. Partial remissions were reported in 16 of 36 evaluable patients overall (44%), including three of the six patients who had advanced disease treated at 980 mg/week. SGN-30 is a humanized antibody that targets the CD30 antigen on subsets of activated T and B cells and in large-cell CD30+ transformed MF. One phase II study demonstrated a 50% response rate in six patients, although administration was limited by immunosuppression.[84]

Cytotoxic Chemotherapy

If the agents described previously fail to control an indolent disease, or with a rapidly progressing or aggressive de novo disease, more potent chemotherapy is warranted. Because of the chronicity of the disease, single-agent chemotherapy that allows the sequential use of these agents is preferred. Gemcitabine (Gemzar) has demonstrated impressive clinical activity in advanced and refractory CTCL, with a 70% response rate when administered on days 1, 8, and 15 of a 28-day schedule at doses of 1000 to 1200 mg/m^2.[88,89] The incidence of grade 3 neutropenia was 25%. Median response duration was 8 months. In a study of chemotherapy-naïve patients treated with 1200 mg/m^2, the response rate was 70% with five CRs.[89,90] Other purine analogues, including fludarabine (Fludara), 2-chlorodeoxyadenosine (2-CDA), and pentostatin (Nipent), also have demonstrated efficacy.[89] Investigators at the MD Anderson Cancer Center reported a response rate of 56% for dose-escalated pentostatin (3–5 mg/m^2/d for 3 days on a 21-day schedule) in 42 patients who had CTCL.[91] The failure-free survival was 2.1 months. Grade 3/4 neutropenia occurred in 21% of patients. The incidence of infectious complications with pentostatin was high initially but subsequently was reduced by prophylactic trimethoprim (Bactrim) and anti-viral therapies. In a combination study of pentostatin at 4 mg/m^2/d × 3 with intermediate-dose interferon-α, the overall response rate was similar, but the median PFS was improved to 13.1 months.[92]

Pegylated liposomal doxorubicin (Doxil) was associated with an overall response rate of 88%, a CR rate of 42%, and a 13-month disease-free survival.[93] In another study at a dose of 20 mg/m^2 every 28 days, there were four CRs, and in a larger study of 34 patients who had CTCL or peripheral T-cell lymphoma who received 20 mg/m^2 every 2 weeks (n = 6), every 2 to 3 weeks (n = 4), or every 4 weeks (n = 23), there were 15 CRs and 15 partial responses, with a median event-free survival of 12.0 months. With the exception of infusion-related events, liposomal doxorubicin was well tolerated. Responding patients received up to 18 cycles of pegylated liposomal doxorubicin.

Bortezomib (Velcade) administered on a weekly schedule has been reported recently to have an impressive response rate of 67% in patients who had relapsed MF/SS.[94] All responses were durable, lasting from 7 to 14 or more months. Overall, the drug was well tolerated, with no grade 4 toxicity. Preclinical studies using bortezomib in Sézary leukemia cells demonstrated inhibition of nuclear factor-κB pathways, thus releasing the block to apoptosis in the cells.

Despite numerous treatment alternatives, many patients who have advanced MF/SS rapidly become refractory to therapy, presumably because of drug resistance. Responses to combination chemotherapy regimens such as cyclophosphamide, doxorubicin, vincristine, and prednisolone are high, but response durations are short. Infusion chemotherapy with etoposide, vincristine, doxorubicin, cyclophosphamide, and oral prednisone was studied in heavily pretreated patients who had CTCL and resulted in an overall response rate of 80%, with a CR rate of 27%.[95] The median progression-free survival was 8 months, and Sézary cells were undetectable in two of six patients who had SS. Other intensive lymphoma salvage regimens likewise have demonstrated responses, albeit with significant toxicity related to immunosuppression.

Hematopoietic Stem Cell Transplantation

Hematopoietic stem cell transplantation has been a very effective treatment for many malignant hematologic disorders that are refractory to conventional treatment. Reports on CTCL remain limited, but transplantation offers patients who have CTCL the chance for long-term cure. High-dose chemotherapy and autologous stem cell transplantation have yielded disappointing results. Most patients studied had highly refractory disease, and high-dose chemotherapy produced only marginal benefit. Almost all patients relapsed with a median duration of response of only 7 months.[96]

Allogeneic stem cell transplantation provides the advantages of a sustained immune-mediated graft-versus-lymphoma effect and a graft that is uncontaminated with tumor cells. The peritransplantation morbidity and mortality are relatively high, however, possibly because of the advanced age of patients who have CTCL as well as the immunosuppressive nature of their disease, which puts them at even higher risk for infection. A review of allogeneic transplantation including reduced-intensity conditioning regimens for MF and SS demonstrates a graft-versus-tumor effect and long-term remissions in a subset of patients.[97] Further, donor lymphocyte infusion was able to induce remissions in patients who had experienced relapse. The timing of allogeneic stem cell transplantation is also an important factor to consider. In patients who have large disease burden or disease with multiple prior relapses, the graft-versus-lymphoma effect may be not be able to overcome the aggressive or resistant nature of disease at that time. An allogeneic transplantation should be considered earlier in the disease course if an HLA-matched donor is identified.

SUMMARY

Although a number of treatments have shown efficacy in the symptomatic management of CTCL, cure remains elusive for most patients. The overall goals of treatment for most patients are to provide palliation for symptoms of pruritus and compromised skin integument and to prevent further immunosuppression. Given the low overall incidence of CTCL, the disease chronicity, the morbidity, and the lack of effective cure, enrollment in clinical trials should be encouraged so that more effective agents with minimal toxicity profiles can be identified.

REFERENCES

1. Girardi M, Heald PW, Wilson LD. The pathogenesis of mycosis fungoides. N Engl J Med 2004;350:1978–88.
2. Criscione VD, Weinstock MA. Incidence of cutaneous T-cell lymphoma in the United States, 1973–2002. Arch Dermatol 2007;143:854–9.
3. Willemze R, Jaffe ES, Burg G, et al. WHO-EORTC classification for cutaneous lymphomas. Blood 2005;105:3768–85.
4. Burg G, Kempf W, Cozzio A, et al. WHO/EORTC classification of cutaneous lymphomas 2005: histological and molecular aspects. J Cutan Pathol 2005;32: 647–74.
5. Lutzner MA, Jordan HW. The ultrastructure of an abnormal cell in Sézary syndrome. Blood 1968;31:719–26.
6. Vonderheid EC, Bernengo MG, Burg G, et al. Update on erythrodermic cutaneous T-cell lymphoma: report of the International Society for Cutaneous Lymphomas. J Am Acad Dermatol 2002;46:95–106.

7. Whittemore AS, Holly EA, Lee IM, et al. Mycosis fungoides in relation to environmental exposures and immune response: a case-control study. J Natl Cancer Inst 1989;81:1560–7.

8. Tuyp E, Burgoyne A, Aitchison T, et al. A case-control study of possible causative factors in mycosis fungoides. Arch Dermatol 1987;123:196–200.

9. Abrams JT, Balin BJ, Vonderheid EC. Association between Sezary T cell-activating factor, Chlamydia pneumoniae, and cutaneous T cell lymphoma. Ann N Y Acad Sci 2001;941:69–85.

10. Rossler MJ, Rappl G, Muche M, et al. No evidence of skin infection with Chlamydia pneumoniae in patients with cutaneous T cell lymphoma. Clin Microbiol Infect 2003;9:721–3.

11. Pancake BA, Wassef EH, Zucker-Franklin D. Demonstration of antibodies to human T-cell lymphotropic virus-I tax in patients with the cutaneous T-cell lymphoma, mycosis fungoides, who are seronegative for antibodies to the structural proteins of the virus. Blood 1996;88:3004–9.

12. Pancake BA, Zucker-Franklin D. The difficulty of detecting HTLV-1 proviral sequences in patients with mycosis fungoides. J Acquir Immune Defic Syndr Hum Retrovirol 1996;13:314–9.

13. Zucker-Franklin D, Hooper WC, Evatt BL. Human lymphotropic retroviruses associated with mycosis fungoides: evidence that human T-cell lymphotropic virus type II (HTLV-II) as well as HTLV-I may play a role in the disease. Blood 1992; 80:1537–45.

14. Zucker-Franklin D, Coutavas EE, Rush MG, et al. Detection of human T-lymphotropic virus-like particles in cultures of peripheral blood lymphocytes from patients with mycosis fungoides. Proc Natl Acad Sci U S A 1991;88:7630–4.

15. Bunn PAJ, Lamberg SI. Report of the Committee on Staging and Classification of Cutaneous T-cell Lymphomas. Cancer Treat Rep 1979;63:725–8.

16. Sausville EA, Worsham GF, Matthews MJ, et al. Histologic assessment of lymph nodes in mycosis fungoides/Sezary syndrome (cutaneous T-cell lymphoma): clinical correlations and prognostic import of a new classification system. Hum Pathol 1985;16:1098–109.

17. Lynch JW Jr, Sausville EA, Eddy J, et al. Prognostic implications of evaluation for lymph node involvement by T-cell antigen receptor gene rearrangement in mycosis fungoides. Blood 1992;79:3293–9.

18. Graham SJ, Sharpe RW, Steinberg SM, et al. Prognostic implications of a bone marrow histopathologic classification system in mycosis fungoides and the Sezary syndrome. Cancer 1993;72:726–34.

19. Sausville EA, Eddy JL, Makuch RW, et al. Histopathologic staging at initial diagnosis of mycosis fungoides and the Sezary syndrome. Definition of three distinctive prognostic groups. Ann Intern Med 1988;109:372–82.

20. Diamandidou E, Colome M, Fayad L, et al. Prognostic factor analysis in mycosis fungoides/Sezary syndrome. J Am Acad Dermatol 1999;40:914–24.

21. Salhany KE, Greer JP, Cousar JB, et al. Marrow involvement in cutaneous T-cell lymphoma. A clinicopathologic study of 60 cases. Am J Clin Pathol 1989;92:747–54.

22. Toro JR, Stoll HL Jr, Stomper PC, et al. Prognostic factors and evaluation of mycosis fungoides and Sezary syndrome. J Am Acad Dermatol 1997;37:58–67.

23. Kim YH, Bishop K, Varghese A, et al. Prognostic factors in erythrodermic mycosis fungoides and the Sezary syndrome. Arch Dermatol 1995;131:1003–8.

24. Diamandidou E, Colome-Grimmer M, Fayad L, et al. Transformation of mycosis fungoides/Sezary syndrome: clinical characteristics and prognosis. Blood 1998;92:1150–9.

25. Dmitrovsky E, Matthews MJ, Bunn PA, et al. Cytologic transformation in cutaneous T cell lymphoma: a clinicopathologic entity associated with poor prognosis. J Clin Oncol 1987;5:208–15.
26. Zackheim HS, Kashani-Sabet M, Amin S. Topical corticosteroids for mycosis fungoides. Experience in 79 patients. Arch Dermatol 1998;134:949–54.
27. Hoppe RT, Abel EA, Deneau DG, et al. Mycosis fungoides: management with topical nitrogen mustard. J Clin Oncol 1987;5:1796–803.
28. Ramsay DL, Halperin PS, Zeleniuch-Jacquotte A. Topical mechlorethamine therapy for early stage mycosis fungoides. J Am Acad Dermatol 1988;19:684–91.
29. Vonderheid EC, Tan ET, Kantor AF, et al. Long-term efficacy, curative potential, and carcinogenicity of topical mechlorethamine chemotherapy in cutaneous T cell lymphoma. J Am Acad Dermatol 1989;20:416–28.
30. Zachariae H, Thestrup-Pedersen K, Sogaard H. Topical nitrogen mustard in early mycosis fungoides. A 12-year experience. Acta Derm Venereol 1985;65:53–8.
31. Zhang C, Duvic M. Treatment of cutaneous T-cell lymphoma with retinoids. Dermatol Ther 2006;19:264–71.
32. Heald P, Mehlmauer M, Martin AG, et al. Topical bexarotene therapy for patients with refractory or persistent early-stage cutaneous T-cell lymphoma: results of the phase III clinical trial. J Am Acad Dermatol 2003;49:801–15.
33. Breneman D, Duvic M, Kuzel T, et al. Phase 1 and 2 trial of bexarotene gel for skin-directed treatment of patients with cutaneous T-cell lymphoma. Arch Dermatol 2002;138:325–32.
34. Berger CL, Hanlon D, Kanada D, et al. The growth of cutaneous T-cell lymphoma is stimulated by immature dendritic cells. Blood 2002;99:2929–39.
35. Querfeld C, Rosen ST, Kuzel TM, et al. Long-term follow-up of patients with early-stage cutaneous T-cell lymphoma who achieved complete remission with psoralen plus UV-A monotherapy. Arch Dermatol 2005;141:305–11.
36. Ramsay DL, Lish KM, Yalowitz CB, et al. Ultraviolet-B phototherapy for early-stage cutaneous T-cell lymphoma. Arch Dermatol 1992;128:931–3.
37. Clark C, Dawe RS, Evans AT, et al. Narrowband TL-01 phototherapy for patch-stage mycosis fungoides. Arch Dermatol 2000;136:748–52.
38. Gathers RC, Scherschun L, Malick F, et al. Narrowband UVB phototherapy for early-stage mycosis fungoides. J Am Acad Dermatol 2002;47:191–7.
39. Hofer A, Cerroni L, Kerl H, et al. Narrowband (311-nm) UV-B therapy for small plaque parapsoriasis and early-stage mycosis fungoides. Arch Dermatol 1999;135:1377–80.
40. Jones G, McLean J, Rosenthal D, et al. Combined treatment with oral etretinate and electron beam therapy in patients with cutaneous T-cell lymphoma (mycosis fungoides and Sezary syndrome). J Am Acad Dermatol 1992;26:960–7.
41. Jones G, Wilson LD, Fox-Goguen L. Total skin electron beam radiotherapy for patients who have mycosis fungoides. Hematol Oncol Clin North Am 2003;17:1421–34.
42. Jones GW, Rosenthal D, Wilson LD. Total skin electron radiation for patients with erythrodermic cutaneous T-cell lymphoma (mycosis fungoides and the Sezary syndrome). Cancer 1999;85:1985–95.
43. Berger CL, Xu AL, Hanlon D, et al. Induction of human tumor-loaded dendritic cells. Int J Cancer 2001;91:438–47.
44. Berger CL, Wang N, Christensen I, et al. The immune response to class I-associated tumor-specific cutaneous T-cell lymphoma antigens. J Invest Dermatol 1996;107:392–7.
45. Edelson R, Berger C, Gasparro F, et al. Treatment of cutaneous T-cell lymphoma by extracorporeal photochemotherapy. Preliminary results. N Engl J Med 1987;316:297–303.

46. Girardi M, Knobler R, Edelson R. Selective immunotherapy through extracorporeal photochemotherapy: yesterday, today, and tomorrow. Hematol Oncol Clin North Am 2003;17:1391–403.

47. Wilson LD, Licata AL, Braverman IM, et al. Systemic chemotherapy and extracorporeal photochemotherapy for T3 and T4 cutaneous T-cell lymphoma patients who have achieved a complete response to total skin electron beam therapy. Int J Radiat Oncol Biol Phys 1995;32:987–95.

48. Saed G, Fivenson DP, Naidu Y, et al. Mycosis fungoides exhibits a Th1-type cell-mediated cytokine profile whereas Sezary syndrome expresses a Th2-type profile. J Invest Dermatol 1994;103:29–33.

49. Fierro MT, Comessatti A, Quaglino P, et al. Expression pattern of chemokine receptors and chemokine release in inflammatory erythroderma and Sezary syndrome. Dermatology 2006;213:284–92.

50. Olsen EA. Interferon in the treatment of cutaneous T-cell lymphoma. Dermatol Ther 2003;16:311–21.

51. Dunn GP, Koebel CM, Schreiber RD. Interferons, immunity and cancer immunoediting. Nat Rev Immunol 2006;6:836–48.

52. Bunn PA Jr, Foon KA, Ihde DC, et al. Recombinant leukocyte A interferon: an active agent in advanced cutaneous T-cell lymphomas. Ann Intern Med 1984; 101:484–7.

53. Olsen EA, Rosen ST, Vollmer RT, et al. Interferon alfa-2a in the treatment of cutaneous T cell lymphoma. J Am Acad Dermatol 1989;20:395–407.

54. Dippel E, Schrag H, Goerdt S, et al. Extracorporeal photopheresis and interferon-alpha in advanced cutaneous T-cell lymphoma. Lancet 1997;350:32–3.

55. Duvic M, Hymes K, Heald P, et al. Bexarotene is effective and safe for treatment of refractory advanced-stage cutaneous T-cell lymphoma: multinational phase II-III trial results. J Clin Oncol 2001;19:2456–71.

56. Hatakeyama M, Minamoto S, Uchiyama T, et al. Reconstitution of functional receptor for human interleukin-2 in mouse cells. Nature 1985;318:467–70.

57. Takeshita T, Asao H, Ohtani K, et al. Cloning of the gamma chain of the human IL-2 receptor. Science 1992;257:379–82.

58. Tsudo M, Kitamura F, Miyasaka M. Characterization of the interleukin 2 receptor beta chain using three distinct monoclonal antibodies. Proc Natl Acad Sci U S A 1989;86:1982–6.

59. Waldmann TA. Anti-Tac (daclizumab, Zenapax) in the treatment of leukemia, autoimmune diseases, and in the prevention of allograft rejection: a 25-year personal odyssey. J Clin Immunol 2007;27:1–18.

60. Foss F. Clinical experience with denileukin diftitox (ONTAK). Semin Oncol 2006; 33:S11–6.

61. Bacha P, Williams DP, Waters C, et al. Interleukin 2 receptor-targeted cytotoxicity. Interleukin 2 receptor-mediated action of a diphtheria toxin-related interleukin 2 fusion protein. J Exp Med 1988;167:612–22.

62. Foss FM. DAB(389)IL-2 (denileukin diftitox, ONTAK): a new fusion protein technology. Clin Lymphoma 2000;1(Suppl 1):S27–31.

63. Olsen E, Duvic M, Frankel A, et al. Pivotal phase III trial of two dose levels of denileukin diftitox for the treatment of cutaneous T-cell lymphoma. J Clin Oncol 2001;19:376–88.

64. Chin KM, Foss FM. Biologic correlates of response and survival in patients with cutaneous T-cell lymphoma treated with denileukin diftitox. Clin Lymphoma Myeloma 2006;7:199–204.

65. Talpur R, Jones DM, Alencar AJ, et al. CD25 expression is correlated with histological grade and response to denileukin diftitox in cutaneous T-cell lymphoma. J Invest Dermatol 2006;126:575–83.

66. Gorgun G, Foss F. Immunomodulatory effects of RXR retinoids: modulation of high-affinity IL-2R expression enhances susceptibility to denileukin diftitox. Blood 2002;100:1399–403.

67. Foss F, Demierre MF, DiVenuti G. A phase-1 trial of bexarotene and denileukin diftitox in patients with relapsed or refractory cutaneous T-cell lymphoma. Blood 2005;106:454–7.

68. Mao X, Lillington D, Scarisbrick JJ, et al. Molecular cytogenetic analysis of cutaneous T-cell lymphomas: identification of common genetic alterations in Sezary syndrome and mycosis fungoides. Br J Dermatol 2002;147:464–75.

69. McGregor JM, Crook T, Fraser-Andrews EA, et al. Spectrum of p53 gene mutations suggests a possible role for ultraviolet radiation in the pathogenesis of advanced cutaneous lymphomas. J Invest Dermatol 1999;112:317–21.

70. Kari L, Loboda A, Nebozhyn M, et al. Classification and prediction of survival in patients with the leukemic phase of cutaneous Tcell lymphoma. J Exp Med 2003;197:1477–88.

71. Shin J, Monti S, Aires DJ, et al. Lesional gene expression profiling in cutaneous T-cell lymphoma reveals natural clusters associated with disease outcome. Blood 2007;110:3015–27.

72. van Doorn R, Zoutman WH, Dijkman R, et al. Epigenetic profiling of cutaneous T-cell lymphoma: promoter hypermethylation of multiple tumor suppressor genes including BCL7a, PTPRG, and p73. J Clin Oncol 2005;23:3886–96.

73. Scarisbrick JJ, Mitchell TJ, Calonje E, et al. Microsatellite instability is associated with hypermethylation of the hMLH1 gene and reduced gene expression in mycosis fungoides. J Invest Dermatol 2003;121:894–901.

74. Scarisbrick JJ, Woolford AJ, Calonje E, et al. Frequent abnormalities of the p15 and p16 genes in mycosis fungoides and Sezary syndrome. J Invest Dermatol 2002;118:493–9.

75. Johnstone RW. Histone-deacetylase inhibitors: novel drugs for the treatment of cancer. Nat Rev Drug Discov 2002;1:287–99.

76. Piekarz RL, Robey R, Sandor V, et al. Inhibitor of histone deacetylation, depsipeptide (FR901228), in the treatment of peripheral and cutaneous T-cell lymphoma: a case report. Blood 2001;98:2865–8.

77. Zhang C, Richon V, Ni X, et al. Selective induction of apoptosis by histone deacetylase inhibitor SAHA in cutaneous T-cell lymphoma cells: relevance to mechanism of therapeutic action. J Invest Dermatol 2005;125:1045–52.

78. Duvic M, Talpur R, Ni X, et al. Phase 2 trial of oral vorinostat (suberoylanilide hydroxamic acid, SAHA) for refractory cutaneous T-cell lymphoma (CTCL). Blood 2007;109:31–9.

79. Olsen EA, Kim YH, Kuzel TM, et al. Phase IIb multicenter trial of vorinostat in patients with persistent, progressive, or treatment refractory cutaneous T-cell lymphoma. J Clin Oncol 2007;25:3109–15.

80. Schramm VL. Development of transition state analogues of purine nucleoside phosphorylase as anti-T-cell agents. Biochim Biophys Acta 2002;1587:107–17.

81. Gandhi V, Balakrishnan K. Pharmacology and mechanism of action of forodesine, a T-cell targeted agent. Semin Oncol 2007;34:S8–12.

82. Duvic M, Forero-Torres A, Foss F, et al. Response to oral forodesine in refractory cutaneous t-cell lymphoma: interim results of a phase I/II study. ASH Annual Meeting Abstracts 2007;110:122.

83. Kim EJ, Hess S, Richardson SK, et al. Immunopathogenesis and therapy of cutaneous T cell lymphoma. J Clin Invest 2005;115:798–812.
84. Whittaker SJ, Foss FM. Efficacy and tolerability of currently available therapies for the mycosis fungoides and Sezary syndrome variants of cutaneous T-cell lymphoma. Cancer Treat Rev 2007;33:146–60.
85. Kennedy GA, Seymour JF, Wolf M, et al. Treatment of patients with advanced mycosis fungoides and Sezary syndrome with alemtuzumab. Eur J Haematol 2003; 71:250–6.
86. Lundin J, Hagberg H, Repp R, et al. Phase 2 study of alemtuzumab (anti-CD52 monoclonal antibody) in patients with advanced mycosis fungoides/Sezary syndrome. Blood 2003;101:4267–72.
87. Kim YH, Duvic M, Obitz E, et al. Clinical efficacy of zanolimumab (HuMax-CD4): two phase II studies in refractory cutaneous T-cell lymphoma. Blood 2006;108: 2731.
88. Duvic M, Talpur R, Wen S, et al. Phase II evaluation of gemcitabine monotherapy for cutaneous T-cell lymphoma. Clin Lymphoma Myeloma 2006;7:51–8.
89. Zinzani PL, Baliva G, Magagnoli M, et al. Gemcitabine treatment in pretreated cutaneous T-cell lymphoma: experience in 44 patients. J Clin Oncol 2000;18: 2603–6.
90. Marchi E, Alinari L, Tani M, et al. Gemcitabine as frontline treatment for cutaneous T-cell lymphoma: phase II study of 32 patients. Cancer 2005;104:2437–41.
91. Kurzrock R, Pilat S, Duvic M. Pentostatin therapy of T-cell lymphomas with cutaneous manifestations. J Clin Oncol 1999;17:3117–21.
92. Foss FM, Ihde DC, Breneman DL, et al. Phase II study of pentostatin and intermittent high-dose recombinant interferon alfa-2a in advanced mycosis fungoides/ Sezary syndrome. J Clin Oncol 1992;10:1907–13.
93. Wollina U, Dummer R, Brockmeyer NH, et al. Multicenter study of pegylated liposomal doxorubicin in patients with cutaneous T-cell lymphoma. Cancer 2003;98: 993–1001.
94. Zinzani PL, Musuraca G, Tani M, et al. Phase II trial of proteasome inhibitor bortezomib in patients with relapsed or refractory cutaneous T-cell lymphoma. J Clin Oncol 2007;25:4293–7.
95. Akpek G, Koh HK, Bogen S, et al. Chemotherapy with etoposide, vincristine, doxorubicin, bolus cyclophosphamide, and oral prednisone in patients with refractory cutaneous T-cell lymphoma. Cancer 1999;86:1368–76.
96. Olavarria E, Child F, Woolford A, et al. T-cell depletion and autologous stem cell transplantation in the management of tumour stage mycosis fungoides with peripheral blood involvement. Br J Haematol 2001;114:624–31.
97. Herbert KE, Spencer A, Grigg A, et al. Graft-versus-lymphoma effect in refractory cutaneous T-cell lymphoma after reduced-intensity HLA-matched sibling allogeneic stem cell transplantation. Bone Marrow Transplant 2004;34:521–5.

Peripheral T-Cell Non-Hodgkin's Lymphoma

Julie M. Vose, MD

KEYWORDS

• T-cell • Non-Hodgkin's lymphoma

T-cell non-Hodgkin's lymphomas (T-NHL) are uncommon malignancies accounting for 10% to 15% of all NHL.[1] Geographic variation has been well documented, ranging from 1.5% in Vancouver to 18.3% of all NHL in Hong Kong.[2] The geographic variation may reflect exposure to specific pathogenic viruses, such as Epstein Barr Virus (EBV) and Human T-cell leukemia virus-1 (HTLV-1) in Asian countries.[3,4] The World Health Organization (WHO) classification specifies 16 major subtypes of T-NHL (**Box 1**).[5] Each of the major subtype of peripheral T-NHL has unique characteristics and are addressed separately in this article.

PERIPHERAL T-CELL LYMPHOMA, NOT OTHERWISE SPECIFIED

Peripheral T-cell lymphoma (PTCL)-not otherwise specified (NOS), is the most common type of peripheral T-cell NHL and is a heterogeneous mix of different types of PTCL. PTCL-NOS is the diffuse large cell equivalent of B-cell NHL. There are two morphologic variants recognized, the T-zone lymphoma variant and the lymphoepithelioid cell variant. Patients with PTCL-NOS have predominantly nodal lymphoma that presents in adults (median age 61 years), with a male:female ratio of 1.5: 1.0.[6] Patients typically have advanced stage disease, with 60% having stage IV disease and many patients having unfavorable characteristics, such as B-symptoms, elevated lactic dehydrogenase (LDH), bulky disease, poor performance status, and extranodal disease so that greater than 50% of patients fall into the unfavorable International Prognostic Index (IPI) category 3 to 5 (**Fig. 1**).[6] Another prognostic model for PTCL-NOS has been used by Gallamini and colleagues,[7] which uses the characteristics of age greater than 60, LDH higher than normal, and performance status greater than or equal to 2. Bone marrow involvement to predict outcome was found to be more discriminatory than the standard IPI for this group of patients (**Fig. 2**).

Treatment for PTCL-NOS with standard NHL regimens, such as cyclophosphamide, hydroxydaunomycin, oncovin, and prednisone (CHOP), produces approximately

Section of Hematology/Oncology, Internal Medicine, University of Nebraska Medical Center, 987680 Nebraska Medical Center, Omaha, NE 68198-7680, USA
E-mail address: jmvose@unmc.edu

Hematol Oncol Clin N Am 22 (2008) 997–1005
doi:10.1016/j.hoc.2008.07.010
0889-8588/08/$ – see front matter

> **Box 1**
> **WHO classification for T/natural killer cell lymphomas**
>
> Nodal
>
>   Anaplastic large cell, naplastic-lymphoma-kinase (ALK)-negative
>
>   Anaplastic large cell, ALK-positive
>
>   Angioimmunoblastic
>
>   Peripheral T-cell lymphoma, unspecified (PTCL-U)
>
> Extranodal
>
>   Nasal, natural killer (NK)/T-cell
>
>   NK/T-cell, extranasal (disseminated)
>
>   Enteropathy associated
>
>   Hepatosplenic γδ
>
>   Subcutaneous panniculitis-like
>
> Leukemia
>
>   T-Prolymphocytic leukemia
>
>   Adult T-cell lymphoma/leukemia
>
>   Large granular lymphocytic leukemia
>
>   Aggressive NK leukemia

a 50% to 60% response rate, but the long-term disease-free survivals are poor, with 10% to 30% of patients surviving long term.[8] Because of these poor results, other regimens have been tried as primary induction regimens, such as HyperCVAD, LNH programs or regimens using platinum compounds. However, these have not had results that were better then the standard CHOP regimen.[9,10]

Other agents that have been found to have some single-agent activity in PTCL include purine analogs, such as 2'deoxycoformin, fludarabine, 2-chlorodeoxyadenosine, which have a response rate of 15% to 80% in several series.[11–13] Other chemotherapy drugs with some documented activity include gemcitabine, which has been

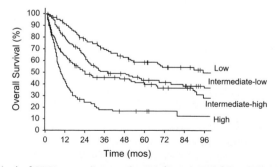

Fig. 1. Overall survival of PTCL according to the IPI. (*Reprinted from* Gallamini A, Stelitano C, Calvi R, et al. Peripheral T-cell lymphoma unspecified (PTCL-U): a new prognostic model from a retrospective multicenter clinical study. Blood 2004;103:2477; with permission. © 2004 American Society of Hematology.)

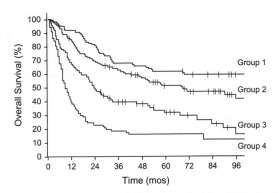

Fig. 2. Overall survival according to the Peripheral T-cell Index (PIT). (*Reprinted from* Gallamini A, Stelitano C, Calvi R, et al. Peripheral T-cell lymphoma unspecified (PTCL-U): a new prognostic model from a retrospective multicenter clinical study. Blood 2004; 103:2477; with permission. © 2004 American Society of Hematology.)

found to have a response rate of approximately 60%,[11] and bortezomib, with a response rate of 30%.[14]

Other classes of agents with activity in PTCL-NOS are immunotherapy, histone deacetylase (HDAC) inhibitors and folate antagonists. Examples of immunotherapy include denileukin diftitox, a recombinant fusion protein consisting of peptide sequences of diphtheria toxin, and recombinant interleukin-2 receptor (CD25), which has a demonstrated 40% response rate in PTCL.[15] Alemtuzumab, a CD52 monoclonal antibody, has a 36% response rate in PTCL-U.[16] More recently HDAC inhibitors, such as depsipeptide and vorinostat, have been found to have activity against PTCL, as well as mycosis fungoides.[17,18] In addition, pralotrexate in phase I/II trials has a documented 45% response rate in T-cell NHL.[19]

High-dose chemotherapy and stem cell transplantation has been proposed in an attempt to improve the poor results of standard chemotherapy. Patients with a chemotherapy-sensitive response to salvage therapy have long-term disease-free survivals of 35% to 45%.[20,21] Because of the poor results with standard therapy, some centers are also using high-dose chemotherapy and autologous stem cell transplant in CR1 patients. In small studies, this strategy demonstrates a high disease-free survival.[22,23] However, this treatment would need to be tested in a large, randomized trial to demonstrate it's efficacy.

The use of an allogeneic stem cell source has been used as an alternative in some small studies. The morbidity and mortality is high in patients receiving a full myeloablative allogeneic transplant; however, patients with PTCL-NOS have a reported 63% 5-year overall survival.[24] More recently, reduced intensity conditioning has emerged as an attractive alternative. A small pilot study of reduced intensity conditioning in PTCL demonstrated 3-year overall and progression-free survival rates of 81% and 64%, respectively.[25] This does appear promising in this highly selected patient population, but will need much further investigation in a larger patient population.

ANGIOIMMUNOBLASTIC T-CELL LYMPHOMA

Angioimmunoblastic T-cell lymphoma (AITL), previously known as angioimmunoblastic lymphadenopathy with dysproteinemia, was the second most common PTCL in the International T-Cell Lymphoma Classification Project.[26] This type accounts for 18.5%

of the PTCLs. The median age at diagnosis is 64 years, with a male predominance and the majority of patients present with advanced-stage disease. Other features include a high percentage of patients with B-symptoms, skin rash, effusions, hypergammaglobulinemia, and other immunologic or rheumatologic abnormalities.[27]

AITL typically has an aggressive clinical course; however, there are occasionally spontaneous regressions that occur. In some studies, high doses of prednisone are used first, followed by standard chemotherapy if the patients progress or relapse. However, treatment of AITL has typically been initiated with an anthracycline-containing regimen which results in CR rates of 50% to 70%, but only 10% to 30% of patients are long-term survivors.[26,28] A recent analysis of AITL patients treated in the Groupe d'Etudes des Lymphomes de L'Adulte (GELA) group with LNH-87 or LNH-93 demonstrated that the only characteristics predictive of a poorer survival included male sex ($P = .004$) and mediastinal lymphadenopathy ($P = .041$). Despite an intensified anthracycline-based regimen, patients in the GELA studies had only a 30% 7-year survival.[29] There are anecdotal reports of patients with relapsed AITL who have responded to immunosuppressive therapy, such as low-dose methotrexate/prednisone, cyclosporine, or purine analogs.[30,31] The results with autologous or allogeneic stem cell transplantation in AITL is similar to PTCL-U.[23–25]

ANAPLASTIC LARGE-CELL LYMPHOMA, T/NULL CELL, PRIMARY SYSTEMIC TYPE

Anaplastic large-cell lymphoma (ALCL), primary systemic type accounts for 2% to 3% of all NHLs[1] and 10.2% of all T/NK-cell lymphomas.[26] This NHL is usually nodal, although extranodal sites can certainly be involved as well. There are two major subtypes of systemic ALCL: ALK-positive and ALK-negative. ALK-positive systemic ALCL is typically diagnosed in younger patients (median age 34 years, with a male predominance) and ALK-negative in older patients (median age 58 years), although this is not an exclusive cutoff.[26,32] The ALK status of patients with systemic ALCL is very important, as patients with ALK-positive ALCL have a 5-year overall survival of 70%, compared with a 5-year overall survival of 49% for ALK-negative ALCL.[26] The chromosomal translocation t(2;5)(p23;q35) is associated with this type of lymphoma and results in the fusion protein NPM-ALK.[33]

Therapy for ALCL, ALK-positive adult patients typically includes an anthracycline-based regimen and usually produces excellent outcomes.[34] However, patients with ALCL, ALK-negative NHL have a worse outcome and some groups add additional agents or advocate high-dose chemotherapy and autologous stem cell transplantation for this subtype.

ANAPLASTIC LARGE-CELL LYMPHOMA, PRIMARY CUTANEOUS

ALCL, primary cutaneous is a rare type of NK/T-cell lymphoma, occurring in 1.7% of the T-cell lymphomas.[26] It typically presents in one or more areas in the skin, often in the same region of the body. It is most frequently ALK-negative but has in general a fairly good prognosis, with 5-year overall survival of 90% and 5-year progression-free survival of 55%.[26] This pattern indicates an indolent-type of lymphoma with relapses and the ability to treat the patient repeatedly with either chemotherapy or radiotherapy.

EXTRANODAL NK/T-CELL LYMPHOMA, NASAL AND EXTRANASAL (NASAL TYPE)

These lymphomas were previously called "angiocentric lymphomas" and are found mostly in Asia and South and Central America.[35] Nasal NK/T-cell lymphoma is typically seen in the nasal and paranasal sinus areas and is associated with EBV infection.[36] These patients often have localized stage I/II disease but an aggressive clinical course. Patients with extranasal NK/T-cell lymphoma (nasal type) typically present with other extranodal sites of disease (skin, respiratory tract, gastrointestinal, and genitourinary).

Treatment for the localized nasal NK/T-cell lymphomas is typically recommended with radiation, an anthracycline-based chemotherapy, and intrathecal prophylaxis.[37] The 5-year overall survival with this type of lymphoma is 42%, from the International T-cell Study.[26] Patients with advanced extranasal NK/T-cell lymphoma are typically treated with aggressive anthracycline-based chemotherapy regimens; however, the 5-year overall survival is 9%.[26] In some young patients, there has been some success with allogeneic stem cell transplantation in NK/T-cell lymphoma.[30]

HEPATOSPLENIC T-CELL LYMPHOMA

This type of lymphoma represents 1.4% of all T-cell lymphomas and is usually seen in young patients (median age 34 years).[26] Patients typically present with B symptoms, hepatosplenomegaly, anemia, neutropenia, thrombocytopenia, lymphadenopathy, and fevers. Most patients typically have an aggressive clinical course despite treatment with aggressive anthracycline-based therapy.[38] In some young selected patients, an allogeneic stem cell transplant may be an option for successful therapy.

ENTEROPATHY TYPE T-CELL LYMPHOMA

Patients with this type of lymphoma often have a pre-existing history of gluten sensitive Enteropathy. The patients usually present with abdominal pain, weight loss, gastrointestinal bleeding, or bowel perforation. Evidence of serologic markers for celiac disease, such as HLA type (DQA1*0501/DQB1*0201/DRB1*0304) may be present.[39] The 5-year overall survival for this type of NHL is only 20%.[26] Treatment for this type of lymphoma is typically with an anthracycline-based regimen along with nutritional support and a gluten-free diet if appropriate.

SUBCUTANEOUS PANNICULITIS-LIKE T-CELL LYMPHOMA

This rare lymphoma infiltrates the subcutaneous fat without epidermal or dermal involvment, which typically causes plaques or violaceous nodules. Patients often also present with fevers, lung infiltrates, hepatosplenomegaly, jaundice, pancytopenia, and hemophagocytosis syndrome.[40] The patients with the $\gamma\delta$ subtype have a more aggressive clinical course and the patients with the $\alpha\beta$ subtype have a more indolent clinical course.[41] When treatment is warranted for the patients presenting with the more aggressive clinical course, combination chemotherapy with an anthracycline is typically used. Outcomes are dependent on the subtype of subcutaneous panniculitis-like T-cell lymphoma.

ADULT T-CELL LEUKEMIA/LYMPHOMA

Adult T-cell leukemia/lymphoma (ATLL) has four subtypes based on clinicopathologic features and prognosis: acute, lymphoma, chronic, and smoldering. Patients with the acute type present with hypercalcemia, leukemic manifestations, bone and tumor lesions, and have a very poor prognosis with a median survival time of 6 months.[42] Patients with the lymphomatous type typically have nodal, hepatosplenic, bone, and gastrointestinal involvement, and a median survival of 10 months. Patients with the chronic and smoldering type have a more indolent course. The retrovirus HTLV-1 is critical to the development of ATLL.[43] In endemic areas such as southern Japan, up to 40% of the population is infected with the virus. However, ATLL develops in only 2% to 3% of the patients who are carriers of the HTLV-1 virus. The virus is transmitted through sexual intercourse, blood products containing white blood cells, shared needles, breast milk, and through child birth.

The median age at presentation is 55 years. The treatment of acute ATLL is difficult. Patients may initially respond to combination chemotherapy but the long-term overall survival is poor, with a 5-year overall survival of 14%.[26] Clinical trials in ATLL are currently adding agents such as arsenic trioxide, retinoid derivatives, bortezomib and high-dose chemotherapy, and autologous or allogeneic stem cell transplantation to conventional chemotherapy regimens.[44]

NOVEL THERAPIES

Because many of the standard chemotherapies used for other types of NHL do not work well for some subtypes of T-cell NHL, new alternatives are currently being explored. In addition to the ones discussed under the PTCL-NOS section, other alternative agents include monoclonal antibodies (mAb) to T-cell antigens. One such example is zanolimumab, a fully human anti-CD4 mAb. This antibody prevents interaction between the CD4 receptor and the major histocompatibility complex class II molecule, thereby interfering with T-cell activation. This agent has been found to have activity in cutaneous T-cell Lymphoma and is currently being studies in PTCL, with 5 out of 21 patients responding.[45] Other antibodies in early phase trials are siplizumab (a humanized anti-CD2 antibody)[46] and KW-0761 (a humanized antibody to CCR4- chemokine receptor 4).[47] CD 30 monoclonal antibodies, SGN 30 and MDX-060, have also been tested in ALCL.[48,49]

Additional agents of interest in PTCL include targeted kinase inhibitors, such as protein kinase C inhibitor, mTOR inhibitors, aurora kinase inhibitors, and tyrosine kinase inhibitors. In addition, a Syk inhibitor may be attractive as it was found to be expressed on greater than 90% of all PTCL samples tested.[50] An oral Syk inhibitor is currently in phase I/II clinical trials. Other novel agents of interest in T-cell lymphomas include lenalidomide as an immunomodulatory agent and bevacizumab, an antibody targeting vascular endothelial growth factor (particularly in Angioimmunoblastic NHL).

SUMMARY

Peripheral T-cell NHL is a rare and heterogeneous entity that has a poor outcome with conventional combination chemotherapy in many histologic subtypes. As molecular and etiologic knowledge of the subtypes is gained, novel therapeutic options may assist with more directed therapy. Because these diseases are so rare, it is important for patients to participate in clinical trials of new agents as they become available.

REFERENCES

1. A clinical evaluation of the International Lymphoma Study Group classification of non-Hodgkin's lymphoma: the Non-Hodgkin's Lymphoma Classification Project. Blood 1997;89:3909–18.
2. Anderson JR, Armitage JO, Weisenburger DD, et al. Epidemiology of the non-Hodgkin's lymphomas: distributions of the major subtypes differ by geographic locations. Ann Oncol 1998;9:717–20.
3. Takatsuki K, Matsuoka M, Yamaguchi K. Adult T-cell leukemia in Japan. J Acquir Immune Defic Syndr Hum Retrovirol 1996;13(Suppl 1):S15–9.

4. Quintanilla-Martinez L, Kumar S, Fend F, et al. Fulminant EBV + T-cell lymphoproliferative disorders following acute/chronic EBV infection: a distinct clinicopathologic syndrome. Blood 2000;96:443–51.
5. Jaffe ES, Harris NL, Stein H, et al. Pathology and genetics of tumours of haematopoietic and lymphoid tissues. Lyon (France): IARC Press; 2001.
6. Rudiger T, Weisenburger DD, Anderson JR, et al. Peripheral T-cell lymphoma (excluding anaplastic large-cell lymphoma): results from the Non-Hodgkin's Lymphoma Classification Project. Ann Oncol 2002;13:140–9.
7. Gallamini A, Stelitano C, Calvi R, et al. Peripheral T-cell lymphoma unspecified (PTCL-U): a new prognostic model from a retrospective multicenter clinical study. Blood 2004;103:2474–9.
8. Savage KJ, Chhanabhai M, Gascoyne RD, et al. Characterization of peripheral T-cell lymphomas in a single North American institution by the WHO classification. Ann Oncol 2004;15:1467–75.
9. Escalon MP, Liu NS, Yang Y, et al. Prognostic factors and treatment of patients with T-cell non-Hodgkin's lymphoma. Cancer 2005;103:2091–8.
10. Gisselbrecht C, Gaulard P, Lepage E, et al. Prognostic significance of T-cell phenotype in aggressive non-Hodgkin's lymphomas. Blood 1998;92:76–82.
11. Tsimberidou AM, Giles F, Duvic M, et al. Phase II study of pentostatin in advanced T-cell lymphoid malignancies: update of an M.D. Anderson Cancer Center series. Cancer 2004;100:342–9.
12. Yamaguchi M, Kotani T, Nakamure Y, et al. Successful treatment of refractory peripheral T-cell lymphoma with a combination of fludarabine and cyclophosphamide. Int J Hematol 2006;83:450–3.
13. Sallah S, Wan JY, Nguyen NP. Treatment of refractory T-cell malignances using gemcitabine. Br J Haematol 2001;113:185–7.
14. Zinzani PL, Musuraca G, Tani M, et al. Phase II trial of proteasome inhibitor bortezomib in patients with relapsed or refractory cutaneous T-cell lymphoma. J Clin Oncol 2007;25:4293–7.
15. Dang NH, Pro B, Hagemeiser FB, et al. Phase II trial of denileukin diftitox for relapsed/refractory T-cell non-Hodgkin's lymphoma. Br J Haematol 2007;136:439–47.
16. Zinzani PL, Alinari L, Tani M, et al. Preliminary observations of a phase II study of reduced-dose alemtuzumab treatment in patients with pretreated T-cell lymphoma. Haematologica 2005;90:702–3.
17. Piekarz RL, Frye R, Turner M, et al. Responses and molecular markers in patients with peripheral T-cell lymphoma treated on a phase II trial of depsipeptide, FK228. J Clin Oncol 2005;23:3061a.
18. Olsen EA, Kim YH, Kuzel TM, et al. Phase IIb multicenter trial of vorinostat in patients with persistent, progressive, or treatment refractory cutaneous T-cell lymphoma. J Clin Oncol 2007;25:3109–15.
19. O'Connor OA, Hamlin PA, Gerecitano J, et al. Pralatrexate (PDX) produces durable complete remissions in patients with chemotherapy resistant precursor and peripheral T-cell lymphomas: results of the MSKCC phase I/II experience. Blood 2006;108:400a.
20. Kewalramani T, Zelenetz AD, Teruya-Feldstein J, et al. Autologous transplantation for relapsed or primary refractory peripheral T-cell lymphoma. Br J Haematol 2006;134:202–7.
21. Chen AI, McMillan A, Nerin RS, et al. Long term results of autologous hematopoietic cell transplantation (AHCT) for peripheral T-cell lymphoma: the Stanford experience. Blood 2007;110:1906a.

22. Rodriguez J, Conde E, Gutierrez A, et al. Frontline autologous stem cell transplantation in high-risk peripheral T-cell lymphoma: a prospective study from the Gel-Tamo-Study Group. Eur J Haematol 2007;79:3–38.

23. Reimer P, Schertlin T, Rudinger T, et al. Myeloablative radiochemotherpy followed by autologous peripheral blood stem cell transplantation as first-line therapy in peripheral T-cell lymphomas: first results of a prospective multicenter study. Hematol J 2004;5:304–11.

24. Le Gouill S, Milpied N, Buzyn A, et al. Graft-versus-lymphoma effect for aggressive T-cell lymphomas in adults: a study by the Societé Francaise of Greffe de Moelle et de Therapie Cellulaire. J Clin Oncol 2008;26:2264–71.

25. Corradini P, Dodero A, Zallio F, et al. Graft-versus-lymphoma effect in relapsed peripheral T-cell non-Hodgkin's lymphomas after reduced intensity conditioning followed by allogeneic transplantation of hematopoietic cells. J Clin Oncol 2004;22:2172–6.

26. Vose JM. International Peripheral T-cell Lymphoma Study: clinical and pathologic review project: poor outcome by prognostic indices and lack of efficacy with anthracylines. Blood 2005;106:811a.

27. Siegert W, Nerl C, Agthe A, et al. Angioimmunoblastic lymphadenopathy (AILD)-type T-cell lymphoma: prognostic impact of clinical observations and laboratory findings at presentation: the Kiel Lymphoma Study Group. Ann Oncol 1995;6: 659–64.

28. Reiser M, Josting A, Soltani M, et al. T-cell non-Hodgkin's lymphoma in adults: clinicopathological characteristics, response to treatment and prognostic factors. Leuk Lymphoma. 2002;43:805–11.

29. Mourad N, Mounier N, Briere J, et al. Clinical, biologic, and pathologic features in 157 patients with angioimmunoblastic T-cell lymphoma treated within the Groupe d'Etude des Lymphomes de l'Adulte (GELA) trials. Blood 2008;111:4463–70.

30. Advani R, Horowitz S, Zelenetz A, et al. Angioimmunoblastic T-cell lymphoma: treatment experience with cyclosporine. Leuk Lymphoma 2007;48:521–5.

31. Quintini G, Iannitto E, Barbera V, et al. Response to low-dose oral methotrexate and prednisone in two patients with angio-immunoblastic lymphadenopathy-type T-cell lymphoma. Hematol J 2001;2:393–5.

32. Falini B, Pileri S, Zinzani PL, et al. ALK+ lymphoma: clinico-pathological findings and outcome. Blood 1999;93:2697–706.

33. Weisenburger DD, Gordon BG, Vose JM, et al. Occurrence of the t(2;5)(p23p35) in non-Hodgkin's lymphoma. Blood 1996;87:3860–8.

34. Zinzani PL, Bendandi M, Martelli M, et al. Anaplastic large-cell lymphoma: clinical and prognostic evaluation of 90 adult patients. J Clin Oncol 1996;14:955–62.

35. Jaffe ES, Chan JK, Su IJ, et al. Report of the workshop on nasal and related extranodal angiocentric T/natural killer cell lymphomas: definitions, differential diagnosis, and epidemiology. Am J Surg Pathol 1996;20:103–11.

36. Cheung MM, Chan JK, Lau WH, et al. Primary non-Hodgkin's lymphoma of the nose and nasopharynx: clinical features, tumor immunphenotype, and treatment outcome of 113 patients. J Clin Oncol 1998;16:70–7.

37. Kim GE, Lee SW, Chang SK, et al. Combined chemotherapy and radiation versus radiation alone in the management of localized angiocentric lymphoma of the head and neck. Radiother Oncol 2001;61:261–9.

38. Belhadj K, Reyes F, Farcet JP, et al. Hepatosplenic γδ T-cell lymphoma is a rare clinicopathologic entity with poor outcome: report on a series of 21 patients. Blood 2003;102:4261–9.

39. Howell WM, Leung ST, Jones DB, et al. HLA-DRB, DQA, and DQB polymorphism in celiac disease and Enteropathy-associated T-cell lymphoma: common features and additional risk factors for malignancy. Hum Immunol 1995;43:29–37.
40. Salhany KE, Macon WR, Choi JK, et al. Subcutaneous panniculitis-like T-cell lymphoma: clinicopathologic, immunophenotypic, and genotypic analysis of alpha/beta and gamma/delta subtypes. Am J Surg Pathol. 1998;22:881–93.
41. Willemze R, Jansen PM, Cerroni L, et al. Subcutaneous panniculitis-like T-cell lymphoma: definition, classification, and prognostic factors: an EORTC Cutaneous Lymphoma Group Study of 83 patients. Blood 2008;111:838–45.
42. Shimoyama M. Diagnostic criteria and classification of clinical subtypes of adult T-cell leukaemia-lymphoma: a report from the Lymphoma Study Group (1984–1987). Br J Haematol 1991;79:428–37.
43. Chen YC, Wang CH, Su IJ, et al. Infection of human T-cell leukemia virus type I and development of human T-cell leukemia lymphoma in patients with hematologic neoplasms: a possible linkage to blood transfusion. Blood 1989;74:388–94.
44. Ishitsuka K, Tamura K. Treatment of adult T-cell leukemia/lymphoma: past, present, and future. Eur J Haematol 2008;80:185–96.
45. d'Amore F, Radford J, Jerkeman M, et al. Zanolimumab (HuMax CD4), a fully human monoclonal antibody: efficacy and safety in patients with relapsed or treatment-refractory non-cutaneous CD4+ T-cell lymphoma. Blood 2007;110:3409a.
46. Casale DA, Barlett NL, Hurd DD, et al. A phase I open label dose escalation study to evaluate MEDI-507 in patients with CD2-positive T-cell lymphoma/leukemia. Blood 2006;108:2727a.
47. Uike N, Tsukasaki K, Utsunomiya A, et al. Phase I study of KW-0761, a humanized anti-CCR4 antibody in patients with relapsed or refractory adult T-cell leukemia/lymphoma (ATLL) and peripheral T-cell lymphoma (PTCL): preliminary results. Blood 2007;110:4492a.
48. Forero-Torres A, Bernstein S, Gopal A, et al. SGN-30 (anti-CD30 monoclonal antibody) is active and well tolerated in patients with refractory or recurrent systemic anaplastic large cell lymphoma. Blood 2004;104:2637a.
49. Ansell SM, Byrd JC, Horwitz SM, et al. Phase I/II open-label dose-escalating study of MDX-060 administered weekly for 4 weeks in subjects with refractory/relapsed CD30 positive lymphoma. Blood 2004;104:2636a.
50. Feldman AL, Sun DX, Law ME, et al. Syk tyrosine kinase is overexpressed in the majority of peripheral T- and NK-cell lymphomas, and represents a potential therapeutic target. Blood 2007;110:690a.

New Drugs for the Treatment of Lymphoma

Luca Paoluzzi, MD[a], Yukiko Kitagawa, MD[a], Matko Kalac, MD[a],
Jasmine Zain, MD[b], Owen A. O'Connor, MD, PhD[b],*

KEYWORDS

• New drugs • Bcl-2 • Lymphoma • Syk • Pralatrexate

During the last decade the development of new drugs for the treatment of hematologic malignancies has come of age. Historically, most drugs developed for treatment of leukemias, lymphomas, and myeloma had already been proven in the solid tumor setting; rarely did the pharmaceutical industry set out to develop a new drug for a hematologic malignancy. This pattern changed when the drug imatinib showed that it was possible to nullify the pathognomic genetic lesion in chronic myelogenous leukemia (CML). Since the approval of imatinib for CML, a host of new drugs have emerged, some of which have a monofocal emphasis in the hematologic malignancies. Some of these drugs represent first-in-class molecules targeting unique biology influenced by conventional agents. Some are promising new chemical platforms modeled after more traditional agents, with the hope of improved efficacy and tolerability. Drugs such as bortezomib, vorinostat, thalidomide, and clofarabine have emerged as agents with proven activity in myeloma, mantle cell lymphoma (MCL), cutaneous T-cell lymphoma, and T-cell lymphoblastic leukemia. Despite their effects on a target theoretically important across many types of cancer, these agents have proven to have minimal activity in the solid tumors. Drugs targeting unique disease-specific pathways also have found potential applicability in treating malignancies such as CML (nilotinib), CD20-positive non-Hodgkin's lymphoma (NHL) (rituximab), follicular lymphoma (Bcl-2-targeted agents), and other B-cell neoplasia (splenic tyrosine kinase [Syk] inhibitors; IkB kinase inhibitors). Finally, many new drugs that represent improvements over older

[a] Herbert Irving Comprehensive Cancer Center, Columbia University, 1130 St. Nicholas Avenue, Room 216, New York, NY 10032, USA
[b] Herbert Irving Comprehensive Cancer Center, College of Physicians and Surgeons, The New York Presbyterian Hospital, Columbia University, 1130 St. Nicholas Avenue, Room 216, New York, NY 10032, USA
* Corresponding author. Lymphoid Development and Malignancy Program, Herbert Irving Comprehensive Cancer Center, College of Physicians and Surgeons, The New York Presbyterian Hospital, Columbia University, New York, NY.
E-mail address: oo2130@columbia.edu (O.A. O'Connor).

Hematol Oncol Clin N Am 22 (2008) 1007–1035
doi:10.1016/j.hoc.2008.07.006
0889-8588/08/$ – see front matter © 2008 Published by Elsevier Inc.
hemonc.theclinics.com

established agents have come of age, such as pralatrexate (a methotrexate derivative) in T-cell lymphoma, clofarabine (a nucleoside analogue) in T-cell acute lymphoblastic leukemia, lenalidomide (a new-generation immunomodulatory drug related to thalidomide) in myeloma and myelodysplastic syndrome, carfilzomib (a new-generation proteasome inhibitor) in myeloma, and a host of histone deacetylase inhibitors (mechanistically similar to vorinostat) in peripheral T-cell lymphoma, Hodgkin's disease, cutaneous T-cell lymphoma, and other hematologic malignancies. These examples demonstrate a new understanding that the hematologic malignancies are a fertile and productive arena for the development of innovative treatment strategies.

This article highlights some of these areas of innovative drug development, when possible emphasizing the biologic basis for the platform and linking this essential biology to the biochemical pharmacology. The article focuses on the many new targets including Syk, Bcl-2, and the phosphoinositide-3 kinase (PI3K)/AKT/mammalian target of rapamycin (mTOR) pathway (**Table 1**).

Table 1
Examples of novel targeted approaches for the treatment of lymphoma

Mechanism	Drugs	Rationale
Inhibit antiapoptotic Bcl-2 family members	ABT-737/263 AT-101 GX015- Oblimersen	Silence the anti-apoptotic influence of Bcl-2, Bcl-xl, Bcl-w, and Mcl-1
Modulate proapoptotic family members and BH3-only proteins	Proteasome inhibitors (Bortezomib, PR-171)	Up-regulating derepression of pro-apoptotic family members will lead to induction of programmed cell death
Down-regulate cyclin D1 and related isoforms	Cyclin D1 antisense (ASDON) Histone deacetylase inhibitors (SAHA)	Down-regulating cyclin D1 and related isoforms will decrease the driving force for cells to transition from G1 into S phase, producing cell-cycle arrest
Increase cell-cycle–dependent kinase inhibitors such as p27/p21	Proteasome inhibitors HDACI	A relative increase in Cdk inhibitors will provide the "breaks" in cell-cycle proliferation, inducing cell cycle arrest
Inhibit pan–cell-cycle–dependent kinases	Flavopiridol AG-024322	Induce cell-cycle arrest
Inhibit selective cell-cycle–dependent kinases	PD-0332991 (cdk4/6) CINK4 (cdk4/6) Seliciclib (cdk2/1) BMS-387,032 (cdk2/1) PNU-252,808 (cdk2/1) PNU-252,808 (cdk2/1) NU6102, NU6140 (cdk2/1)	Inhibit specific phase transitions of cell-cycle progression
Inhibit protein translation and signaling pathways mediated through tyrosine kinase receptors and Ras	mTOR inhibitors (most derived from rapamycin, including temsirolimus), AKT inhibitor	Associated with a broad effect on cancer cell biology, including translation, NF-kB, transcription factors, and apoptosis

TARGETING SURVIVAL PATHWAYS
Biology of Apoptosis

In the early 1970s, apoptosis was recognized as an intrinsic cellular program that was thought to play a complementary role in mitosis in regulating tissue homeostasis.[1] About 15 years later, the Bcl-2 gene was discovered in a B-cell lymphoma, which was associated with the promotion of cell survival. The inhibition of apoptosis was recognized as a central step in tumor development, and the demonstration that Bcl-2 cooperated with the transcription factor Myc to affect transformation established the importance of both proliferation and survival defects in oncogenesis.[2] During the 1990s, several sentinel studies established (1) the marked evolutionary conservation of the apoptotic machinery; (2) the central role of cysteine proteases, later called "caspases," in the apoptotic cascade; (3) the existence of pro- and anti-apoptotic relatives of Bcl-2 which, through specific interactions, modulate the balance of pro- and anti-apoptotic fates; and (4) the existence of at least two distinct pathways leading to apoptosis in mammalian cells, one involving the mitochondria (the intrinsic pathway) and the other involving cell-surface death receptors (the extrinsic pathway).[3-6] During a relatively short period of time, most of the elements required to appreciate the importance of these survival pathways in cancer biology were elucidated, laying the groundwork for rational therapeutic intervention.

All Bcl-2 family members contain characteristic regions of homology termed "Bcl-2 homology" (BH) domains. Members of this family can be divided into three groups based on their structures and functions. The anti-apoptotic (pro-survival) group, BH1, including Bcl-2, Bcl-X$_L$, Mcl-1, Bcl-w, and A1, contains four BH domains. The second group, BH2, including BAX and BAK, is pro-apoptotic and contains multiple BH domains.[7] The third group is more commonly referred to as the "BH3-only proteins" and includes at least eight members (Bad, BID, Bik, Bim, Bmf, Hrk, Noxa, and PUMA). These proteins display sequence homology with other Bcl-2 family members only within the amphipathic and α-helical BH3 segments.[8] Structural studies revealed that the BH1, BH2, and BH3 domains in the anti-apoptotic proteins fold into a globular domain containing a hydrophobic groove on its surface.[9] The α-helical BH3 domains of pro-apoptotic proteins bind to this hydrophobic groove and neutralize the anti-apoptotic proteins.[10] In healthy cells, basal levels of anti-apoptotic proteins prevent BAX and BAK from being activated. Upon the induction of apoptotic signals, BH3-only proteins are activated and bind competitively to the hydrophobic grooves of the anti-apoptotic proteins through their BH3 domain.[11] This action displaces BAX and BAK and allows them to form multimers that permeabilize the mitochondrial outer membrane. Most, if not all, apoptotic signals transmitted by BH3 domains converge through BAX and BAK.[12]

Once a cell becomes committed to apoptosis, a cascade of downstream events is triggered to execute cell death, including collapse of the mitochondrial membrane potential, release of the apoptogenic mitochondrial proteins such as cytochrome c, SMAC/Diablo, and apoptosis inducing factor, and activation of caspases.[13,14] The relative levels of BH3-only proteins and their pro-survival relatives is crucial in establishing the threshold for commitment of a cell to undergo programmed cell death and therefore for the control of tissue homeostasis.[15]

The extrinsic pathway of apoptosis is centered on the role of tumor necrosis factor–related apoptosis-inducing ligand (TRAIL) and its receptors. TRAIL induces apoptosis by binding to the DR4 and DR5 receptors, causing the intracellular death domains of these receptors to trimerize, leading to the recruitment of Fas-associated protein with death domain molecule and activation of caspase 8, caspase 3, and caspase 7. Caspase 8 activation further amplifies the death signal by activating the intrinsic apoptosis pathway by cleaving the Bcl2 family member BID (**Fig. 1**). Cleaved BID binds to BAX and BAK, causing the release of cytochrome *c* and SMAC from the mitochondria, activating caspase 9 and other downstream caspases. Clearly, a detailed understanding of this complicated biology has created enormous opportunity for adjusting the threshold required for the induction of apoptosis in tumor cells.

Pharmacologic Modulation of Apoptotic Pathways

The following sections introduce the major molecules moving through early-phase clinical trials (**Table 2**). During the past several decades, an understanding of the complexities of the survival pathways has provided a fertile arena for formulating new strategies for targeting these pathways in human cancer. The experimental therapies

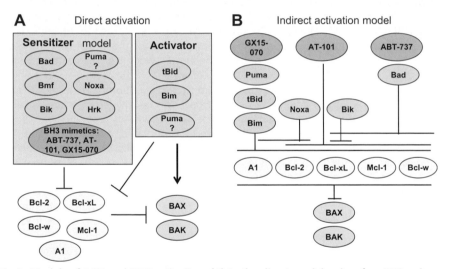

Fig. 1. Models of BAX and BAK activation. (*A*) In the direct model only a few BH3-only proteins (activators) are able to bind and activate BAX and BAK directly; most of BH3-only proteins can bind only to the pro-survival proteins and act as sensitizers, displacing the activators and allowing them to interact with BAX and BAK. (*Data from* Letai A, Bassik MC, Walensky LD, et al. Distinct BH3 domains either sensitive or activate mitochondrial apoptosis, serving as prototype cancer therapeutics. Cancer Cell 2002;2:183–92; and Kuwana T, Bouchier-Hayes L, Chipuk JE, et al. BH3 domains of BH3-only proteins differentially regulate BAX-mediated mitochondrial membrane permeabilization both directly and indirectly. Mol Cell 2005;17:525–35; and Certo M, Del Gaizo Moore V, Nishino M, et al. Mitochondria primed by death signals determine cellular addiction to antiapoptotic BCL-2 family members. Cancer Cell 2006;9(5):351–65.) (*B*) In the indirect activation model BH3-only proteins have a binding profile that is different from that of the pro-apoptotic proteins; the BH3-only proteins that are able to engage all the pro-survival proteins are the most potent inducers of apoptosis. (*Data from* Chen L, Willis SN, Wei A, et al. Differential targeting of prosurvival Bcl-2 proteins by their BH3-only ligands allows complementary apoptotic function. Mol Cell 2005;17(3):393–403; and Willis SN, Chen L, Dewson G, et al. Proapoptotic BAK is sequestered by Mcl-1 and Bcl-xL, but not Bcl-2, until displayed by BH3-only proteins. Genes Dev 2005;19(11):1294-305; and Willis SN, Fletcher JI, Kaufmann T, et al. Apoptosis initiated when BH3 ligands engage multiple Bcl-2 homologs, not BAK or BAK. Science 2007;315(5813):856–9.)

Table 2
Bcl-2–targeted agents in clinical trials

Agent	Development Status	Dose and Schedule	Dose-Limiting Toxicities/Toxicities	Activity
ABT-263[47]	Phase I and II (hematologic malignancies)	Escalating	DLTs: elevated liver function tests, thrombocytopenia arrhythmia	OR = 3/23(SLL/ CLL, 1 NK-T)
Obatoclax mesylate (GX15-070)[30,31]	Phase 1 and 2 (hematologic malignancies)	Up to 60 mg, 24-h infusion, every 2 weeks or 45 mg/d on days 1, 4, 8, and 11	DLT: QT prolongation. Other toxicities: neurologic (euphoria, gait disturbance, headache, dizziness), gastrointestinal (nausea, diarrhea), edema, weight loss, chills, hyperhydrosis, febrile neutropenia, cough, chest pain	1 complete response (acute myeloid leukemia) 1 partial response (myelodys-plastic syndrome)
AT-101[26]	Phase II (+ rituximab, CLL)	AT-101 intermittent (80 mg on days 1–3 and 15–17 every 28 days) versus continuous (30 mg/d for 3 weeks)	DLTs: none Other toxicities: gastrointestinal (liver function tests)	Intermittent: partial response = 3/6 Continuous: partial response = 5/12

Abbreviations: NK-T, natural killer T-cell; OR, overall response.

focused on this biology are directed toward the following major areas of basic and translational research: (1) the synthesis and development of new small molecules capable of nullifying the anti-apoptotic effects of Bcl-2 family members; (2) the development of TRAIL receptor agonists that stimulate the extrinsic apoptotic pathways; and (3) the development of X-linked inhibitor of apoptosis protein (XIAP) inhibitors.

Recently, many small-molecule inhibitors of anti-apoptotic family members have begun to emerge. A number of compounds targeting anti-apoptotic proteins such as Bcl-2 and Bcl-X_L have been identified through a variety of methods, including computational modeling, structure-based design, and high-throughput screening of natural products and synthetic libraries. The following sections introduce the major molecules moving through early-phase clinical trials.

Biochemical pharmacology of gossypol derivatives

Gossypol is an orally available compound found in cottonseeds originally used as an herbal medicine in China.[16] The (-)-enantiomer ((-)-gossypol; AT-101), binds to the BH3-binding grooves of Bcl-2, Bcl-X_L, and Mcl-1, displacing BH3 peptides with a sub-micromolar concentration of (IC_{50}).[17] This enantiomer promotes an allosteric conformational change in Bcl-2 and loss of mitochondrial membrane potential in a BAX/BAK–independent fashion.[18] (-)-Gossypol induces cytochrome *c* release from mitochondria and activation of several caspases and recently has been demonstrated to improve the efficacy of a combination chemotherapy regimen (cyclophosphamide, doxorubicin, vincristine, and prednisolone) as well as a biochemotherapy-based regimen in lymphoma xenograft models.[19,20] Several attempts have been made to generate semi-synthetic analogues of gossypol with improved pharmacologic properties. Apogossypol was synthesized and characterized using a combination of approaches including molecular modeling, magnetic resonance-based structural analysis, fluorescence polarization assays, and cell-based assays.[21] Apogossypol binds to and inhibits Bcl-2, Bcl-X$_L$, Mcl-1, Bcl-w, and Bcl-B with high affinity, inducing apoptosis in tumor cell lines in the submicromolar range, and is active in transgenic mouse models of follicular lymphoma.[22]

TW-37 is another rationally designed gossypol derivative based on computer modeling of the BH3 domain of Bim.[23] It binds to Bcl-2, Bcl-X$_L$, and Mcl-1 with high affinity. Preclinical studies have shown that TW-37 is effective against a variety of NHL and leukemia cell lines with minimal toxicity to normal peripheral blood lymphocytes.[24,25]

Clinical pharmacology of AT-101 A phase II open-label trial presently is evaluating the efficacy of AT-101 in combination with rituximab in patients who have relapsed or refractory chronic lymphocytic leukemia (CLL).[26] Previous experiences have compared high area under the curve (AUC) exposures (treatment on days 1, 3, 5, 8, 15, 22, 29, 31, 33, 40, 57, 59, 61) with high maximum plasma concentration (C$_{max}$) or pulse schedules (80 mg/d on days 1–3 and 15–17 of each 28-day cycle), in combination with weekly rituximab. Gastrointestinal toxicity, the most notable adverse effect of AT-101 with daily administration, seemed to be reduced with intermittent exposures. Apoptosis of primary CLL cells was seen in 18% to 45% of cells in four of the six patients at the C$_{max}$ after a single 80-mg dose of AT-101. By comparison, apoptosis after a 30-mg dose of AT-101 was detected in approximately 1% to 15% of cells. After 80 mg of AT-101, plasma concentrations of up to 6.6 μM were observed, compared with concentrations of approximately 0.8 to 1.8 μM after a 30-mg dose in the cohort of patients receiving a daily dose. In the cohort of patients receiving pulse AT-101, partial responses were observed in three of six patients; the other three patients are still undergoing treatment. Five of 12 patients in the previously reported group receiving continuous-exposure AT-101 had a partial response. The authors concluded that intermittent administration of AT-101 with a pulsed dose exposure was associated with higher C$_{max}$, leading to an increased pro-apoptotic effect in vivo, with less toxicity than seen with daily dosing. Enrollment continues to confirm these observations and to assess the merits of combining AT-101 with rituximab.

Biochemical pharmacology of obatoclax Obatoclax (GX015-070) is an indole derivative and a broad-spectrum inhibitor of pro-survival Bcl-2 family proteins.[27] It activates the mitochondrial apoptotic pathway by displacing BAK from Mcl-1 and Bcl-X$_L$, upregulating Bim, and inducing BAX and BAK conformational changes, mitochondrial depolarization, and caspase activation. It synergizes with the proteasome inhibitor bortezomib in MCL cells without enhancing cytotoxicity to peripheral blood mononuclear cells from healthy donors.[28] As a single agent or in combination with melphalan, dexamethasone, or bortezomib, GX015-070 is effective against cultured or patient-derived multiple myeloma cells.[29]

Clinical pharmacology of obatoclax A multicenter study is exploring a prolonged infusion schedule to minimize toxicities while maintaining clinical activity.[30] Twenty-one patients received obatoclax in doses between 20 and 28 mg/m^2/24 h weekly (n = 9) or 20 mg/m^2/24 h for 2, 3, or 4 consecutive days every 2 to 3 weeks (n = 12). The cohort treated at the final dose level of 28 mg/m^2/24 h for 4 days is accruing now. The most common adverse events were euphoric mood (57%), fatigue (57%), febrile neutropenia (43%), gait disturbance (43%), chills (33%), diarrhea (33%), nausea (33%), somnolence (33%), and dizziness (29%). All were of grade 1 or 2 except for grade 3 febrile neutropenia in seven patients, and grade 3 diarrhea, fatigue, and gait disturbance, each in one patient. Interestingly, no dose-limiting toxicities (DLTs) were observed. Plasma concentrations of obatoclax reached a steady state before end of infusion. Mean C_{max} values at 20 mg/m^2/24 h during 1 × 24, 2 × 24, 3 × 24, 4 × 24 h, and 28 mg/m^2/24 h during 1 × 24 h infusions were 15.3, 8.4, 10.1, 15.7, and 10.8 ng/mL, respectively. The mean $AUC_{(0-tlast)}$ values at 20 mg/m^2/24 h associated with 1 × 24, 2 × 24, 3 × 24, 4 × 24 h, and 28 mg/m^2/24 h associated with 1 × 24 h infusions were 264.3, 396.9, 624.3, 1109.3, and 211.1 ng · hr/mL, respectively, increasing proportionately as a function of dose and duration of the infusion. One patient who had treatment-related acute myelogenous leukemia (AML) achieved a cytogenetic complete response with complete hematologic recovery and transfusion independence on day 9 after the start of weekly 24-h infusions of obatoclax. This complete response was sustained for more than 8 months while the patient received a total of 35 weekly infusions of 20 mg/m^2 without cumulative toxicities. The infusional schedules described here will be attractive for combining with standard chemotherapy regimens for AML.

Borthakur and colleagues[31] recently reported the results of a phase I trial of obatoclax administered by a 24-hour infusion every 2 weeks to patients who had myeloid malignancies and CLL. This trial was designed to evaluate the potential of prolonged infusions to minimize toxicities while maintaining optimal clinical activity. Fourteen patients (three to six patients in each cohort) have been treated at doses ranging from 7 to 40 mg/m^2 over 24 hours every 2 weeks using a modified accelerated-titration design doubling the dose to a maximum of 28 mg/m^2. At doses of 28 mg/m^2 or less, low-grade toxicities included dizziness (2/9), headache (2/9), euphoric mood (2/9) (all < grade 1) and grade 2 somnolence (2/9). At the dose level of 40 mg/m^2, DLTs of grade 3 QTc prolongation with no accompanying arrhythmias were reported in two of five patients, both of whom had QTc prolongation at baseline. Other toxicities included grade 2 somnolence (4/5), grade 1 euphoric mood (3/5), grade 1 anxiety (2/5), and single episodes of dizziness, dysarthria, dysphasia, confusion, hallucination, and disorientation. The pharmacokinetic profile of obatoclax following a 24-h intravenous infusion was dose proportional for both C_{max} and AUC_{24h}. Induction of apoptosis was monitored quantitatively with serial determinations of plasma concentration of histone-oligonucleosomal DNA complexes. An early release of oligonucleosomal DNA greater than fourfold over baseline occurred in 10 of 14 patients by the midpoint of the infusion and was sustained through the end of the infusion. The rapid elimination of the plasma obatoclax concentration immediately after the end of infusion was associated with a decline in the plasma oligonucleosomal DNA level; however, multiple additional peaks of oligonucleosomal DNA concentrations occurring over days following the infusion were detected in 9 of 14 patients. Three of eight patients who had myelodysplastic syndrome showed hematologic improvement with independence from red blood cell or platelet transfusion. Bone marrow blasts were reduced from 14% to 4% in another patient who had secondary myelodysplastic syndrome. The authors concluded that single-agent obatoclax is well tolerated when administered as a 24-h continuous infusion, with abrogation of previously noted infusional central nervous system toxicities. Biologic and clinical activity were retained. Further prolongation of the infusion may lead to more robust activity and will be explored. Phase II single-agent trials using doses of 28 mg/m^2 over 24 hours every 2 weeks have been initiated in patients who have myelofibrosis and previously untreated myelodysplastic syndrome with anemia and/or thrombocytopenia to evaluate further the potential for hematologic improvement in response to obatoclax.

Biochemical pharmacology of 1-aminobenzotriazole derivatives

Aminobenzotriazole (ABT)-737 is a synthetic small molecule that may be the most potent and specific Bcl-2/Bcl-X_L inhibitor in development to date.[32] ABT-737 has extremely high affinity for Bcl-X_L, Bcl-2, and Bcl-w, with a dissociation constant below 1 nM for each Bcl family member, although it binds poorly to Mcl-1 and A1. Mechanistic studies reveal that ABT-737 is similar to the BH3 domain of Bad. By itself ABT-737 does not bind to BAX, but it disrupts the complex of BAX and Bcl-2 and triggers conformational alteration of BAX. ABT-737 also displaces BH3-only proteins such as Bim from its binding partners. Importantly, the effects of ABT-737 are completely abrogated in BAX- and BAK-deficient cells.[33] This strict dependence on BAX and BAK distinguishes ABT-737 from other small-molecule Bcl-2/Bcl-X_L inhibitors and substantiates its function as an authentic BH3 mimetic. As a single agent, ABT-737 is efficacious against small-cell lung carcinoma (SCLC) and several lymphoid malignancies including follicular lymphoma, diffuse large B-cell lymphoma (DLBCL), CLL, acute lymphocytic leukemia, and acute myeloid leukemia with IC_{50s} in the nanomolar range and in multiple myeloma with IC_{50s} in the micromolar range. Apoptosis induced by ABT-737 is associated with dissociation of pro-apoptotic and anti-apoptotic Bcl-2 family members, conformational change of BAX, cytochrome c release from the mitochondria, and activation of caspases.[34–37]

ABT-737 exhibits striking synergy when combined with γ-irradiation and with a variety of anticancer agents including etoposide, doxorubicin, cisplatin, melphalan, ara-C, paclitaxel, vincristine, dexamethasone, thalidomide, and bortezomib.[38,39] It also has been shown to enhance the anticancer effects of several investigational agents, such as the cyclin-dependent kinase inhibitor roscovitine and the MDM2 inhibitor Nutlin-3a.[40] Like other Bcl-2–targeted agents, ABT-737 seems to have minimal toxicity against normal hematopoietic cells and bone marrow cells.

Interestingly, Mcl-1 expression plays a major role in causing ABT-737 resistance. Leukemia and SCLC cells expressing relatively higher levels of Bcl-2 and Bcl-X_L and lower levels of Mcl-1 were found to be most sensitive to ABT-737. Conversely, cells expressing high levels of Mcl-1 were resistant to ABT-737.[41,42] Unbiased genomic analysis and siRNA library screening also identified Mcl-1 and Noxa as modulators of ABT-737 sensitivity.[43] Furthermore, combining ABT-737 with agents that decrease Mcl-1 expression, such as the cyclin-dependent kinase inhibitor roscovitine and protein synthesis inhibitor cycloheximide, markedly boosted the effects of ABT-737 in human leukemia and SCLC cell lines. These studies validated the specificity and molecular mechanisms of ABT-737 and provided a rationale for targeting Mcl-1 to improve its therapeutic effects. ABT-737 is likely to be most efficacious as a single agent for targeting tumors in which Mcl-1 expression is low, absent, or inactivated, such as follicular lymphoma, CLL, and SCLC. For tumors in which Mcl-1 is the predominant survival protein, ABT-737 is unlikely to be effective as a single agent but may serve to enhance therapies that down-regulate Mcl-1. Combination therapies using genotoxic agents and ABT-737 could be particularly effective, because many genotoxic drugs induce Mcl-1 degradation.[44] Furthermore, the rapid turnover of *Mcl-1* mRNA and protein provide the rationale for combining ABT-737 with inhibitors of transcription or translation, such as cyclin-dependent kinase inhibitors and multi-kinase inhibitors. Mcl-1 degradation is regulated by the ubiquitin E3 ligase Mule,[45] which theoretically could be manipulated to enhance the therapeutic effects of ABT-737. Although ABT-737 seems to be well tolerated in animals, its ability to inhibit several pro-survival proteins in normal cells might be a concern for causing adverse effects. For example, ABT-737 causes dose-dependent acute thrombocytopenia by reducing the number of circulating platelets, whose turnover is regulated by apoptosis.[46] Platelets are particularly sensitive to ABT-737, perhaps because of BAK-dependent apoptosis that normally is constrained by Bcl-X$_L$ in these cells. Avoiding unwanted apoptosis in normal cells will be a major issue confronted in future clinical applications of this and related drugs.

Clinical development of ABT-263 ABT-263 is being investigated in three phase I/IIa studies in patients who have lymphoid malignancies, SCLC/solid tumors, and CLL. In a multicenter study, patients who had lymphoid malignancies were enrolled to determine first the maximum tolerated dose, the DLT, and the recommended phase II dose.[47] For each 21-day cycle, patients received ABT-263 orally each day for 14 consecutive days followed by 7 days off drug. The phase IIa portion of the study is evaluating ABT-263 in up to 40 subjects who have follicular and aggressive NHL to obtain additional safety information and a preliminary assessment of efficacy. Presently, 17 subjects have been enrolled in the lymphoma study. Cohorts of three subjects each have completed the 10-, 20-, 40-, and 80-mg dose levels thus far. A grade 3 DLT occurred in the 160-mg cohort, so that cohort was expanded to six participants. Two patients in the 40- and 160-mg cohorts who had bulky CLL/small lymphocytic lymphoma (SLL) experienced 95% and 64% tumor reductions after cycles four and two, respectively, and continue on treatment. The pharmakinetic profile of ABT-263 is linear between the 10-mg and 160-mg dose levels. The average terminal half-life of ABT-263 varies between 14 and 25 hours across all dose levels, and ABT-263 reduces the platelet level in a dose-dependent manner. These studies have established that ABT-263 is a novel, orally bioavailable, and active small-molecule Bcl-2 family protein inhibitor with preliminary evidence of activity in lymphoid malignancies.

Targeting the tumor necrosis factor–related apoptosis-inducing ligand receptors
The death receptors of the tumor necrosis factor super-family represent potential targets for promoting apoptosis in cancer. Because death receptor–mediated apoptosis is thought to be independent of *p53*, cancers with inactivating *p53* mutations may be susceptible to this targeted approach. In an attempt to develop effective agents for the treatment of cancer by triggering TRAIL receptors, agonistic antibodies against DR4[48] and DR5[49,50] have been generated. These antibodies induce apoptosis in cancer cells, but not in normal cells, and in xenograft tumor models slow the growth of tumors with minimal systemic toxicity. Antibodies have the advantage of having a relatively long half-life and can exploit additional mechanisms for cell killing through antibody-dependent cellular cytotoxicity and complement-dependent cytotoxicity.[51] Approaches for targeting TRAIL receptors currently are being tested in the clinic with phase I and/or phase II clinical trials exploring recombinant TRAIL and the agonistic antibodies targeting DR4 (mapatumumab) and DR5 (lexatumumab). A phase II study with mapatumumab in patients who had relapsed or refractory NHL reported three responses in 14 patients who had follicular lymphoma including one complete response.[52] Another approach for pharmacologically triggering the TRAIL receptors involves the use of soluble truncated versions of TRAIL that contain the extracellular domain. In preclinical studies, recombinant TRAIL induced apoptosis in various cancer cell lines, including those with *p53* mutations, without affecting normal cells. In addition, chemotherapeutic drugs and histone deacetylase inhibitors were shown to augment the apoptotic activity of TRAIL.[53,54] When given as a single agent, TRAIL also displayed anti-tumor activity in vivo in mouse models of multiple myeloma.[55]

Although some recombinant forms of TRAIL have been shown to be toxic to hepatocytes and other normal cells, these effects are thought to be related to the particular recombinant forms of the protein rather than to TRAIL itself.[56] Safety evaluations in primates with TRAIL that did not contain extraneous amino acid residues showed no toxicities related to TRAIL exposure.[57]

Targeting the inhibitors of apoptosis

The inhibitors of apoptosis (IAPs) are important regulators of apoptosis that function by binding to and inhibiting caspases.[58] The most comprehensively studied IAP, XIAP, inhibits caspase 3, caspase 7, and caspase 9.The inhibition of XIAP and other IAPs represents a potential mechanism for inducing apoptosis and treating cancer.[59] The XIAP protein is overexpressed in many cancers, and the expression of XIAP correlates with apoptotic resistance. Knockdown of *XIAP* by antisense oligonucleotides or RNA interference induces apoptosis in cancer cell lines and promotes the synergistic killing of cancer cells by TRAIL and actinomycin D. In addition to using antisense oligonucleotides for targeting *XIAP*, peptidic and non-peptidic inhibitors of XIAP have been studied. Cell-permeable SMAC peptides can enhance the apoptotic effects of chemotherapeutic agents in vitro and in vivo. SMAC peptidomimetics have been shown to induce caspase activation and apoptosis potently in cancer cells and to inhibit the growth of tumors in xenograft mouse models.[60,61] All-molecule inhibitors of XIAP that induce apoptosis and small molecules that disrupt the XIAP–caspase 3 interaction have been described also.[62,63] At present, however, it is unclear how they disrupt this interaction. A different member of the IAP family is survivin,[64] the smallest member of this family. In addition to inhibiting apoptosis (probably by a mechanism different from that used by XIAP), survivin has an important function in mitosis. Survivin is expressed during mitosis and binds to various components of the mitotic apparatus. Except for its cell-cycle–dependent expression, survivin is not present in most normal adult tissues but is overexpressed in many different tumors and is important for tumor cell viability.[65] Approaches for inhibiting survivin include the use of antisense oligonucleotides, vaccination strategies against survivin-bearing tumor cells, and inhibiting the phosphorylation of survivin to create a dominant-negative phenotype.[66]

Conclusion

Clearly, the complex biology that contributes to the survival advantage of transformed cells represents one of the most exciting opportunities for treating many human cancers. The lymphoid neoplasias commonly are characterized by defects in various Bcl-2 family members. A plethora of novel small molecules, each with its own distinct pharmacology, represent a potentially important strategy for modulating the threshold required to induce programmed cell death. Without question, most investigators believe the real value of these agents will be in combination with other DNA-damaging agents: in theory, the potential of the Bcl-2–targeted drugs to lower the threshold required to induce apoptosis could improve the efficiency of tumor cell kill.

TARGETING B-CELL RECEPTOR SIGNALING PATHWAYS

B-Cell Receptor Signaling

The B-cell antigen receptor is a hallmark of B lymphocytes and is central to their development and immune response.[67] Tyrosine kinases are essential for transducing signals from the cell-surface receptors on B and T cells after receptor activation (**Fig. 2**). B-cell ontogeny is a multistep process that begins with the sequential rearrangements of the immunoglobulin heavy- and light-chain locus and the expression of the B-cell receptor (BCR) on the cell surface, which defines a B lymphocyte. The

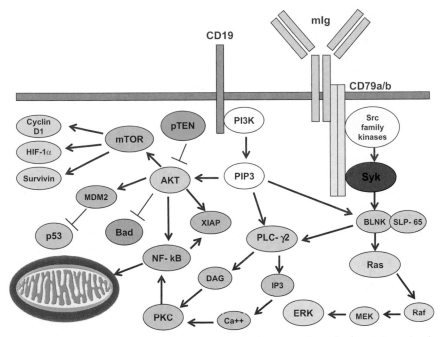

Fig. 2. A simplified account of known signaling pathways activated after BCR activation. CD19 is an important co-receptor that is activated in response to BCR ligation. Cell growth and proliferation, angiogenesis, and inhibition of apoptosis result from the activation of multiple intracellular pathways including the PI3K/AKT/mTor and NF-kB pathways.

signaling ability of this receptor seems to be mandatory for developmental progression of the B cell into a memory cell or a mature plasma cell.

A functional BCR is composed of an antigen-binding component produced by rearrangements of heavy- and light-chain genes noncovalently linked to the signal-transducing elements Igα (CD79a) and Igβ (CD79b). Antigen binding leads to receptor aggregation and phosphorylation of tyrosine-based activation motifs present in the cytoplasmic domain of the receptor complex, aided by the Scr family of kinases including Lyn, Fyn, and Blk. These kinases in turn recruit another tyrosine kinase, Syk, which leads to downstream events that include phosphorylation and activation of several adaptor molecules, including B-cell linker (BLNK)/SLP65, phosphoinositide 3-kinase (PI3K), Btk, phospholipase C-2, AKT, and protein kinase C. This activation then leads to activation of the Ras/Raf/extracellular signal-regulated kinase and p38/mitogen-activated protein kinase (MAPK) signaling pathway and transcriptional activation of nuclear factor-κB and nuclear factor of activated T cells.[68] These signals are imperative for the growth and survival of B cells.

Splenic Tyrosine Kinase Pathways in Lymphomagenesis

DLBCL are clinically and genetically heterogeneous lymphomas with a variable clinical history and response to therapy. Molecular profiling studies have been used to classify DLBCL to delineate further the heterogeneity within this group.[69] Using clustering algorithms, the transcriptional profiles of two large series of DLBCL have led to the subclassification of this disease, highlighting the importance of the different genetic mechanisms involved in the pathogenesis of large-cell lymphoma. This understanding has helped paved the way for new rationally designed therapeutic agents targeting specific pathogenetic mechanisms.

Recent insights into the molecular heterogeneity of DLBCL have been based on gene-expression profiling, which successfully stratified patients who had relatively favorable and unfavorable disease based on signatures obtained from significant gene-profiling experiences. For example, Alizadeh and colleagues[70] reported the application of gene-expression profiling on tissue from patients who had DLBCL, proposing a molecular classification that subcategorized DLBCL into subtypes based on the cell of origin: a germinal center subtype and an activated B-cell or postgerminal center subtype. A favorable outcome was seen in lymphomas arising from the germinal center. Subsequently, using a slightly different platform, Monti and colleagues[69] applied similar approaches in molecular profiling, subclassifying DLBCL based on clustering of consensus genes into three groups: (1) DLBCL with genes over-representing metabolic pathways involved in oxidative phosphorylation (ie, the Ox Phos phenotype); (2) DLBCL with genes over-represented in the B-cell receptor signaling pathway (ie, the BCR phenotype), and (3) DLBCL with genes over-representing the host response. The Ox Phos phenotypes displayed increased expression of genes regulating mitochondrial function, electron transport, and proteosomes. These tumors were more likely to exhibit genetic changes that affect apoptotic pathways (including both the intrinsic and extrinsic pathways and the FAS death domain). The host-response DLBCLs exhibit a rich host immune and inflammatory response. They have a prominent T-cell and dendritic cell infiltrate and may be more responsive to immunomodulation.

The BCR large B-cell lymphomas have increased expression of the multiple components of the BCR complex including over-expression of Syk, the B-cell–specific transcription factors such as Bcl-6, and cell-cycle regulatory and DNA repair genes. The tumors in the BCR category exhibited a higher incidence of translocations involving Bcl-6 and are known to be addicted to tonic BCR survival signals, suggesting they may be sensitive to pharmacologic inhibition of BCR pathways and Bcl-6 inhibitors (histone deacetylase inhibitors). In fact, stimulation of the BCR is a potent mitogenic stimulus for B cells, and the tonic stimulation through dysregulated downstream effectors leads to a potentially uninterrupted growth stimulus.

These important observations, directly translated from the experience with gene-expression profiling, have led to the identification of a completely new class of drugs targeting this specific biology, the Syk inhibitors. This information is being used to understand better the molecular pathogenesis of these diseases, creating a new platform for a new generation of targeted therapies for all forms of lymphoma.

The importance of Syk in propagating intracytoplasmic signaling in immune and some non-immune cells has been demonstrated.[70] Syk is expressed in normal hematopoietic tissue, and although its activation is controlled by BCR signaling, it is kept in its normal inactivated state by protein tyrosine phosphatase (PTP). Syk is an important substrate for a lymphoid-specific PTP, PTP receptor type O truncated (PTPROt), that is tightly regulated in developing B cells.[71] It is highly expressed in naïve B cells, is reduced in antigen-activated and actively proliferating germinal center cells, and is up-regulated in memory B cells. Overexpression of PTPROt correlates with decreased Syk phosphorylation and its associated downstream events.

The importance of Syk as a regulator of B-cell development has led some to suggest it may be a potential oncogene. Wossning and colleagues[72] have shown that deregulated Syk allows growth factor–independent growth of pre-B cells and that Syk-transformed pre-B cells show increased *myc* expression and defective differentiation and can induce leukemia in mice. Furthermore R406/R788, a unique inhibitor of Syk, can reverse the developmental block and allow differentiation of

Syk-transformed cells into immature B cells. DNA and tissue microarray analyses of tumor cell lines and tissue samples have confirmed that Syk is over represented in DLBCL, splenic marginal zone lymphoma, primary mediastinal lymphoma, and MCL as compared with normal lymphoid tissue. These observations have led to the hypothesis that Syk and its regulator PTPROt are important for BCR signaling and tumor cell survival in B-cell malignancies.

In vitro data by Chen and colleagues[71] have confirmed that there is tonic BCR signaling in DLBCL cell lines as shown by basal phosphorylation of Syk and the Syk-dependent linker protein BLNK. R406 blocks the phosphorylation of Syk and can lead to apoptosis via the intrinsic apoptotic pathway. This effect is dependent on an intact BCR signaling pathway and is seen in cell lines that belong to the BCR cluster using cell-line transcriptional profiles. Remarkably, none of the non-BCR tumor cell lines showed sensitivity to the drug. It also was shown that R406-sensitive cell lines with intact BCR signaling system demonstrated an increased expression of surface IgM or IgG. These findings were validated in cell suspensions from 10 primary DLBCL tumors and also demonstrated that primary DLBCLs differ in their expression of surface immunoglobulins. There was clear correlation between the high level of surface IgG or IgM and detectable Syk352 at baseline in the tumors exhibiting tonic BCR signaling. R406 treatment was shown to inhibit the Syk-dependent phosphorylation of BLNK.

Syk also has been shown to be potentially important in other forms of DLBCL. Gene-expression profiling and comparative genomic hybridization studies on MCL cell lines have identified overexpression of Syk at the DNA, RNA, and protein level.[73] Leseux and colleagues[74] have shown that Syk is highly expressed in follicular lymphoma cells as compared with normal B cells, existing predominantly in the activated phosphorylated form, and operates through PLD- and p13K/AKT–independent pathways. It involves activation of mTOR by a yet-unknown mechanism, possibly through the tuberous sclerosis complex 1/2 tumor suppressor, another upstream regulator of mTOR. Piceatannol and small interfering RNAs that interfere with the activity of Syk can down-regulate mTOR, thus proving a direct link between the two. Therefore Syk is an attractive target for the treatment of B-cell malignancies.

Pharmacologic Modulation of Splenic Tyrosine Kinase Pathways

R788/406 was developed as an oral agent that binds to the ATP-binding pocket of Syk and inhibits its kinase activity as an ATP-competitive inhibitor (dissociation constant = 30 nM). R406 inhibits phosphorylation of Syk substrate BLNK/SLP65 in B cells. Furthermore, R406 blocked Syk-dependent Fc receptor–mediated activation of monocytes/macrophages and neutrophils and BCR-mediated activation of B lymphocytes.[75] Consistent with Syk inhibition, oral administration of R406 to mice reduced immune complex–mediated inflammation.[76] The phase I study of this drug was completed in patients who had rheumatoid arthritis. Syk-dependent survival signals may play an important role in other B-cell lymphomas including MCL (JEKO-1) and follicular lymphoma. Other compounds such as piceatannol and curcumin also inhibit Syk and decrease the proliferation of DLBCL cell lines. Clinical trials in the treatment of B-cell lymphomas are underway. **Table 3** summarizes the available data for Syk inhibitors.

Clinical Activity of R406 in B-Cell Lymphomas

The results of a phase I/II clinical trial of R406 (tamatinib fosdium, previously known as R406/788) in B-cell lymphoma were reported recently by Friedberg and colleagues.[77] The first part of the trial was designed as a phase I trial and explored two different doses of tamatinib fosdium given on a twice-daily schedule. Thirteen patients (five of whom had follicular lymphoma, two of whom had CLL, three of whom had MCL,

Table 3
Syk inhibitors in development

Agent	In vitro	Mechanism of action	Effect	Clinical trials
R406/788[122–125]	BCR cluster cell lines, primary tumor suspensions from DLBCLs	BCR signaling pathway	Inhibited phophorylation of Syk 352, Syk 525/526 and BLNK Cleavage of caspase 3,9 activation of intrinsic apoptotic pathway	Phase I/II in B cell lymphoma-ongoing
Curcurmin[126–128] (diferuloylmethane)	Murine and human lymphoma cell lines	Inhibits Syk phosphorylaion	Inhibits AKT and its target Bad Apoptosis	N/A
3-(1-Methyl-1H-indol-3-yl-methylene)-2-oxo-2,3-dihydro-1H-indole-5-sulfonamide spleen tyrosine kinase inhibitor[129,130]	Rat basophilic leukemia cell lines	Inhibits FcR mediated degranulation	N/A	N/A

Abbreviation: NA, not applicable.

and three of whom had DLBCL), all heavily pretreated with a median of five prior therapies, were enrolled. Response was evaluated at day 57 and included one partial response in a patient who had follicular lymphoma. The DLT was neutropenia, leading to identification of the 200-mg twice-daily dose as the recommended phase II dose. Following the initial phase of study, 59 patients (17 DLBCL, 20 follicular lymphoma, 8 MCL, 3 marginal zone lymphoma of mucosa-associated lymphoid tissue, 10 CLL, and 1 other) were enrolled in the phase II portion of the trial. Response evaluation was performed at day 57 and revealed 11 partial remissions, including 6 of the 10 patients who had CLL; 18 patients had stable disease after 2 months of therapy. The most common side effects were diarrhea, infection, and cytopenias, but there were no grade 3 or grade 4 toxicities, and 44% of the patients remained on trial for up to 224 days without progression. This trial demonstrates that inhibiting BCR signaling has a clear therapeutic benefit in B-cell lymphomas, particularly in low-grade disease, and justifies further development of this agent as therapy for B-cell malignancies.

THE PHOSPHOINOSITIDE-3 KINASE/AKT/MAMMALIAN TARGET OF RAPAMYCIN SIGNALING PATHWAY
Biologic Rationale

Signal transduction in cancer cells frequently involves the conditional or constitutive activation of receptor tyrosine kinases that trigger multiple cytoplasmic kinases, which often are serine/threonine kinases. Three major signaling pathways that have been identified as important in multiple cancers are the PI3K/AKT kinase cascade,[78,79] the protein kinase C family,[80,81] and the MAPK/Ras signaling cascades.[82] mTOR has been identified as a key kinase acting downstream of the activation of PI3K.[83] Cumulative evidence supports the hypothesis that mTOR acts as a master switch of cellular catabolism and anabolism, thereby determining whether cells—and in particular tumor cells—grow and proliferate. In addition, mTOR has profound effects on the regulation of apoptotic cell death, which is dictated mainly by the cellular context and downstream targets including p53, Bcl-2, Bad, p21, p27, and c-Myc.[84] Activation of various receptor tyrosine kinases leads to autophosphorylation of the intracellular portion of these receptors; in particular, phosphorylated tyrosine residues of the receptor tyrosine kinase interact with PI3K, which can transfer the γ-phosphate group from ATP to phosphatidylinositol-4,5-bisphosphate (PtdIns(4,5)P$_2$), thereby generating phosphatidylinositol-3,4,5-trisphosphate (PtdIns(3,4,5)P$_3$) and ADP. Receptor tyrosine kinases also can activate PI3K indirectly by activating Ras, which in turn binds to and activates PI3K. To regulate PI3K negatively, cells contain phosphatase and tensin homologue deleted on chromosome 10 (PTEN) as well as other phosphatases that dephosphorylate PtdIns(3,4,5)P$_3$ back to PtdIns(4,5)P$_2$. A reduction in PTEN expression indirectly stimulates PI3K activity (and PtdIns(3,4,5)P$_3$ concentrations), thereby contributing to oncogenesis in humans. PtdIns(3,4,5)P$_3$ serves as a ligand to recruit AKT to the plasma membrane. Once at the inner leaflet of the plasma membrane, AKT becomes phosphorylated by the serine/threonine kinase, phosphatidylinositol 3–dependent kinase 1, resulting in AKT activation. Activated AKT, itself a serine/threonine kinase, promotes cell proliferation, growth, and survival and other processes involved in oncogenesis by phosphorylating various intracellular proteins. Of particular interest among the AKT targets is the downstream effector mTOR (see **Table 4**).

The proteins in the TOR family have pleiotropic functions, participate in the regulation of the initiation of mRNA transcription and protein translation, and influence the organization of the actin cytoskeleton, membrane trafficking, protein degradation, protein kinase C signaling, and ribosome biogenesis.[85,86] mTOR is involved in coupling growth stimuli to cell-cycle progression. In response to growth-inducing signals,

Table 4
New drugs targeting the PI3K/AKT/mTOR pathway in clinical trials

Agent	Development Status	Dose and Schedule	Dose-Limiting Toxicities/Toxicities	Activity
CCI-779 (temsirolimus)[111,130]	Phase I and II (MCL)	25–250 mg/week	DLT: mucositis, thrombocytopenia hyperlipemia Other toxicities: hyperglycemia, anemia, neutropenia, fatigue, rash, weight loss, aspartate aminotransferase elevation, abnormal taste, loss of appetite, sensory neuropathy	OR = 24/61 (39%) TTP = 6–6.5 months
RAD001 (everolimus)[112]	Phase I and II (hematologic malignancies)	10 mg/day	Toxicities: hyperglycemia, hypophosphatemia, fatigue, anorexia, diarrhea	OR = 2/27 (myelodysplastic syndrome)
AP23573 (deferolimus)[113]	Phase I and II (hematologic malignancies)	12.5 mg/day for 5 days every 2 weeks	DLT: Mouth sores Other toxicities: fatigue, nausea, thrombocytopenia, rash	OR = 5/52 (3 MCL)

Abbreviations: OR, overall response; TTP, time to progression.

quiescent cells increase the translation of a subset of mRNAs, the protein products of which are required for progression through the G1 phase of the cell cycle. PI3K and AKT are the key elements of the upstream pathway that links the ligation of growth factor receptors to the phosphorylation and activation state of mTOR.[87,88] After phosphorylation, mTOR modulates two distinct downstream signaling pathways that control the translation of specific subsets of mRNAs, including the serine/threonine kinase S6K1 and the small protein *4EBP1* that acts as a repressor of protein translation. Additionally, several elements of the PI3K/AKT/mTOR pathway have been shown to be constitutionally activated in malignancies.[89–91] The hyperactivation of PI3K/AKT/mTOR signaling elements in PTEN-deficient malignancies suggests that cancers often depend on this pathway for growth and sustenance.[92]

A plethora of mechanisms can result in the constitutive activation of the PI3K/AKT/mTOR pathway in cancer cells. Cell-intrinsic processes resulting in mTOR activation involve loss of PTEN function, mutation or amplification of the PI3K subunits, amplification of AKT isoenzymes, and inactivation or mutations of AKT-associated mTOR-regulatory proteins. The mTOR pathway also can be activated by exogenous oncogenes, including overexpressed or mutated tyrosine kinase receptors such as human epidermal growth factor receptors 1–4, platelet-derived growth factor receptor/kinase tyrosine, and insulin-like growth factor (IGF) receptor. Ras directly binds PI3K,[93] an interaction that is important for membrane anchoring. Downstream of mTOR, the overexpression and/or amplification of S6K1 or eIF4E also could contribute to oncogenesis. No mutation of mTOR itself has been described. There is another rationale for mTOR activation in cancer, however.

Activated p53 acts as a negative regulator of mTOR (eg, in conditions of glucose deprivation).[94] p53 function often is lost in cancer, and in theory this loss of function could favor the constitutive activation of mTOR. The role of these signal transduction proteins in carcinogenesis has been studied extensively in a number of cellular and animal models, suggesting that activation of the PI3K/AKT/mTOR pathway alone is not sufficient to induce cancer; rather, a second oncogenic event is required to induce cellular transformation. PI3K/AKT/mTOR activation affects many tumor types, activation of receptor tyrosine kinase is frequent in malignancies, and the loss of PTEN function via gene mutation or deletion or promoter methylation has been reported in different subsets of solid tumors. Tumors associated with PTEN inactivation are particularly susceptible to the therapeutic effects of mTOR inhibitors.

Biochemical Pharmacology of Mammalian Target of Rapamycin Inhibitors

To date, four mTOR inhibitors are being studied in clinical trials: the prototype, rapamycin, and three rapamycin derivatives, CCI-779 (temsirolimus), RAD001 (everolimus), and AP23573 (deforolimus) (**Table 4**). Each of these inhibitors forms a complex with the small intracellular protein FKBP12; the resulting complex interacts with and inhibits mTOR. No other proteins have been identified as rapamycin targets, and the requirement of a cofactor makes the mTOR–rapamycin interaction very specific. Rapamycin (also known as "sirolimus") is a macrocyclic lactone produced by *Streptomyces hygroscopicus* that was developed initially as an antifungal drug.[95] When rapamycin was evaluated by the National Cancer Institute, it was identified as a non-cytotoxic agent that had cytostatic activity against several human cancers in vitro and in vivo. Rapamycin also inhibits T-cell proliferation as well as proliferative responses induced by several cytokines, including interleukin (IL)-1, IL-2, IL-3, IL-4, IL-6, IGF, platelet-derived growth factor, and colony-stimulating factors. Rapamycin was approved in the United States in 1999 (and in Europe in 2000) for the prevention of acute organ rejection in combination with cyclosporine and steroids. Rapamycin, unlike cyclosporine, does not increase the risk of malignancy but rather decreases the risk of posttransplantation lymphopro-liferative disorders.[96] Recently, rapamycin has been shown to inhibit the growth of sev-eral murine and human cancer cell lines in a concentration-dependent manner, both in tissue culture and in xenograft models including P388 leukemia.[97,98] In the 60 tumor cell line screen by the National Cancer Institute, the spectrum of activity of rapamycin was different from that of other anticancer agents in leukemia and solid tumor cell lines. In addition, rapamycin inhibits the oncogenic transformation of human cells induced by either PI3K or AKT and inhibits metastatic tumor growth and tumor vascularization in vivo in murine models.[99] Direct exposure of cancer cells to rapamycin and to rapamycin derivatives results in several effects that depend on specific cellular characteristics and drug concentration. In cancer cells possessing an activated PI3K/AKT/mTOR pathway, rapamycin and its derivatives block the binding of the mTOR-associated protein raptor to mTOR, which is required for downstream phosphorylation of 4EBP1 and S6K1. This effect restores the proper control of the activated PI3K/AKT/mTOR signaling pathway and can be viewed as a gain of function rather than a straightforward inhibitory effect on protein function. After even short exposures to rapamycin, molecular interactions be-tween rapamycin, FKBP12, and mTOR can persist for about 72 hours, blocking mTOR function for several days. Chemical inactivation of mTOR in hypoxia-activated endo-thelial cells and pericytes can induce a G0–G1 cell-cycle block (associated with re-duced expression of cyclin D1 and accumulation of p27) rather than apoptosis.[100] Consistently, rapamycin induces a decrease in cyclin D1 expression and can lead to an increase in p27 that can result in late G1/S cell-cycle arrest.

In some tumor models, rapamycin has been shown to induce cancer cell death by inducing either apoptosis or autophagy. The molecular mechanisms leading to apo-ptosis in cancer cells have not yet been deciphered fully. One link between mTOR in-hibition and apoptosis induction is thought to be mediated by the downstream target S6K1, which can phosphorylate the pro-apoptotic molecule Bad, a reaction that dis-rupts Bad's binding to the mitochondrial death inhibitors Bcl-xL and Bcl-2 and thereby inactivating Bad.[101,102] In this scenario, rapamycin-mediated S6K1 inactivation indi-rectly causes Bad activation. In addition, two recent studies have suggested that members of the Bcl-2 family could be downstream mediators of the IGF-1–stimulated, PI3K-dependent survival of cells.[103,104] Furthermore, several growth factors that acti-vate the PI3K and S6K1 pathways have been shown to increase expression of Bcl-2, thereby promoting cell survival in myeloid progenitor cells.[105]

In addition to inducting apoptosis, rapamycin also activates autophagic pro-cesses.[106] Surprisingly, cell death induced by rapamycin and its derivatives does not seem to be dose dependent. Preclinical activity of mTOR inhibitors recently has been established in a variety of different lymphoproliferative malignancies, including Hodgkin's lymphoma, anaplastic large cell lymphoma, MCL, CLL/SLL, acute lympho-blastic leukemia/lymphoma, DLBCL, plasma cell myeloma, and posttransplantation lymphoproliferative disorders.[107] On the basis of these preclinical results, studies of rapamycin as an anticancer drug have been launched, and rapamycin derivatives with improved pharmacokinetic profiles and reduced immunosuppressive effects have been developed. Unlike rapamycin, the three rapamycin derivatives do not me-diate any substantial immunosuppression when administered intermittently in clinical settings. CCI-779 is administered either orally or intravenously, RAD001 is available as an oral formulation, and AP23573 is given either orally or intravenously.

Clinical Development of Rapamycin Derivatives

To date, most clinical investigations of mTOR inhibitors have focused on the ra-pamycin derivatives CCI-779 (temsirolimus), RAD001 (everolimus), and AP23573 (deforolimus). These compounds were studied in the clinic using three primary oral and intravenous schedules: (1) daily dosing for 5 days every 2 weeks; (2) once-weekly dosing or, (3) daily oral continuous dosing until tumor progression.[108–111] DLTs in the three compounds are similar and typically include reversible mucositis, asthenia, and thrombocytopenia, most commonly observed with the five-times daily dosing schedule. Severe psychiatric disorders have been seen at very high doses on the weekly schedule of CCI-779. No significant immunosuppression was observed for CCI-779, RAD001, or AP23573, and at the recommended dose the most prevalent toxic effects were reversible cutaneous herpes lesions, aseptic acne-like rash, maculopapular rash, and nail disorders, which occurred in about 75% of patients. At the recommended doses, these compounds display a side-effect profile that renders them potentially amenable to combination with cytotoxic agents or other targeted therapies.

One of the most promising results published to date regarding the use of mTOR inhibitors in hematologic malignancies comes from a phase II trial using CCI-779 in the treatment of patients who had MCL.[112] In this study, 35 patients who had refractory or relapsed disease received a weekly dose of CCI-779 at 250 mg as a single agent. The overall response rate was 38% with one complete response; the median duration of responses was 6.9 months, and the median time to progression in all patients was 6.5 months. Hematologic toxicities were the most common, with 71% of patients (25/35) experiencing grade 3 events and 11% of patients (4/35) experiencing grade 4 toxicities. Thrombocytopenia was the most frequent cause of dose reductions but was of short duration, typically resolving within 1 week. An additional phase II trial tested low-dose temsirolimus (25 mg weekly) in 29 patients who had relapsed MCL. The overall response rate was 41% (11 of 27 patients) with one complete response and 10 partial responses. The median time to progression was 6 months, and the median duration of response for the 11 responders was 6 months. Hematologic toxicities were the most common, with grade 3 toxicities seen in 50% of patients (14/28) and grade 4 toxicities observed in 4% of patients (1/28). Thrombocytopenia was the most frequent cause of dose reduction. Interestingly, the 25-mg dose level retained the antitumor activity of the 250-mg dose with less myelosuppression.

In a phase I/II trial, 27 patients who had relapsed or refractory hematologic malignancies received RAD001 (everolimus) at two dose levels (5 or 10 mg orally once daily continuously). Everolimus was well tolerated at 10 mg daily and showed promising activity in patients who had myelodysplastic syndromes.[113] Deforolimus (AP23573) has been tested in a phase II trial to determine its efficacy and safety in patients who have relapsed or refractory hematologic malignancies.[114] Deforolimus was given at 12.5 mg as a 30-minute infusion once daily for 5 days every 2 weeks. Of the 52 evaluable patients, partial responses were noted in 5 (10%) cases, specifically in two of seven patients who had angiogenic myeloid metaplasia and in three of nine patients who had MCL. Hematologic improvement/stable disease was observed in 21 patients (40%). Common treatment-related adverse events, which generally were mild and reversible, were mouth sores, fatigue, nausea, and thrombocytopenia.

PRALATREXATE

Methotrexate, an antifolate used for decades in the treatment of lymphoma, is used under very select situations, most commonly for aggressive acute lymphoblastic lymphoma/leukemia, and to a lesser extent in cutaneous T-cell disorders in low doses.[115] Given their established synergistic relationship with cytidine analogues, antifolates represent potential natural partners for agents like gemcitabine, which have clear activity in DLBCL, Hodgkin's disease, and select forms of T-cell lymphoma. Pralatrexate is a novel antifolate with properties that differ from those of methotrexate and, as described in the following section, also possesses unusual activity against T-cell lymphomas.

Pralatrexate is a member of the 10—deazaaminopterins, a class of folate analogues that demonstrates greater antitumor effects than the other antifolates in a variety of murine animal models.[116–118] The improved activity results from more effective internalization by the 1-carbon, reduced folate transporter (RFC) and the subsequent accumulation in tumor cells. Once in the intracellular compartment, the drug is polyglutamylated, which increases its intracellular retention. In contrast to the many generations of antifolates developed historically, pralatrexate was designed to have very high affinity for the RFC transporter, effecting high intracellular concentrations of pralatrexate.

RFC is a fetal oncoprotein expressed on fetal and malignant tissue. This transporter represents the principal means through which pralatrexate, although not necessarily all antifolates, enters the cell. This transporter has evolved to transport reduced natural folates efficiently into highly proliferative cells to meet the demands for purine and pyrimidine nucleotides during DNA synthesis. In fact, the influx V_{max}/K_m data reveal that pralatrexate is transported far more efficiently, being incorporated at a rate nearly 14 times greater than that seen for methotrexate. Similarly, the V_{max}/K_m for the folylpolyglutamyl synthetase (FPGS)-mediated glutamylation reactions suggest that pralatrexate also is polyglutamylated 10 times more efficiently than methotrexate, a favorable pharmacologic feature. These biochemical behaviors suggest that pralatrexate should be a more potent antineoplastic agent than methotrexate and could overcome known mechanisms of methotrexate resistance in which down-regulation of RFC-1 and/or FPGS leads to frank methotrexate resistance.

In preclinical xenograft models of lymphoma, pralatrexate is markedly superior to methotrexate and, in fact, is superior to many standard agents used in the treatment of lymphoma. Across a large panel of lymphoma cell lines, pralatrexate is at least one-log more potent in enzymatic assays, cytotoxicity assays, and xenograft models of both B- and T-cell lymphoma.[119,120] To date, there does not seem to be a significant difference between pralatrexate activity in B- and T-cell lymphoma lines. In fact, in virtually all cell lines studied, pralatrexate is at least the one-log more potent than methotrexate. Recent data also have confirmed that that across preclinical models of T- and B-cell lymphoma pralatrexate seems to synergize with nucleoside analogues such as gemcitabine.[119] These data, which have demonstrated that combinations of pralatrexate and gemcitabine in low concentrations induce apoptosis, now have led to a combination phase I study in patients who have either B- or T-cell lymphoma.

In the clinic, pralatrexate has proven to be remarkably active in patients who have T-cell lymphoma, even in those who are frankly resistant to conventional chemotherapy.[121] The available data suggest an overall response rate of approximately 50% in patients who have primarily refractory disease. In addition, these responses have been very durable, in general lasting at least 6 months and with some responses lasting up to 1 year. The major adverse effects of the drug include thrombocytopenia and mucositis; the latter seems to be influenced favorably by normalized homocysteine and methylmalonic acid. Based on the promising activity seen in phase II studies, an international multicenter, registration-directed study (PROPEL) was launched to confirm the activity in T-cell lymphoma. An interim analysis of the data reported by the trial sponsors in May 2008 indicates that 29% of the first 65 evaluable patients enrolled in the study experienced a complete or a partial response, as assessed by central independent oncology review. The response rate based on independent investigator review was 45%. As expected, the most common drug-related grade 3 or grade 4 adverse events were mucositis and thrombocytopenia, which were seen in 14% and 23% of patients, respectively. Although the results of the single-agent phase II and registration-directed study are expected within the next year, the early data in T-cell lymphoma have led to the hope that a new strategy for treating T-cell lymphoma can begin to crystallize around these newly identified agents.

FUTURE DIRECTIONS

The increasing realization that cancer is a complex and heterogenous disease has provided an opportunity to dissect the molecular basis for these different subsets of disease, in the process exposing new opportunities for targeting cancer at its most fundamental level. During the past decade the lymphoid neoplasia have provided a platform for thinking about the stratification of these diseases based on molecular signatures and about the use of this information in translating these discoveries into rational therapeutic approaches. The sheer volume of new targets and agents makes it impossible to discuss all of them with any clarity in this article. This discussion has been limited to four very specific examples of how the understanding of lymphoma biology has translated into new, albeit early, opportunities to treat lymphoma subtypes in a biologically focused and directed manner. Targeting of Bcl-2, Syk, and the PI3K/AKT/mTOR pathway has well-established biologic rationales and has achieved proof of principle, but a new set of challenges has emerged. No longer is the rate-limiting step identifying the next target, or even identifying the best agent. The challenge now is to identify the best combination.

No one expects that any of these new targets will in and of itself be the cure for any disease, let alone a complicated one like lymphoma. The challenge is to identify precisely what combination of agents will perturb or inhibit the central signaling hubs in these diseases in a fashion that pre-empts the emergence of acquired drug resistance. In fact, new concepts in understanding the gene-expression profile in the context of complex signaling networks have begun to pave a new path that could guide the rational selection of the most complementary of agents. Computer based identification of oncogenic lesions using a systems biology approach is beginning to identify new genetic lesions and also can provide a framework for thinking about how lymphoma cells circumnavigate the lethal effects of cytotoxic chemotherapy and even targeted agents. These strategies, which are based on the analysis of molecular interactions that become dysregulated in specific tumor phenotypes, will provide essential guidance about how best to combine the panoply of new agents, moving investigators away from the realm of empirically based drug development. What remains indisputable in the efforts to develop new agents and strategies for treating the lymphoid neoplasia is the urgent need to enroll patients in clinical trials; regrettably, patient accrual has become the rate-limiting step in advancing most promising new ideas for treating lymphoma into practice.

REFERENCES

1. Kerr JFR, Wyllie AH, Currie AR. Apoptosis: a basic biological phenomenon with wide-ranging implications in tissue kinetics. Br J Cancer 1972;26:239–57.
2. Vaux DL, Cory S, Adams JM. Bcl-2 gene promotes haemopoietic cell survival and cooperates with c-Myc to immortalize pre-B cells. Nature 1988;335:440–2.
3. Vaux DL, Weissman IL, Kim SK. Prevention of programmed cell death in Caenorhabditis elegans by human BCL-2. Science 1992;258:1955–7.

4. Yuan J, Shaham S, Ledoux S, et al. The C. Elegans cell death gene ced-3 encodes a protein similar to mammalian interleukin-1β-converting enzyme. Cell 1993;75:641–52.

5. Li P, Nijhawan D, Budihardjo I, et al. Cytochrome c and dATP-dependent formation of Apaf-1/caspase-9 complex initiates an apoptotic protease cascade. Cell 1997;91:479–89.

6. Oltvai ZN, Milliman CL, Korsmeyer SJ. Bcl-2 heterodimerizes in vivo with a conserved homolog, BAX, that accelerates programmed cell death. Cell 1993;74: 609–19.

7. Adams JM, Cory S. The Bcl-2 apoptotic switch in cancer development and therapy. Oncogene 2007;26:1324–37.

8. Huang DC, Strasser A. BH3-only proteins-essential initiators of apoptotic cell death. Cell 2000;103:839–42.

9. Sattler M, Liang H, Nettesheim D, et al. Structure of Bcl-XL-BAK peptide complex: recognition between regulators of apoptosis. Science 1997;275:983–6.

10. Petros AM, Nettesheim DG, Wang Y, et al. Rationale for Bcl-XL/Bad peptide complex formation from structure, mutagenesis, and biophysical studies. Protein Sci 2000;9:2528–34.

11. Cheng EH, Wei MC, Weiler S, et al. BCL-2, BCL-X(L) sequester BH3 domain-only molecules preventing BAX- and BAK-mediated mitochondrial apoptosis. Mol Cell 2001;8:705–11.

12. Zong WX, Lindsten T, Ross AJ, et al. BH3-only proteins that bind pro-survival Bcl-2 family members fail to induce apoptosis in the absence of BAX and BAK. Genes Dev 2001;15:1481–6.

13. Green DR, Kroemer G. The pathophysiology of mitochondrial cell death. Science 2004;305:626–9.

14. Wang X. The expanding role of mitochondria in apoptosis. Genes Dev 2001;15: 2922–33.

15. Bouillet P, Cory S, Zhang L-C, et al. Degenerative disorders caused by Bcl-2 deficiency are prevented by loss of its BH3-only antagonist Bim. Dev Cell 2001;1:645–53.

16. Pellecchia M, Reed JC. Inhibition of anti-apoptotic Bcl-2 family proteins by natural polyphenols: new avenues for cancer chemoprevention and chemotherapy. Curr Pharm Des 2004;10(12):1387–98 [review].

17. Kitada S, Leone M, Sareth S, et al. Discovery, characterization, and structure-activity relationships studies of proapoptotic polyphenols targeting B-cell lymphocyte/leukemia-2 proteins. J Med Chem 2003;46(20):4259–64.

18. Lei X, Chen Y, Du G, et al. Gossypol induces BAX/BAK-independent activation of apoptosis and cytochrome c release via a conformational change in Bcl-2. FASEB J 2006;20(12):2147–9 [Epub 2006 Aug 25].

19. Mohammad RM, Wang S, Aboukameel A, et al. Preclinical studies of a nonpeptidic small-molecule inhibitor of Bcl-2 and Bcl-X(L) [(-)-gossypol] against diffuse large cell lymphoma. Mol Cancer Ther 2005;4(1):13–21.

20. Paoluzzi L, Gonen M, Gardner JR, et al. Targeting Bcl-2 family members with the BH3 mimetic AT-101 markedly enhances the therapeutic effects of chemotherapeutic agents in in vitro and in vivo models of B-cell lymphoma. Blood 2008; 111(11):5350–8 [Epub 2008 Feb 21].

21. Becattini B, Kitada S, Leone M, et al. Rational design and real time, in-cell detection of the proapoptotic activity of a novel compound targeting Bcl-X(L). Chem Biol 2004;11(3):389–95.

22. Kitada S, Kress CL, Krajewska M, et al. Bcl-2 antagonist apogossypol (NSC736630) displays single-agent activity in Bcl-2-transgenic mice and has superior efficacy with less toxicity compared with gossypol (NSC19048). Blood 2008;111(6):3211–9 [Epub 2008 Jan 17].
23. Wang G, Nikolovska-Coleska Z, Yang CY, et al. Structure-based design of potent small-molecule inhibitors of anti-apoptotic Bcl-2 proteins. J Med Chem 2006; 49(21):6139–42.
24. Mohammad RM, Goustin AS, Aboukameel A, et al. Preclinical studies of TW-37, a new nonpeptidic small-molecule inhibitor of Bcl-2, in diffuse large cell lymphoma xenograft model reveal drug action on both Bcl-2 and Mcl-1. Clin Cancer Res 2007;13(7):2226–35.
25. Mohammad RM, Sun Y, Wang S, et al. Evaluation of TW-37, a pan Bcl-2 proteins small-molecule inhibitor, against spectrum of human B-cell lines and patient-derived samples. Blood (ASH Annual Meeting Abstracts) 2007;110:4521.
26. Castro JE, Loria OJ, Aguillon RA, et al. A phase II, open label study of AT-101 in combination with rituximab in patients with relapsed or refractory chronic lymphocytic leukemia. Evaluation of two dose regimens. Blood (ASH Annual Meeting Abstracts) 2007;110:3119.
27. Shore GC, Viallet J. Modulating the Bcl-2 family of apoptosis suppressors for potential therapeutic benefit in cancer. Hematology (Am Soc Hematol Educ Program) 2005;226–30.
28. Pérez-Galán P, Roué G, Villamor N, et al. The BH3-mimetic GX15-070 synergizes with bortezomib in mantle cell lymphoma by enhancing Noxa-mediated activation of BAK. Blood 2007;109(10):4441–9 [Epub 2007 Jan 16].
29. Trudel S, Li ZH, Rauw J, et al. Preclinical studies of the pan-Bcl inhibitor obatoclax (GX015-070) in multiple myeloma. Blood 2007;109(12):5430–8.
30. Schimmer AD, Brandwein J, O'Brien SM, et al. A phase I trial of the small molecule pan-Bcl-2 family inhibitor obatoclax mesylate (GX15-070) administered by continuous infusion for up to four days to patients with hematological malignancies. Blood (ASH Annual Meeting Abstracts) 2007;110:892.
31. Borthakur G, O'Brien S, Ravandi-Kashani F, et al. A phase I trial of the small molecule pan-Bcl-2 family inhibitor obatoclax mesylate (GX15-070) administered by 24 hour infusion every 2 weeks to patients with myeloid malignancies and chronic lymphocytic leukemia (CLL). Blood (ASH Annual Meeting Abstracts) 2006;108:2654.
32. Oltersdorf T, Elmore SW, Shoemaker AR, et al. An inhibitor of Bcl-2 family proteins induces regression of solid tumours. Nature 2005;435(7042):677–81 [Epub 2005 May 15].
33. van Delft MF, Wei AH, Mason KD, et al. The BH3 mimetic ABT-737 targets selective Bcl-2 proteins and efficiently induces apoptosis via BAK/BAX if Mcl-1 is neutralized. Cancer Cell 2006;10(5):389–99.
34. Deng J, Carlson N, Takeyama K, et al. BH3 profiling identifies three distinct classes of apoptotic blocks to predict response to ABT-737 and conventional chemotherapeutic agents. Cancer Cell 2007;12(2):171–85.
35. Konopleva M, Contractor R, Tsao T, et al. Mechanisms of apoptosis sensitivity and resistance to the BH3 mimetic ABT-737 in acute myeloid leukemia. Cancer Cell 2006;10(5):375–88.
36. Chauhan D, Velankar M, Brahmandam M, et al. A novel Bcl-2/Bcl-X(L)/Bcl-w inhibitor ABT-737 as therapy in multiple myeloma. Oncogene 2007;26(16): 2374–80 [Epub 2006 Oct 2].

37. Kline MP, Rajkumar SV, Timm MM, et al. ABT-737, an inhibitor of Bcl-2 family proteins, is a potent inducer of apoptosis in multiple myeloma cells. Leukemia 2007;21(7):1549–60 [Epub 2007 Apr 26].

38. Kang MH, Kang YH, Szymanska B, et al. Activity of vincristine, L-ASP, and dexamethasone against acute lymphoblastic leukemia is enhanced by the BH3-mimetic ABT-737 in vitro and in vivo. Blood 2007;110(6):2057–66 [Epub 2007 May 29].

39. Paoluzzi L, Gonen M, Bhagat G, et al. The BH3-only mimetic ABT-737 synergizes the anti-neoplastic activity of proteasome inhibitors in lymphoid malignancies. Blood 2008 [Epub ahead of print].

40. Chen S, Dai Y, Harada H, et al. Mcl-1 down-regulation potentiates ABT-737 lethality by cooperatively inducing BAK activation and BAX translocation. Cancer Res 2007;67(2):782–91.

41. Del Gaizo Moore V, Schlis KD, Sallan SE, et al. BCL-2 dependence and ABT-737 sensitivity in acute lymphoblastic leukemia. Blood 2008;111(4):2300–9.

42. Tahir SK, Yang X, Anderson MG, et al. Influence of Bcl-2 family members on the cellular response of small-cell lung cancer cell lines to ABT-737. Cancer Res 2007;67(3):1176–83.

43. Lin X, Morgan-Lappe S, Huang X, et al. 'Seed' analysis of off-target siRNAs reveals an essential role of Mcl-1 in resistance to the small-molecule Bcl-2/Bcl-XL inhibitor ABT-737. Oncogene 2007;26(27):3972–9 [Epub 2006 Dec 18].

44. Nijhawan D, Fang M, Traer E, et al. Elimination of Mcl-1 is required for the initiation of apoptosis following ultraviolet irradiation. Genes Dev 2003;17(12):1475–86 [Epub 2003 Jun 3].

45. Zhong Q, Gao W, Du F, et al. Mule/ARF-BP1, a BH3-only E3 ubiquitin ligase, catalyzes the polyubiquitylation of Mcl-1 and regulates apoptosis. Cell 2005;121(7):1085–95.

46. Mason KD, Carpinelli MR, Fletcher JI, et al. Programmed anuclear cell death delimits platelet life span. Cell 2007;128(6):1173–86.

47. Wilson WH, Tulpule A, Levine AM, et al. A phase 1/2a study evaluating the safety, pharmacokinetics, and efficacy of ABT-263 in subjects with refractory or relapsed lymphoid malignancies. Blood (ASH Annual Meeting Abstracts) 2007;110:1371.

48. Chuntharapai A, Dodge K, Grimmer K, et al. Isotype-dependent inhibition of tumor growth in vivo by monoclonal antibodies to death receptor 4. J Immunol 2001;166:4891–8.

49. Ichikawa K, et al. Tumoricidal activity of a novel anti-human DR5 monoclonal antibody without hepatocyte cytotoxicity. Nature Med 2001;7:954–60.

50. Takeda K, Yamaguchi N, Akiba H, et al. Induction of tumor-specific T cell immunity by anti-DR5 antibody therapy. J Exp Med 2004;199:437–48.

51. Presta LG. Engineering antibodies for therapy. Curr Pharm Biotechnol 2002;3:237–56.

52. Younes A, Vose JM, Zelenetz AD, et al. Results of a phase 2 trial of HGS-ETR1 (agonistic human monoclonal antibody to TRAIL receptor 1) in subjects with relapsed/refractory non-Hodgkin's lymphoma (NHL). Blood (ASH Annual Meeting Abstracts) 2005;106:489.

53. Shankar S, Chen X, Srivastava RK. Effects of sequential treatments with chemotherapeutic drugs followed by TRAIL on prostate cancer in vitro and in vivo. Prostate 2005;62:165–86.

54. Inoue S, MacFarlane M, Harper N, et al. Histone deacetylase inhibitors potentiate TNF-related apoptosis-inducing ligand (TRAIL)-induced apoptosis in lymphoid malignancies. Cell Death Differ 2004;11:S193–206.
55. Mitsiades CS, Treon SP, Mitsiades N, et al. TRAIL/Apo2L ligand selectively induces apoptosis and overcomes drug resistance in multiple myeloma: therapeutic applications. Blood 2001;98:795–804.
56. Ashkenazi A, et al. Safety and antitumor activity of recombinant soluble Apo2 ligand. J Clin Invest 1999;104:155–62.
57. Kelley SK, et al. Preclinical studies to predict the disposition of Apo2L/tumor necrosis factor-related apoptosis-inducing ligand in humans: characterization of in vivo efficacy, pharmacokinetics, and safety. J Pharmacol Exp Ther 2001;299:31–8.
58. Deveraux QL, Takahashi R, Salvesen GS, et al. X-linked IAP is a direct inhibitor of cell-death proteases. Nature 1997;388(6639):300–4.
59. LaCasse EC, Baird S, Korneluk RG, et al. The inhibitors of apoptosis (IAPs) and their emerging role in cancer. Oncogene 1998;17(25):3247–59 [review].
60. Sun H, Nikolovska-Coleska Z, Yang CY, et al. Structure-based design, synthesis, and evaluation of conformationally constrained mimetics of the second mitochondria-derived activator of caspase that target the X-linked inhibitor of apoptosis protein/caspase-9 interaction site. J Med Chem 2004;47(17):4147–50.
61. Oost TK, Sun C, Armstrong RC, et al. Discovery of potent antagonists of the anti-apoptotic protein XIAP for the treatment of cancer. J Med Chem 2004;47(18): 4417–26.
62. Nikolovska-Coleska Z, Xu L, Hu Z, et al. Discovery of embelin as a cell-permeable, small-molecular weight inhibitor of XIAP through structure-based computational screening of a traditional herbal medicine three-dimensional structure database. J Med Chem 2004;47(10):2430–40.
63. Li L, Thomas RM, Suzuki H, et al. A small molecule Smac mimic potentiates TRAIL- and TNFalpha-mediated cell death. Science 2004;305(5689):1471–4.
64. Ambrosini G, Adida C, Altieri DC. A novel anti-apoptosis gene, survivin, expressed in cancer and lymphoma. Nat Med 1997;3(8):917–21.
65. Altieri DC. Survivin, versatile modulation of cell division and apoptosis in cancer. Oncogene 2003;22(53):8581–9.
66. Congmin G, Mu Z, Yihui M, et al. Survivin—an attractive target for RNAi in non-Hodgkin's lymphoma, Daudi cell line as a model. Leuk Lymphoma 2006;47(9): 1941–8.
67. Turner M, Schweighoffer E, Colucci F, et al. Tyrosine kinase Syk: essential functions for immunoreceptor signaling. Immunol Today 2000;21:148–54.
68. Stephen Gauld, Cambier J. B cell antigen receptor signaling: roles in cell development and disease. Science 2002;296:1641–2.
69. Monti S, Shipp M. Molecular profiling of diffuse large B cell lymphomas identifies robust subtypes including one characterized by host inflammatory response. Blood 2005;105:1851–61.
70. Alizadeh AA, Eisen MB, Davis RE, et al. Distinct types of diffuse large B-cell lymphoma identified by gene expression profiling. Nature 2000;403(6769):503–11.
71. Chen L, Shipp M. Syk dependent tonic B cell receptor signalling is a rational treatment target in diffuse large B cell lymphoma. Blood 2008;111:2230–7.
72. Wossning T, Jumaa H. Deregulated Syk inhibits differentiation and induces growth factor- independent proliferation of pre-B cells. J Exp Med 2006;203: 2829–40.

73. Rinasldi A, Bertoni F. Genomic and expression profiling identifies the B cell associated Syk as a possible therapeutic target in mantle cell lymphoma. Br J Haematol 2005;132:303–16.
74. Leseux I, Bezombes C. Syk dependent m TOR activation in follicular lymphoma cells. Blood 2006;108:4156–62.
75. Braselmann S, Taylor V, Zhao H, et al. R406, an orally available spleen tyrosine kinase inhibitor blocks Fc receptor signaling and reduces immune complex mediated inflammation. J Pharmacol Exp Ther 2006;319:998–1008.
76. Vasileois C, Tsokos G. Syk kinase as a treatment target for therapy/in autoimmune diseases. Clin Immunol 2007;124:235–7.
77. Friedberg J, Sharman J, Schaefer-Curillo J, et al. Tamatinib fosdium (TAMF), an oral Syk inhibitor, has significant clinical activity in B-cell non-Hodgkin's lymphoma (NHL). 10th International Conference on Malignant Lymphoma, Lugano, Switzerland, 2008.
78. Vignot S, Faivre S, Aguirre D, et al. mTOR-targeted therapy of cancer with rapamycin derivatives. Ann Oncol 2005;16:525–37.
79. Larue L, Bellacosa A. Epithelial-mesenchymal transition in development and cancer: role of phosphatidylinositol 3' kinase/AKT pathways. Oncogene 2005; 24:7443–54.
80. Gschwendt M. Protein kinase C. Eur J Biochem 1999;259:555–64.
81. Steinberg SF. Distinctive activation mechanisms and functions for protein kinase C. Biochem J 2004;384:449–59.
82. Fang JY, Richardson BC. The MAPK signalling pathways and colorectal cancer. Lancet Oncol 2005;6:322–7.
83. Hay N. The Akt-mTOR tango and its relevance to cancer. Cancer Cell 2005;8: 179–83.
84. Castedo M, Ferri KF, Kroemer G. Mammalian target of rapamycin (mTOR): pro- and anti-apoptotic. Cell Death Differ 2002;9:99–100.
85. Thomas G, Hall MN. TOR signaling and control of control of cell growth. Curr Opin Cell Biol 1997;9:782–7.
86. Schmelzle T, Hall MN. TOR, a central controller of cell growth. Cell 2000;103:253–62.
87. Scott PH, Brunn GJ, Kohn AD, et al. Evidence of insulin-stimulated phosphorylation and activation of the mammalian target of rapamycin mediated by a protein kinase B signaling pathway. Proc Natl Acad Sci U S A 1998;95:7772–7.
88. Nave BT, Ouwens M, Withers DJ, et al. Mammalian target of rapamycin is a direct target for protein kinase B: identification of a convergence point for opposing effects of insulin and amino-acid deficiency on protein translation. Biochem J 1999;344:427–31.
89. Cheng JQ, Godwin AK, Bellacosa A, et al. Akt2, a putative oncogene encoding a member of a subfamily of serine/threonine kinases, is amplified in human ovarian carcinomas. Proc Natl Acad Sci U S A 1992;89:9267–71.
90. Cheng JQ, Ruggeri B, Klein WM, et al. Amplification of AKT 2 in human pancreatic cells and inhibition of Akt 2 expression and tumorigenicity by antisense RNA. Proc Natl Acad Sci U S A 1996;93:3636–41.
91. Bellacosa A, dee Feo D, Gowin AK, et al. Molecular alterations of the AKT2 oncogene in ovarian and breast carcinomas. Int J Cancer 1995;64:280–5.
92. Neshat MS, Mellinghoff IK, Tran C, et al. Enhanced sensitivity of PTEN-deficient tumors to inhibition of FRAP/mTOR. Proc Natl Acad Sci U S A 2001;98:10314–9.
93. Rodriguez-Viciana P. Phosphatidylinositol-3-OH kinase as a direct target of Ras. Nature 1994;370:527–32.

94. Feng Z, Zhang H, Levine AJ, et al. The coordinate regulation of the p53 and mTOR pathways in cells. Proc Natl Acad Sci U S A 2005;102:8204–9.
95. Vezina C, Kudelski A, Sehgal SN. Rapamycin (AY-22,989), a new antifungal antibiotic. Taxonomy of the producing streptomycete and isolation of the active principle. I. J Antibiot (Tokyo) 1975;28(10):721–6.
96. Kauffman HM, Cherikh WS, Cheng Y, et al. Maintenance immunosuppression with target-of-rapamycin inhibitors is associated with a reduced incidence of de novo malignancies. Transplantation 2005;80:883–9.
97. Busca R, Bertolotto C, Ortonne JP, et al. Inhibition of the phosphatidylinositol 3-kinase/p70(S6)-kinase pathway induces B16 melanoma cell differentiation. J Biol Chem 1996;271:31824–30.
98. Grewe M, Gansauge F, Schmid RM, et al. Regulation of cell growth and cyclin D1 expression by the constitutively active FRAP–p70s6K pathway in human pancreatic cancer cells. Cancer Res 1999;59:3581–7.
99. Humar R, Kiefer FN, Berns H, et al. Hypoxia enhances vascular cell proliferation and angiogenesis in vitro via rapamycin (mTOR)-dependent signaling. FASEB J 2002;16:771–80.
100. Costa LF, Balcells M, Edelman ER, et al. Pro-angiogenic stimulation of bone marrow endothelium engages mTOR, and is inhibited by simultaneous blockade of mTOR and NF-B. Blood 2006;107:285–92.
101. Castedo T, et al. Sequential involvement of Cdk1, mTOR and p53 in apoptosis induced by the HIV-1 envelope. EMBO J 2002;21:4070–80.
102. Decaudin D, Geley S, Hirsch T, et al. Bcl-2 and Bcl-XL antagonize the mitochondrial dysfunction preceding nuclear apoptosis induced by chemotherapeutic agents. Cancer Res 1997;57:62–7.
103. Zangemeister-Wittke U, Leech SH, Olie RA, et al. A novel bispecific antisense oligonucleotide inhibiting both BCL-2 and BCL-XL expression efficiently induces apoptosis in tumor cells. Clin Cancer Res 2000;6:2547–55.
104. Shinjyo T, et al. Down regulation of Bim, a proapoptotic relative of Bcl-2, is a pivotal step in cytokine-initiated survival signaling in murine hematopoietic progenitors. Mol Cell Biol 2001;21:854–64.
105. Li X, Alafuzoff I, Soininen H, et al. Levels of mTOR and its downstream targets 4E-BP1, eEF2, and eEF2 kinase in relationships with tau in Alzheimer's disease brain. FEBS J 2005;272:4211–20.
106. Kroemer G, Jaattela M. Lysosomes and autophagy in cell death control. Nature Rev Cancer 2005;11:886–97.
107. Drakos E, Rassidakis GZ, Medeiros LJ. Mammalian target of rapamycin (mTOR) pathway signalling in lymphomas. Expert Rev Mol Med 2008;10:e4 [review].
108. Raymond E, et al. Safety and pharmacokinetics of escalated doses of weekly intravenous infusion of CCI-779, a novel mTOR inhibitor, in patients with cancer. J Clin Oncol 2004;16:2336–47.
109. Hidalgo M, Rowinsky E, Erlichman C, et al. CCI-779, a rapamycin analog and multifaceted inhibitor of signal transduction: a phase I study. 187a. Proc Am Soc Clin Oncol 2000;19:A726.
110. O'Donnell A, Faivre S, Burris HA 3rd, et al. Phase I pharmacokinetic and pharmacodynamic study of the oral mammalian target of rapamycin inhibitor everolimus in patients with advanced solid tumors. J Clin Oncol 2008;26(10):1588–95 [Epub 2008 Mar 10].
111. Mita MM, Mita AC, Chu QS, et al. Phase I trial of the novel mammalian target of rapamycin inhibitor deforolimus (AP23573; MK-8669) administered

intravenously daily for 5 days every 2 weeks to patients with advanced malignancies. J Clin Oncol 2008;26(3):361–7.

112. Witzig TE, Geyer SM, Ghobrial I, et al. Phase II trial of single-agent temsirolimus (CCI-779) for relapsed mantle cell lymphoma. J Clin Oncol 2005;23:5347–56.

113. Yee KW, Zeng Z, Konopleva M, et al. Phase I/II study of the mammalian target of rapamycin inhibitor everolimus (RAD001) in patients with relapsed or refractory hematologic malignancies. Clin Cancer Res 2006;12(17):5165–73.

114. Rizzieri DA, Feldman E, Dipersio JF, et al. A phase 2 clinical trial of deforolimus (AP23573, MK-8669), a novel mammalian target of rapamycin inhibitor, in patients with relapsed or refractory hematologic malignancies. Clin Cancer Res 2008;14(9):2756–62.

115. Abd-el-Baki J, Demierre MF, Li N, et al. Transformation in mycosis fungoides: the role of methotrexate. J Cutan Med Surg 2002;6:109–16.

116. Schmid FA, Sirotnak FM, Otter GM, et al. New folate analogs of the 10-deaza-aminopterin series: markedly increased antitumor activity of the 10-ethyl analog compared to the parent compound and methotrexate against some human tumor xenografts in nude mice. Cancer Treat Rep 1985;69:551–3.

117. Sirotnak FM, DeGraw JI, Moccio DM, et al. New folate analogs of the 10-deaza-aminopterin series. Basis for structural design and biochemical and pharmacologic properties. Cancer Chemother Pharmacol 1984;12:18–25.

118. Sirotnak FM, DeGraw JI, Schmid FA, et al. New folate analogs of the 10-deaza-aminopterin series. Further evidence for markedly increased antitumor efficacy compared with methotrexate in ascitic and solid murine tumor models. Cancer Chemother Pharmacol 1984;12:26–30.

119. Toner LE, Vrhovac R, Smith EA, et al. The schedule-dependent effects of the novel antifolate pralatrexate and gemcitabine are superior to methotrexate and cytarabine in models of human non-Hodgkin's lymphoma. Clin Cancer Res 2006;12:924–32.

120. Wang ES, O'Connor O, She Y, et al. Activity of a novel anti-folate (PDX, 10-propargyl 10-deazaaminopterin) against human lymphoma is superior to methotrexate and correlates with tumor RFC-1 gene expression. Leuk Lymphoma 2003;44:1027–35.

121. O'Connor OA, Hamlin P, Portlock C, et al. Pralatrexate, a novel class of antifol with high affinity for the reduced folate carrier type-1, produces marked complete and durable remissions in a diversity of chemotherapy refractory cases of T-cell lymphoma. Br J Haematol 2007;139(3):425–8.

122. Braselmann S, Taylor V, Zhao H, et al. R406, an orallyt available spleen tyrosine kinase inhibitor blocks receptor signaling and reduces immune complex-mediated inflammation. J Pharmacol Exp Ther 2006;319:998–1008.

123. Zhu Y, Herlaar E, Masuda ES, et al. Immunotoxicity assessment for the novel spleen tyrosine kinase inhibitor R406. Toxicol Appl Pharmacol 2007;221(3):267–77.

124. Wossning T, Herzog S, Köhler F, et al. Deregulated Syk inhibits differentiation and induces growth factor-independent proliferation of pre-B cells. J Exp Med 2006;203(13):2829–40.

125. Wossning L, Monti S, Juszcynski P, et al. Syk-dependent tonic B-cell receptor signaling is a rationL treatment target in diffuse large B-cell lymphoma. Blood 2008;111(4):2230–7.

126. Aggarwal BB, Bannerjee S, Bharadwaj U, et al. Curcumin induces the degradation of cyclin E expression through ubiquitin-dependent pathway and up-regulates

cyclin-dependent kinase inhibitors p21 and p27 in multiple human tumor cell lines. Biochem Pharmacol 2007;73(7):1024–32.

127. Mackenzie GG, Queisser N, Wolfson ML, et al. Curcumin induces cell-arrest and apoptosis in association with the inhibition of constitutively active NF-κB and STST3 pathways in Hodgkin's lymphoma cells. Int J Cancer 2008;123(1):56–65.

128. Gururajan M, Dasu T, Shahidain S, et al. Spleen tyrosine kinase (Syk), a novel target of curcumin, is required for B lymphoma growth. J Immunol 2007; 178(1):11–121.

129. Speich HE, Grgurevich S, Kueter TJ, et al. Platelets undergo phosphorylation of Syk at Y525/526 and Y352 in response to pathophysiological shear stress. Am J Physiol Cell Physiol 2008; [Epub ahead of print].

130. Bhavaraju K, Kim S, Daniel JL, et al. Evaluation of [3-(1-methyl-1H-indol-3-yl-methylene)-2-oxo-2, 3-dihydro-1H-indole-5-sulfonamide] (OXSI-2), as a Syk-selective inhibitor in platelets. Eur J Pharmacol 2008;580(3):258–90.

New Biologic Agents and Immunologic Strategies

Rebecca L. Elstrom, MD, Peter Martin, MD, John P. Leonard, MD*

KEYWORDS

- Lymphoma • Monoclonal antibody • Immunomodulatory

The treatment of non-Hodgkin's lymphoma (NHL) has traditionally consisted of cytotoxic chemotherapy, which can frequently induce remissions but less reliably delivers long-term disease-free survival. The last two decades have heralded an era of increasing exploration of therapies derived from improved biologic understanding of tumors and tumor-host interactions, including the development of therapeutic tactics that take advantage of immune mechanisms to target and kill tumors. Foremost among these has been the development of monoclonal antibodies, including rituximab, which has significant single-agent antitumor activity and can improve survival of patients with follicular lymphoma (FL) and diffuse, large B-cell lymphoma (DLBCL) who receive it in combination with chemotherapy. There is, however, clearly room for improvement in the case of primary and secondary resistance, because many patients still die of NHL. Currently, there is an array of novel therapeutics in development that may improve outcomes further. These include novel monoclonals and other agents that take advantage of or optimize immune system function in the treatment of lymphoma or that provide other mechanisms of antitumor activity.

MONOCLONAL ANTIBODY THERAPY
Unconjugated Antibodies

The activity of monoclonal antibodies as therapeutic agents is dependent on characteristics of both the target antigen and the antibody. An optimal target antigen is expressed on all malignant cells, but minimally or not at all on normal cells to minimize toxicity. The antigen should not be shed either on binding of the antibody, or over time with clonal evolution of the tumor, suggesting an important biologic relationship between the target and the cell. Internalization of a target antigen on antibody binding may provide a delivery mechanism for toxins or radioisotopes that may be bound to

Division of Hematology/Oncology, Weill Cornell Medical College, 520 East 70th Street, Starr 340, New York, NY 10021, USA
* Corresponding author.
E-mail address: jpleonar@med.cornell.edu (J.P. Leonard).

Hematol Oncol Clin N Am 22 (2008) 1037–1049
doi:10.1016/j.hoc.2008.07.003   hemonc.theclinics.com
0889-8588/08/$ – see front matter © 2008 Elsevier Inc. All rights reserved.

the antibody, however, making this mode of modulation a potentially attractive characteristic in specific circumstances.

Several potential mechanisms by which antibodies induce antitumor activity have been described.[1] A significant portion of the activity of many therapeutic antibodies depends on the interaction of the antibody with the host's intrinsic immune system. Antibody-dependent cellular cytotoxicity (ADCC) is induced through binding of the Fc portion of the antibody to Fc receptors on cytolytic effector cells, particularly natural killer (NK) cells.

Complement-dependent cytoxicity (CDC) is induced by promoting complement fixation at the cell surface, leading to complement-dependent lysis of target cells. The ability of certain anti-CD20 monoclonal antibodies to trigger CDC seems to relate to their ability to segregate CD20 into low-density, detergent-insoluble lipid rafts.[2] Although an apparent mechanism of antitumor activity, complement fixation and CDC have also been implicated as causative factors in some of the infusion-related side effects associated with certain antibody therapies, such as rituximab.[3]

The ability of some monoclonal antibodies to induce cell death independent of the host immune system seems to be caused by direct induction of apoptosis. This mechanism is dependent on characteristics of both the antibody and the target antigen. Rituximab, for example, seems to induce a signal through CD20, which alters the ratio of proapoptotic and antiapoptotic Bcl-2 family proteins,[4,5] leading to induction of programmed cell death.

Targeting CD20

Rituximab is a chimeric IgG1 kappa monoclonal antibody that binds to CD20, inducing cell death in both normal and neoplastic B cells. The proposed mechanisms by which rituximab exerts these effects include direct induction of apoptosis and induction of ADCC and CDC. Rituximab was approved by the Food and Drug Administration (FDA) in 1997 for treatment of relapsed or refractory CD20-positive follicular or indolent B-cell NHL, and subsequent studies have shown that rituximab is effective in many B-cell NHL subtypes alone and in combination with chemotherapy. Addition of rituximab to chemotherapeutic regimens has also been associated with improved survival of patients with both FL and DLBCL.[6–8] Rituximab also has a modest toxicity profile. Although rituximab induces infusion reactions in many patients especially during the first infusion, these effects are manageable in most patients and decrease with subsequent infusions. Although rituximab depletes normal B cells, infectious complications attributable to rituximab are unusual and occur mostly in patients who are otherwise immunosuppressed. Nevertheless, JC virus infection and reactivation of hepatitis B virus have been recognized as rare but potentially life-threatening complications of rituximab therapy. Late, self-limited neutropenia is increasingly recognized as a potential side effect of rituximab.[9,10]

Although rituximab is a valuable addition to the treatment armamentarium for B-cell NHL, the drug has some shortcomings and there is great interest in the development of newer anti-CD20 targeted agents. Toxicity of rituximab is manageable in most patients, but infusion reactions can be very uncomfortable, and in some cases severe or life-threatening. Furthermore, efficacy of rituximab may be limited by several factors intrinsic to the molecule. Rituximab is chimeric, containing murine sequences that may be immunogenic, and uncommonly induces human antichimera antibodies. Human antichimera antibodies potentially reduce the half-life of the antibody, compromising efficacy. Furthermore, the foreign component of the molecule might contribute to the severity of infusion reactions. These drawbacks of the chimeric molecule have led to the investigation of humanized antibodies, which do not contain any foreign protein components. It is hoped that such constructs will be associated with decreased infusion reactions and immunogenicity, and possibly an improved pharmacokinetic profile because of decreased immune-mediated clearance of the drug. The clinical benefit of these modifications, however, remains to be determined.

Other factors that may influence the efficacy of rituximab include its interaction with the patient's intrinsic immune system, including induction of ADCC, through binding of the Fc portion of the antibody to Fc receptors on effector cells, and fixation of complement leading to complement-dependent lysis. Both of these activities could be affected by alterations of the structure of the antibody. Cartron and colleagues[11] first demonstrated that FcgRIII polymorphisms affect responses to rituximab, with previously untreated patients with FL who were homozygous for valine at position 158 (158 V/V) having an overall response rate (ORR) of 100% to single-agent rituximab, whereas only 67% of those who carried at least one phenylalanine allele (158F) responded. Similar findings have been demonstrated in DLBCL, where Kim and colleagues[12] demonstrated that patients with the FcgRIIIA 158 V/V polymorphism had an 88% ORR with the combination of rituximab, cyclophosphamide, doxorubicin, and prednisone (R-CHOP), whereas only 50% of individuals with the FcgRIIIA 158 F/F polymorphism responded.

Newer-generation anti-CD20 antibodies designed to improve on rituximab are in development. In general, modification strategies include humanization of the molecule to decrease infusion reactions and immunogenicity, enhancement of binding affinity, and modification of the Fc portion of the molecule to optimize effector functions, particularly ADCC.

Ofatumumab is a fully human IgG1 kappa antibody that binds to CD20 at an epitope distinct from that of rituximab. It mediates both ADCC and CDC, and has a slow off rate from CD20, which may enhance complement fixation.[13] Ofatumumab has shown activity in two phase I/II trials of patients with recurrent FL[14] and in patients who have chronic lymphocytic leukemia.[15] In patients with FL, infusion reactions were observed, but were for the most part mild. The median half-life of atumumab was 342 hours as compared with 205 hours reported for rituximab, suggesting a more favorable circulation of the drug. Responses were seen in 60% of patients with FL and 52% of patients who have chronic lymphocytic leukemia at the highest dose levels in each study. A trial of ofatumumab in patients with rituximab-refractory NHL is underway.

Other novel anti-CD20 antibodies are also under investigation. Veltuzumab (hA20) is a humanized antibody that targets the same epitope as rituximab.[16] A phase I/II study of veltuzumab in patients with B-cell NHL who had previously been treated with rituximab showed responses at lower doses than those standardly used with rituximab, suggesting the possibility of more potency or improved pharmacokinetics.[17] This antibody is currently being explored in subcutaneous dosing.

Ocrelizumab is a humanized IgG1 anti-CD20 antibody whose Fc portion has been optimized for improved binding to the low-affinity variant of the FcgRIII molecule and improved ADCC.[18] A phase I/II trial in patients with relapsed and refractory FL recently reported in abstract form demonstrated good tolerability, with infusion-related reactions common but for the most part mild. A modest response rate was observed (36% overall) in this pretreated population without a clear dose-response relationship.[19]

Other anti-CD20 molecules with enhanced FcgRIII binding and ADCC are in development, and other approaches, such as conjugation to interleukin (IL)-2 to create an immunocytokine,[20] are under investigation. A major issue in moving forward with these novel anti-CD20 antibodies is the identification of an appropriate niche for their use. Rituximab has become nearly ubiquitous in the treatment of B-cell NHL, and proving superiority in specific instances is a challenge. Demonstration of significant activity in patients with rituximab-refractory disease would provide a clear and exciting role for these novel approaches.

Other Targets for Unconjugated Antibodies

CD22

CD22 is an immunoglobulin superfamily molecule expressed exclusively on B cells. It contains immunoreceptor tyrosine-based inhibitory motifs, leading to negative regulation of B-cell receptor signaling. CD22 is internalized on binding of ligand or antibody, making it potentially useful as a target for a conjugated antibody, as discussed later. Epratuzumab is a humanized anti-CD22 IgG1 antibody that exerts antilymphoma effects through promotion of ADCC and direct induction of cell death. Phase I/II clinical studies have shown excellent tolerability and modest single-agent activity in patients with relapsed and refractory indolent and aggressive NHL.[21,22] Two phase II studies evaluating the combination of epratuzumab and rituximab have shown responses, including complete responses (CR), both in rituximab-naive patients and patients previously treated with rituximab.[23,24] Determination of whether these findings represent an improvement over rituximab alone requires a phase III randomized trial. Ongoing studies are evaluating the use of epratuzumab plus rituximab as initial treatment in FL, and in combination with CHOP chemotherapy in DLBCL.

CD30

CD30 is a tumor necrosis factor receptor family molecule expressed in specific circumstances on T cells, B cells, NK cells, and eosinophils. It is also expressed on many T-cell lymphomas and Hodgkin's lymphoma cells, where it has been implicated in induction of ligand-independent NF-kB signaling, possibly contributing to oncogenesis.[25] The anti-CD30 antibody SGN-30 is currently being investigated in patients with Hodgkin's and CD30[+] T-cell lymphomas. A phase I study demonstrated good tolerability with no objective responses, but several patients with stable disease.[26] Phase II studies of the combination of SGN-30 with chemotherapy are ongoing.

CD40

CD40 is a tumor necrosis factor receptor family molecule expressed on normal B cells, B- and T-cell lymphomas, Reed-Sternberg cells, and plasma cells in multiple myeloma, and many other normal and malignant nonhematopoietic cell types. CD40 signaling promotes B-cell activation and proliferation, and may be relevant in promoting survival.[27] SGN-40 is a humanized IgG1 antibody that binds to CD40, inhibiting proliferation and directly inducing apoptosis in B-cell lymphoma cell lines in vitro. A recent phase I study of SGN-40 showed good tolerability and objective responses in patients with recurrent B-cell NHL.[28] Phase II studies of SGN-40 both alone and in combination with chemotherapy are currently in progress.

CD80

CD80 is a cell surface protein expressed on antigen-presenting cells, including B cells. CD80 interacts with the T-cell costimulatory molecule CD28 and the inhibitory molecule CTLA-4, modulating T-cell activation, IL-2 production, and proliferation. Not only does CD80 act as a ligand for T-cell signaling molecules, influencing T-cell function, but it also mediates signal transduction in B cells. CD80 is constitutively expressed in many B-cell NHLs, making it a target of interest for antibody therapy. Cross-linking of CD80 on B cells and B-cell lymphoma cell lines leads to up-regulation of proapoptotic molecules, such as caspases 3 and 8, Fas, Fas ligand, Bak, and Bax, and down-regulation of the antiapoptotic molecule Bcl-X_L.[29] Galiximab is a chimeric anti-CD80 IgG1 antibody that is currently in clinical trials for B-cell lymphomas.

A phase I/II study of galiximab in relapsed and refractory FL showed excellent tolerability with a modest response rate of 11%.[30] A phase II study of the combination of galiximab and rituximab in patients with relapsed and refractory FL demonstrated a response rate of 64%,[31] and further studies of this combination are ongoing.

Vascular endothelial growth factor

Angiogenesis is increasingly recognized as an important pathogenic factor in solid tumor growth and survival, and strategies to inhibit this process, such as interfering with vascular endothelial growth factor, have shown clinical promise. Bevacizumab is a monoclonal antibody against vascular endothelial growth factor that is approved for use in combination with chemotherapy in patients with metastatic colon cancer and non–small cell lung cancer. More recently, investigations of the relevance of angiogenesis in lymphoma have demonstrated that aggressive lymphoma subtypes are characterized by heightened stromal hemangiogenesis.[32] Further study has demonstrated the autocrine proliferation and survival of lymphoma tumor cells by the vascular endothelial growth factor–vascular endothelial growth factor receptor axis, and recruitment of bone marrow–derived hemangiogenesis to support neovascular assembly and metastasis. A by-product of traditional full-dose chemotherapy is promotion of angiogenesis. Bevacizumab has shown modest activity as a single agent in NHL,[33] and is currently under investigation in the treatment of NHL in combination with chemotherapy.

Conjugated Antibodies

Another mechanism by which monoclonal antibodies may be useful in the treatment of cancer is through targeted delivery of cytotoxic substances, such as radiation or toxins. Conjugates of monoclonal antibodies with such cytotoxins have shown significant promise in inducing clinical responses in patients with lymphoma.

Radioimmunotherapy

Conjugation of various monoclonal antibodies with radioisotopes has been under investigation for decades. Two such radioimmunoconjugates are currently approved by the FDA for use in recurrent indolent B-cell lymphomas: ^{90}Y-ibritumomab tiuxetan and ^{131}I-tositumomab. Both are CD20-targeted, and show response rates in the range of 50% to 75% in patients with previously treated B-cell NHL, including patients with chemotherapy- and rituximab-refractory disease.[34–37] Toxicity consists mainly of myelosuppression, which tends to be delayed until 6 to 9 weeks following treatment. ^{131}I-tositumomab has also been studied as initial therapy in patients with FL, with 95% of patients responding, 75% with CR.[38] The rate of human antimouse antibody formation was high in this study, and efforts are under way to identify a strategy to minimize this effect in first-line radioimmunotherapy. Other strategies to incorporate radioimmunotherapy into first-line therapy include use of the radioimmunoconjugate as consolidation following chemotherapy in FL[39,40] and DLBCL,[41] and alone or in combination with high-dose chemotherapy in regimens using autologous stem cell transplantation.[42–44]

Epratuzumab is also being explored as a platform for radioimmunotherapy because its target, CD22, is internalized on antibody binding, facilitating delivery of the radioisotope directly into the cell. To this end, ^{90}Y is more likely to be retained intracellularly following antigen modulation than ^{131}I, allowing increased radiation exposure of the target cell. A recent phase I/II trial of fractionated dosing of ^{90}Y-epratuzumab in patients with previously treated B-cell NHL suggested a dose-response relationship, with 90% ORR at the highest dose level, including 60% CR.[45]

Concerns about radiation safety, need for treatment in specialized centers, and economic issues have limited the dissemination of radioimmunotherapy as a standard treatment regimen. The efficacy seen in these studies, and the potential for beneficial responses in wider circumstances, increases the urgency to ensure that this treatment strategy remains viable into the future.

Immunotoxins

The conjugation of potent cytotoxins to monoclonal antibodies allows the delivery of these toxic agents directly to target tissues, allowing potentially therapeutic dosing of substances that is intolerable for nonspecific systemic delivery.

CMC-544

In addition to being used as a target for unconjugated and radioconjugated antibodies, CD22 is also the target for an immunoconjugate bearing the potent antitumor agent calicheamicin. Calicheamicin has shown significant activity in acute myelogenous leukemia as a CD33-antibody conjugate. The internalization of CD22 on antibody binding allows internalization and delivery of the calicheamicin into CD22$^+$ lymphoma cells. A recent phase I study of CMC-544 identified a maximum tolerated dose of 1.8 mg/m^2, and major toxicities included myelosuppression, asthenia, and liver function abnormalities.[46] The investigators reported activity of the drug in an expanded cohort at the maximum tolerated dose, demonstrating responses of 69% in FL and 33% in DLBCL in a very heavily pretreated patient population.

SGN-35

SGN-35 is an antibody-drug conjugate comprised of an anti-CD30 antibody linked to the antitubulin drug monomethylauristatin E. On CD30 binding, the complex is internalized, and lysosomal degradation releases the toxin inside the cell, disrupting tubulin networks. A phase I study of this conjugate is underway, and a preliminary report has suggested activity in CD30$^+$ lymphomas at submaximum tolerated dose doses.[47]

Denileukin diftitox

A third immunoconjugate is a nonantibody recombinant protein that fuses IL-2 with diphtheria toxin. The IL-2 component of this conjugate binds to the IL-2 receptor on target cells, such as many T- and B-cell lymphomas, targeting the toxin specifically to those cells. On internalization, the toxin binds to and inactivates elongation factor-2, disrupting translation and leading to cell death. Denileukin diftitox is approved by the FDA for use in cutaneous T-cell lymphoma. This drug is under investigation with promising results in peripheral T-cell lymphomas and B-cell lymphomas, and immunomodulatory a phase I trial evaluating combination with CHOP chemotherapy showed good tolerability.[48] Determination of whether denileukin diftitox adds significant activity to CHOP alone requires further study.

IMMUNOMODULATING AGENTS

Immunomodulating agents are drugs with limited effect on tumor cells as single agents, but that promote antitumor immune activity through a range of potential mechanisms. These agents include both native biologic substances, such as cytokines, and drugs, such as IMiDs. Because most monoclonal antibodies exert antilymphoma effects through immune-dependent mechanisms, such as ADCC, the integration of immunomodulatory agents with monoclonal antibodies presents a rational approach in exploring new therapeutic combinations.

Granulocyte-Macrophage Colony–Stimulating Factor

Granulocyte-macrophage colony–stimulating factor induces development and activation of myeloid cells. It also promotes the generation of monocytes and myeloid dendritic cells, which can enhance immune responses. A study in a murine model aimed at identification of components of the immune system that are important for the B-cell depletion activity of rituximab demonstrated a critical role for monocytes as effector cells.[49] This suggests that enhancing the development and activation of effector cells may improve responses and long-term outcomes with rituximab therapy. A phase II clinical study of the combination of rituximab and granulocyte-macrophage colony–stimulating factor in patients with relapsed and refractory FL demonstrated a response rate of 70%, with 45% CR and progression-free survival of 16.7 months.[50] These results are promising, and clinicians can look forward to a comparison study with rituximab alone to determine whether this strategy represents a true improvement.

Interleukin-2

IL-2 is a cytokine with wide-ranging immunoregulatory effects. In vivo, IL-2 promotes cellular immunity through enhancement of T cell and NK cell cytotoxicity, including ADCC, and promotion of the production of cytokines, such as tumor necrosis factor, IL-1, and interferon-γ. These effects of IL-2 could promote rituximab activity, and this possibility has been explored in clinical trials. A phase I study showed that the combination was feasible, and demonstrated expansion of NK cell numbers and ADCC, which correlated with clinical response.[51] A phase II study in patients with relapsed or refractory FL treated with the combination of IL-2 and rituximab showed an ORR of 55% and median progression-free survival of greater than 13 months. Although these end points are not clearly improved over results expected with rituximab alone, the authors do report that 3 of the 20 patients experienced extended remissions, remaining progression free at 41, 49, and 84 months.[52]

Interleukin-21

The receptor for the cytokine IL-21 shares a common gamma chain with IL-2. Like IL-2, IL-21 activates NK cells and cytotoxic T lymphocytes and enhances ADCC, but unlike IL-2, it is able to promote resistance of cytotoxic T cells to suppression by regulatory T cells. In addition, IL-21 has direct antitumor effects against malignant B cells. A preliminary report of a phase I study of the combination of IL-21 and rituximab in patients with relapsed and refractory indolent lymphomas demonstrated objective responses in 5 of 15 patients, including two with rituximab-refractory disease.[53] This study is ongoing, with an expansion cohort planned at the maximum tolerated dose to assess better the activity of the combination.

CpG Oligonucleotides

CpG DNA oligonucleotides are short sequences of DNA containing unmethylated CpG dimers. These sequences were initially identified to have immunostimulatory properties through study of bacterial DNA, which has a high frequency of unmethylated CpG dimers as compared with eukaryotic DNA. The immunostimulatory properties of bacterial DNA can be mimicked by synthetic CpG DNA oligonucleotides, which have been shown to promote both innate and adaptive immune functions in mammals, promoting enhanced ADCC and promotion of effector cell function. Furthermore, CpG oligonucleotides induce up-regulation of CD20 expression on B cells,[54] providing clear rationale for combination with rituximab. A recent phase II study demonstrated feasibility of the combination in patients with relapsed and refractory FL, and responses in 45% of treated patients.[55] The authors showed evidence of immune stimulation in a subset of patients including enhanced ADCC and T-cell infiltration of tumor sites. A preliminary report of a phase I study of CpG oligonucleotides in combination with rituximab and ^{90}Y-ibritumomab tiuxetan showed good tolerability and response rates of greater than 90% in patients with previously treated CD20[+] B-cell lymphomas.[56] This seems to be a very promising strategy, and further study will clarify the role of this approach.

Lenalidomide

Lenalidomide is a member of a novel class of therapeutic agents, known as "immuno-modulatory drugs," which includes thalidomide. Lenalidomide is more potent than thalidomide and is approved by the FDA for treatment of myelodysplastic syndromes and multiple myeloma. The major side effect of lenalidomide is myelosuppression.

The mechanisms by which lenalidomide induces tumor regression are actively under exploration. Proposed mechanisms include inhibition of angiogenesis; direct induction of apoptosis in tumors through inhibition of prosurvival factors, such as Akt; and modulation of immune function. Lenalidomide has been shown to have multiple immunomodulatory effects in vitro and in vivo, including inhibition of proin-flammatory cytokines, such as tumor necrosis factor-α, IL-1β, IL-6, and IL-12. It pro-motes production of IL-2 and interferon-γ, and enhances T cell– and NK cell–mediated killing of tumor cells.[57,58] In vitro studies demonstrated improved ADCC in response to antibodies, such as rituximab, galixumab, and alemtuzumab in the presence of lenalidomide.[59] Preliminary investigations of this finding suggest that these effects are mediated through promotion of costimulatory molecule expression and effector T-cell and NK-cell activity.

Clinical studies have demonstrated activity of lenalidomide as a single agent in sev-eral lymphoid malignancies in addition to multiple myeloma.[60] Responses, including CR, have been observed in chronic lymphocytic leukemia, cutaneous T-cell lym-phoma, and indolent and aggressive systemic NHL. In an ongoing study, Witzig and colleagues[61] reported that 11 of 43 evaluable patients with recurrent indolent lymphoma treated with lenalidomide showed objective responses (two CR, one CR unconfirmed, and eight partial responses), and seven demonstrated stable disease. Wiernik and colleagues[62] have reported on 49 patients with relapsed and refractory aggressive NHL, with 17 objective responses (2 CR, 4 CR unconfirmed, and 11 partial responses) and 6 patients demonstrating stable disease.

Lenalidomide is also being studied in combination with rituximab and other mono-clonal antibodies. In an ongoing study of lenalidomide in combination with rituximab in relapsed and refractory mantle cell lymphoma, the maximum tolerated dose of lena-lidomide in the combination was found to be 20 mg for 21 days of a 28-day cycle. Of 10 evaluable patients at this dose, seven achieved objective responses, including three CR and four partial response.[63] The preliminary efficacy and tolerability results of the combination in this difficult group of patients raises significant interest in pursuing its evaluation in other settings.

SUMMARY

The development of monoclonal antibodies, such as rituximab, and their increasing incorporation into therapy has already significantly impacted both therapeutic out-comes and the approach to lymphoma therapy in general, specifically demonstrating that minimally toxic agents used alone or in combination can contribute important benefits to patients with lymphoma. The success of rituximab has led to increased research to understand better how monoclonal antibodies affect their antilymphoma activity. One research direction has been the development of second- and third-generation anti-CD20 antibodies designed to optimize these therapeutic mechanisms. Furthermore, improved understanding of the mechanistic basis of antibody activity has allowed the rational development of combination approaches designed to optimize the activity of monoclonal antibody therapy, such as the addition of cytokines and other immune modulators. Although this article concentrates on agents that interact with and promote specific immune system functions, combinations using other strategies are also under study with promising results. These include agents that enhance the apoptotic function of monoclonal antibodies through modulation of specific apoptotic regulators, and agents with specific targets but more generalized cellular effects, such as bortezomib. A major challenge in moving forward with these novel antibodies is to identify appropriate clinical settings for their use, either concentrating on patients who do not tolerate or respond poorly to rituximab, or demonstrating significantly improved therapeutic characteristics over rituximab. Likewise, the incorporation of other novel biologic therapies into treatment requires judicious investigation of appropriate patient groups and clinical settings optimally to exploit their activity.

REFERENCES

1. Cartron G, Watier H, Golay J, et al. From the bench to the bedside: ways to improve rituximab efficacy. Blood 2004;104(9):2635–42.
2. Cragg MS, Morgan SM, Chan HT, et al. Complement-mediated lysis by anti-CD20 mAb correlates with segregation into lipid rafts. Blood 2003;101(3):1045–52.
3. van der Kolk LE, Grillo-Lopez AJ, Baars JW, et al. Complement activation plays a key role in the side-effects of rituximab treatment. Br J Haematol 2001;115(4): 807–11.
4. Alas S, Bonavida B. Rituximab inactivates signal transducer and activation of transcription 3 (STAT3) activity in B-non-Hodgkin's lymphoma through inhibition of the interleukin 10 autocrine/paracrine loop and results in down-regulation of Bcl-2 and sensitization to cytotoxic drugs. Cancer Res 2001;61(13):5137–44.
5. Byrd JC, Kitada S, Flinn IW, et al. The mechanism of tumor cell clearance by rituximab in vivo in patients with B-cell chronic lymphocytic leukemia: evidence of caspase activation and apoptosis induction. Blood 2002;99(3):1038–43.
6. Feugier P, Van Hoof A, Sebban C, et al. Long-term results of the R-CHOP study in the treatment of elderly patients with diffuse large B-cell lymphoma: a study by the Groupe d'Etude des Lymphomes de l'Adulte. J Clin Oncol 2005;23(18): 4117–26.
7. Habermann TM, Weller EA, Morrison VA, et al. Rituximab-CHOP versus CHOP alone or with maintenance rituximab in older patients with diffuse large B-cell lymphoma. J Clin Oncol 2006;24(19):3121–7.
8. van Oers MH, Klasa R, Marcus RE, et al. Rituximab maintenance improves clinical outcome of relapsed/resistant follicular non-Hodgkin lymphoma in patients both with and without rituximab during induction: results of a prospective randomized phase 3 intergroup trial. Blood 2006;108(10):3295–301.
9. Chaiwatanatorn K, Lee N, Grigg A, et al. Delayed-onset neutropenia associated with rituximab therapy. Br J Haematol 2003;121(6):913–8.
10. Nitta E, Izutsu K, Sato T, et al. A high incidence of late-onset neutropenia following rituximab-containing chemotherapy as a primary treatment of CD20-positive B-cell lymphoma: a single-institution study. Ann Oncol 2007;18(2):364–9.

11. Cartron G, Dacheux L, Salles G, et al. Therapeutic activity of humanized anti-CD20 monoclonal antibody and polymorphism in IgG Fc receptor FcgammaRIIIa gene. Blood 2002;99(3):754–8.

12. Kim DH, Jung HD, Kim JG, et al. FCGR3A gene polymorphisms may correlate with response to frontline R-CHOP therapy for diffuse large B-cell lymphoma. Blood 2006;108(8):2720–5.

13. Teeling JL, French RR, Cragg MS, et al. Characterization of new human CD20 monoclonal antibodies with potent cytolytic activity against non-Hodgkin lymphomas. Blood 2004;104(6):1793–800.

14. Hagenbeek A, Plesner T, Johnson P, et al. HuMax-CD20, a novel fully human anti-CD20 monoclonal antibody: results of a phase I/II trial in relapsed or refractory follicular Non-Hodgkin's lymphoma. ASH Annual Meeting Abstracts 2005;106: 4760.

15. Coiffier B, Lepretre S, Pederson L, et al. Safety and efficacy of ofatumumab, a fully human monoclonal anti-CD20 antibody, in patients with relapsed or refractory B-cell chronic lymphocytic leukemia: a phase 1,2 study. Blood 2008;111:1094.

16. Stein R, Qu Z, Chen S, et al. Characterization of a new humanized anti-CD20 monoclonal antibody, IMMU-106, and Its use in combination with the humanized anti-CD22 antibody, epratuzumab, for the therapy of non-Hodgkin's lymphoma. Clin Cancer Res 2004;10(8):2868–78.

17. Morshhauser F, Leonard JP, Coiffier B, et al. Phase I/II results of a second-generation humanized anti-CD20 antibody, IMMU-106 (hA20), in NHL. ASCO Meeting Abstracts 2006;24:7530.

18. Vugmeyster Y, Beyer J, Howell K, et al. Depletion of B cells by a humanized anti-CD20 antibody PRO70769 in Macaca fascicularis. J Immuno Ther 2005;28(3): 212–9.

19. Morschhauser F, Marlton P, Vitolo U, et al. Interim results of a phase I/II study of ocrelizumab, a new humanised anti-CD20 antibody in patients with relapsed/refractory follicular non-Hodgkin's lymphoma. ASH Annual Meeting Abstracts 2007; 110:645.

20. Gillies SD, Lan Y, Williams S, et al. An anti-CD20-IL-2 immunocytokine is highly efficacious in a SCID mouse model of established human B lymphoma. Blood 2005;105(10):3972–8.

21. Leonard JP, Coleman M, Ketas JC, et al. Phase I/II trial of epratuzumab (humanized anti-CD22 antibody) in indolent non-Hodgkin's lymphoma. J Clin Oncol 2003;21(16):3051–9.

22. Leonard JP, Coleman M, Ketas JC, et al. Epratuzumab, a humanized anti-CD22 antibody, in aggressive non-Hodgkin's lymphoma: phase I/II clinical trial results. Clin Cancer Res 2004;10(16):5327–34.

23. Leonard JP, Coleman M, Ketas J, et al. Combination antibody therapy with epratuzumab and rituximab in relapsed or refractory non-Hodgkin's lymphoma. J Clin Oncol 2005;23(22):5044–51.

24. Strauss SJ, Morschhauser F, Rech J, et al. Multicenter phase II trial of immunotherapy with the humanized anti-CD22 antibody, epratuzumab, in combination with rituximab, in refractory or recurrent non-Hodgkin's lymphoma. J Clin Oncol 2006;24(24):3880–6.

25. Watts TH. TNF/TNFR family members in costimulation of T cell responses. Annu Rev Immunol 2005;23:23–68.

26. Bartlett NL, Younes A, Carabasi MH, et al. A phase 1 multidose study of SGN-30 immunotherapy in patients with refractory or recurrent CD30+ hematologic malignancies. Blood 2008;111(4):1848–54.

27. Vonderheide RH. Prospect of targeting the CD40 pathway for cancer therapy. Clin Cancer Res 2007;13(4):1083–8.
28. Forero-Torres A, Furman RR, Rosenblatt JD, et al. A humanized antibody against CD40 (SGN-40) is well tolerated and active in non-Hodgkin's lymphoma (NHL): results of a phase I study. ASCO Meeting Abstracts 2006;24:7534.
29. Suvas S, Singh V, Sahdev S, et al. Distinct role of CD80 and CD86 in the regulation of the activation of B cell and B cell lymphoma. J Biol Chem 2002;277(10): 7766–75.
30. Czuczman MS, Thall A, Witzig TE, et al. Phase I/II study of galiximab, an anti-CD80 antibody, for relapsed or refractory follicular lymphoma. J Clin Oncol 2005;23(19):4390–8.
31. Friedberg JW, Leonard JP, Younes A, et al. Updated results from a phase II study of galiximab (anti-CD80) in combination with rituximab for relapsed or refractory, follicular NHL. ASH Annual Meeting Abstracts 2005;106:2435.
32. Ruan J, Hyjek E, Kermani P, et al. Magnitude of stromal hemangiogenesis correlates with histologic subtype of non-Hodgkin's lymphoma. Clin Cancer Res 2006; 12(19):5622–31.
33. Stopeck A, Bellamy W, Unger J, et al. Phase II trial of single agent bevacizumab (Avanti) in patients with relapsed, aggressive non-Hodgkin's lymphoma (NHL): southwest oncology group study S0108. ASCO Meeting Abstracts 2005;23: 6592.
34. Davies AJ, Rohatiner AZ, Howell S, et al. Tositumomab and iodine I 131 tositumomab for recurrent indolent and transformed B-cell non-Hodgkin's lymphoma. J Clin Oncol 2004;22(8):1469–79.
35. Fisher RI, Kaminski MS, Wahl RL, et al. Tositumomab and iodine-131 tositumomab produces durable complete remissions in a subset of heavily pretreated patients with low-grade and transformed non-Hodgkin's lymphomas. J Clin Oncol 2005;23(30):7565–73.
36. Horning SJ, Younes A, Jain V, et al. Efficacy and safety of tositumomab and iodine-131 tositumomab (Bexxar) in B-cell lymphoma, progressive after rituximab. J Clin Oncol 2005;23(4):712–9.
37. Kaminski MS, Zelenetz AD, Press OW, et al. Pivotal study of iodine I 131 tositumomab for chemotherapy-refractory low-grade or transformed low-grade B-cell non-Hodgkin's lymphomas. J Clin Oncol 2001;19(19):3918–28.
38. Kaminski MS, Tuck M, Estes J, et al. 131I-tositumomab therapy as initial treatment for follicular lymphoma. N Engl J Med 2005;352(5):441–9.
39. Press OW, Unger JM, Braziel RM, et al. Phase II trial of CHOP chemotherapy followed by tositumomab/iodine I-131 tositumomab for previously untreated follicular non-Hodgkin's lymphoma: five-year follow-up of Southwest Oncology Group Protocol S9911. J Clin Oncol 2006;24(25):4143–9.
40. Hagenbeek A, Bischof-Delaloye A, Radford JA, et al. 90Y-ibritumomab tiuxetan (Zevalin) consolidation of first remission in advanced stage follicular non-Hodgkin's lymphoma: first results of the international randomized phase 3 first-line indolent trial (FIT) in 414 patients. ASH Annual Meeting Abstracts 2007;110:643.
41. Zinzani P-L, Tani M, Fanti S, et al. A phase II trial of chop chemotherapy followed by yttrium 90 (90Y) ibritumomab tiuxetan (zevalin) for previously untreated elderly diffuse large B-cell lymphoma (DLBCL) patients. ASH Annual Meeting Abstracts 2006;108:2431.
42. Liu SY, Eary JF, Petersdorf SH, et al. Follow-up of relapsed B-cell lymphoma patients treated with iodine-131-labeled anti-CD20 antibody and autologous stem-cell rescue. J Clin Oncol 1998;16(10):3270–8.

43. Press OW, Eary JF, Appelbaum FR, et al. Radiolabeled-antibody therapy of B-cell lymphoma with autologous bone marrow support. N Engl J Med 1993;329(17): 1219–24.

44. Vose JM, Bierman PJ, Enke C, et al. Phase I trial of iodine-131 tositumomab with high-dose chemotherapy and autologous stem-cell transplantation for relapsed non-Hodgkin's lymphoma. J Clin Oncol 2005;23(3):461–7.

45. Morschhauser F, Kraeber-Bodere F, Petillon M, et al. Fractionated radioimmunotherapy with ^{90}Y-epratuzumab. EHA Annual Meeting Abstracts 2007;45222.

46. Fayad L, Patel H, Verhoef G, et al. Clinical activity of the immunoconjugate CMC-544 in B-cell malignancies. ASH Annual Meeting Abstracts 2006;108:2711.

47. Younes A, Ferrero-Torres A, Bartlett N, et al. Phase I study of SGN-35 in CD30+ malignancies. Presented at 7th International symposium on HL 11/2007. Haematologica 92(S5) P099bis.

48. Foss F, Sjak-Shie N, Goy A, et al. A phase II Study of denileukin diftitox (Ontak) with CHOP chemotherapy in patients with newly-diagnosed aggressive T-cell lymphomas, the CONCEPT trial: interim analysis. ASH Annual Meeting Abstracts 2007;110:2461.

49. Uchida J, Hamaguchi Y, Oliver JA, et al. The innate mononuclear phagocyte network depletes B lymphocytes through Fc receptor-dependent mechanisms during anti-CD20 antibody immunotherapy. J Exp Med 2004;199(12):1659–69.

50. Rossi JF, Lu ZY, Quittet P, et al. Rituximab activity is potentiated by GM-CSF in patients with relapsed, follicular lymphoma. ASH Annual Meeting Abstracts 2005;106:2432.

51. Gluck WL, Hurst D, Yuen A, et al. Phase I studies of interleukin (IL)-2 and rituximab in B-cell non-Hodgkin's lymphoma: IL-2 mediated natural killer cell expansion correlations with clinical response. Clin Cancer Res 2004;10(7):2253–64.

52. Friedberg JW, Freedman AS. Antibody and immunomodulatory agents in treatment of indolent non-Hodgkin's lymphoma. Curr Treat Options Oncol 2006;7(4): 276–84.

53. Timmerman J, Byrd J, Andorsky D, et al. Recombinant interleukin-21 plus rituximab: clinical activity in a phase 1, dose-finding trial in relapsed low-grade b cell lymphoma. ASH Annual Meeting Abstracts 2007;110:2577.

54. Nijmeijer B, Van Schie M, Willemze R, et al. Upregulation of cd20 on human acute lymphoblastic leukemia cells by IL-4 and CpG motif containing oligonucleotides increases susceptibility to rituximab. ASH Annual Meeting Abstracts 2007;110: 1879.

55. Friedberg J, Kelly J, Kutok J, et al. combination immunotherapy with a cpg oligonucleotide and rituximab augments the immunological response and favorably alters the malignant microenvironment of follicular lymphoma. ASH Annual Meeting Abstracts 2007;110:2713.

56. Witzig T, Wiseman G, Weiner G, et al. A phase I trial of CpG-7909, rituximab immunotherapy and y90 Zevalin radioimmunotherapy for patients with previously treated CD20+ non-Hodgkin lymphoma. ASH Annual Meeting Abstracts 2007; 110:124.

57. Chang DH, Liu N, Klimek V, et al. Enhancement of ligand-dependent activation of human natural killer T cells by lenalidomide: therapeutic implications. Blood 2006; 108(2):618–21.

58. Davies FE, Raje N, Hideshima T, et al. Thalidomide and immunomodulatory derivatives augment natural killer cell cytotoxicity in multiple myeloma. Blood 2001; 98(1):210–6.

59. Reddy N, Cruz R, Hernandez-Ilizaliturri F, et al. Lenalidomide enhances monoclonal antibody-associated ant-tumor activity against rituximab-sensitive and rituximab-resistant B cell lymphoma cell lines. ASH Annual Meeting Abstracts 2006; 108:2522.
60. Richardson PG, Blood E, Mitsiades CS, et al. A randomized phase 2 study of lenalidomide therapy for patients with relapsed or relapsed and refractory multiple myeloma. Blood 2006;108(10):3458–64.
61. Witzig TE, Vose JM, Kaplan HP, et al. Early results from a phase II study of lenalidomide monotherapy in relapsed/refractory indolent non-Hodgkin's lymphoma. ASH Annual Meeting Abstracts 2007;110:2560.
62. Wiernik PH, Lossos I, Tuscano J, et al. Preliminary results from a phase II study of lenalidomide monotherapy in relapsed/refractory aggressive non-Hodgkin's lymphoma. ASH Annual Meeting Abstracts 2007;110:2565.
63. Wang M, Fayad L, Hagemeister F, et al. Lenalidomide (Len) in combination with rituximab (r) demonstrated early evidence of efficacy in a phase I/II study in relapsed/refractory mantle cell lymphoma (MCL). ASH Annual Meeting Abstracts 2007;110:2565.

Stem Cell Transplantation for Non-Hodgkin's Lymphoma

David Wrench, MB, MRCP[a], John G. Gribben, MD, DSc, FMedSci[b],*

KEYWORDS

• Non-Hodgkin's lymphoma • Aggressive
• Indolent • Stem cell transplant • Allogeneic • Autologous

Non-Hodgkin's lymphoma (NHL) includes a diverse set of conditions ranging from high-grade aggressive to more indolent low-grade disease. Hematopoietic stem cell transplantation (HSCT) has a valuable role in the management of these conditions and can provide long-term remission in selected cases. HSCT usually is performed with curative intent but requires judicious use because it is associated with considerable morbidity and mortality, which vary considerably between procedures and clinical situations. In addition, most studies assessing HSCT in NHL were initiated in the era before monoclonal antibody therapy was available, and the impact of anti-CD20 monoclonal antibody (rituximab) therapy on HSCT in NHL has not been established fully. Consequently, the optimal role of HSCT in NHL remains the subject of much ongoing study.

AUTOLOGOUS AND ALLOGENEIC HEMATOPOIETIC STEM CELL TRANSPLANTATION

Autologous HSCT (auto-HSCT) enables the application of high-dose chemotherapy (HDT) by subsequent rescue of hematopoiesis by infusion of previously harvested hematopoietic progenitor cells. The most common source of these cells is peripheral blood stem cells mobilized following the use of recombinant growth factors with or without chemotherapy. The toxicity of auto-HSCT continues to fall with improvements in supportive care. Although this approach has a relatively low toxicity compared with allogeneic HSCT (allo-HSCT), there is a persistent risk of tumor cells being present within the harvest and there is no graft-versus-lymphoma (GvL) effect. Consequently, auto-SCT is associated with an increased risk of relapsing disease postprocedure.

This work was supported by a Grant from Cancer Research UK.
[a] Centre for Medical Oncology, Barts and The London School of Medicine, Charterhouse Square, London EC1M 6BQ, UK
[b] Centre for Experimental Cancer Medicine, Barts and The London School of Medicine, Charterhouse Square, London EC1M 6BQ, UK
* Corresponding author.
E-mail address: john.gribben@cancer.org.uk (J.G. Gribben).

Hematol Oncol Clin N Am 22 (2008) 1051–1079
doi:10.1016/j.hoc.2008.07.007
0889-8588/08/$ – see front matter © 2008 Elsevier Inc. All rights reserved.

hemonc.theclinics.com

Recent efforts to improve the outcome of HSCT in NHL by reducing relapse include the addition of radio-immunoconjugates to conditioning regimens and the use of rituximab for "in vivo purging" around the time of stem cell harvesting and also as maintenance therapy after HSCT.

Allo-HSCT uses hematopoietic stem cells obtained from bone marrow or peripheral blood from siblings or unrelated donors or from cord blood. Allo-HSCT removes the risk of infusing disease present in an autologous harvest and allows exploitation of the GvL effect, whereby donor-derived immune cells can recognize the lymphoma as "non-self." Allo-HSCT has a higher morbidity and mortality, largely resulting from the risk of graft-versus-host disease (GvHD), which may negate the additive effect of GvL. The greater toxicities associated with allo-HSCT have led investigators to explore reducing the intensity of conditioning regimens and increasing the use of reduced-intensity conditioning allo-HSCT (RIC-allo). The loss of the potent anti-lymphoma effect of intensive-conditioning regimens may be abrogated by the effect of GvL and lower treatment-related toxicity and mortality.

AGGRESSIVE NON-HODGKIN'S LYMPHOMA
Autologous Hematopoietic Stem Cell Transplantation

Relapsed aggressive lymphoma
The most established use of auto-HSCT in NHL is its application in patients who have relapsed chemosensitive diffuse large B-cell lymphoma (DLBCL) (**Table 1**). A number of phase II studies suggested good outcome for patients who had relapsed disease that responded to salvage therapy (sensitive relapse),[1,2] and the beneficial effect of autologous stem-cell transplantation (auto-SCT) in this disease setting was demonstrated in the Parma International prospective multicenter trial.[3] In this study 109 of 215 patients who had relapsed NHL responded to two courses of salvage chemotherapy and were assigned randomly to receive either four further courses of chemotherapy or HDT with auto-HSCT. At 5 years, event-free survival rates (EFS) were 46% and 12%, respectively, and overall survival (OS) rates were 53% and 32%, respectively, for the transplantation and chemotherapy groups.

Refractory/chemo-resistant disease
Patients who undergo auto-SCT who have primary refractory disease or who have relapsed disease that does not respond to salvage chemotherapy have poor outcomes.[2] A number of studies have explored the use of HDT and auto-SCT in this setting (see **Table 1**). Chemoresistant patients whose disease subsequently is sensitive to second-line chemotherapy may achieve 3-year OS and EFS rates of 52.5% and 44.2%, respectively, if they receive auto-HSCT.[4] Improvements in salvage regimens to achieve better response rates and less toxicity might make more patients who have relapsed disease candidates for auto-HSCT. Promising data show that the addition of rituximab to salvage remission-induction chemotherapy improves the response rate from 54% to 75% and improves progression-free survival (PFS) and OS.[5] Of note, in this study only 4% of patients had prior rituximab therapy. Other studies have suggested that in these patients alternative intensive salvage chemotherapy regimens may be associated with improved outcome.[6]

Predicting which poor-risk patients might benefit most from auto-HSCT would enable appropriate targeting of this therapy, and those unlikely to benefit could be offered alternative experimental therapies. In patients who have relapsed or primary refractory DLBCL treated with auto-HSCT, the age-adjusted international prognostic index (IPI) predicts both PFS and OS.[7] Germinal center immunophenotype on immunohistochemical analysis and low (< 10%) BCL-2 expression retain their prognostic significance in patients who have poor-risk DLBCL treated with auto-HSCT in first remission,[8] but the cell of origin does not predict outcome in patients who have relapsed and refractory DLBCL and who are eligible for auto-HSCT.[9]

Because of the poor response rates and outcomes reported to date, auto-HSCT is not recommended in primary refractory or relapsed/refractory aggressive NHL not responding to salvage chemotherapy. Alternative treatment strategies are required in these cases, and, wherever possible, patients should be enrolled in clinical trials assessing new treatment regimens and novel therapeutic agents.

First-line therapy

Auto-HSCT has been studied as a first-line treatment modality in first complete remission in patients who have high-risk DLBCL (ie, disease that is unlikely to achieve long-term remission with conventional first-line chemotherapy) (see **Table 1**). Such treatment includes anthracycline-based regimens, commonly cyclophosphamide, doxorubicin, vincristine, and prednisolone (CHOP) or CHOP-like combination chemotherapy with rituximab. For patients at high risk as classified by the IPI[10] the long-term outcome is poor, with a 5-year OS rate of 32%. Auto-HSCT has been evaluated in such patients as a means of enabling the early administration of more intensive chemotherapy with the potential for greater anti-lymphoma effect. The German High-Grade NHL Study Group conducted a randomized study comparing five cycles of CHOP-like chemotherapy with three cycles of the same chemotherapy followed by bischloroethylnitrosourea, etoposide, ara-c, and melphalan (BEAM) and auto-HSCT as primary therapy in 312 patients aged 60 years or younger who had aggressive NHL.[11] OS and EFS were not significantly different between the two groups, and early relapse after auto-HSCT predicted worse survival than if it occurred after chemotherapy alone. A randomized, multicenter study comparing methotrexate-leucovorin, doxorubicin, cyclophosphamide, vincristine, prednisone, bleomycin (MACOP-B) chemotherapy with attenuated MACOP-B chemotherapy followed by HDT and auto-HSCT as first-line therapies in 150 patients who had high-intermediate or high-risk aggressive NHL found no benefit of induction auto-HSCT.[12] A recent systematic review and meta-analysis of 15 randomized, controlled trials comparing conventional chemotherapy versus HDT with auto-HSCT as first-line treatment of adults who had aggressive NHL (n = 3079) found no benefit for auto-SCT.[13] Treatment-related mortality (TRM) at 6% in the group receiving HDT with auto-SCT was not significantly different from that seen with conventional chemotherapy. The use of auto-SCT was associated with higher complete remission (CR) rates in 13 studies that included 2018 patients, but it did not affect OS when compared with conventional chemotherapy, and there was no difference in EFS. Analysis of prognostic groups based on the IPI in 12 of the trials showed no difference in survival between the HDT with auto-SCT and conventional chemotherapy groups, confirming the results of a previous meta-analysis that had shown that first-line auto-HSCT improves CR rates but does not provide benefits in OS or EFS when compared with conventional chemotherapy overall or in patients at good risk.[14] In addition, evidence is lacking that patients at poor risk might benefit from this approach.

Although auto-SCT presently cannot be recommended as first-line therapy for aggressive NHL, improvements in first-line therapy and conditioning regimens might benefit the 40% to 50% of patients who do not achieve a satisfactory response with standard first-line chemotherapy. Intensified first-line chemotherapy followed by auto-SCT has been assessed in various nonrandomized trials. In two phase II trials using first-line auto-SCT in poor-risk, aggressive NHL, the Dutch-Belgian Hemato-Oncology Cooperative Group showed that adding dose-intensified CHOP

Table 1
Studies of autologous hematopoietic stem cell transplantation in diffuse large B-cell lymphoma

Source	Patients (n)	Intervention	Median Follow-up (Months)	Age (Years)	OS	PFS	TRM
Relapsed disease							
Takvorian et al[1]	49	Auto-HSCT	> 11	—	—	Disease-free remission, 2 to > 52 months	4% (2/49)
Gribben et al[2]	50 (20[a])	Auto-HSCT	Minimum 12	—	—	—	—
Philip et al[3]	109	Chemosensitive: then four rounds of chemotherapy or auto-HSCT	63	18–60	53% (5 years) P = .038	EFS 46% (5 years) P = .001	5% (3/55)
Refractory/resistant disease							
Kewalramani et al[4]	85 (42[b])	Three rounds of ICE + auto-HSCT	—	20–66	53% (3 years)	EFS 44% (3 years)	100-day mortality 9.5%
Vellenga et al[5]	225	DHAP + auto-HSCT versusR-DHAP + auto-HSCT	31	18–65	59% (2 years) P = .15	PFS 52% (2 years) P < .002	—
Front-line standard dose conditioning							
Kaiser et al[11]	312	Three rounds of CHOEP versus three rounds of CHOEP + BEAM auto-HSCT	46	15–60	62% (3 years) P = ns	EFS 59% (auto-HSCT) P = ns	—
Martelli et al[12]	150	12 weeks MACOP-B versus 8 weeks MACOP-B + BEAC auto-HSCT	24	19–60	64% (5 years) P = ns	61% (5 yr) P = ns	—
Meta-analyses							
Greb et al[13] (15 RCTs)	3079	Conventional chemotherapy versus HDT and auto-HSCT	—	—	P = ns	EFS P = ns	—

Study	No.	Treatment	Age			
Greb et al[14] (15 RCTs)	2728	Conventional chemotherapy versus HDT and auto-HSCT	—	P = ns (subgroup difference: good versus poor risk)	EFS P = ns	—
Front Line Escalated dose conditioning						
van Imhoff et al[15]	66 (HOVON 27) 81 (HOVON 40)	Chemotherapy + auto-HSCT versus intensified chemotherapy + auto-HSCT	16–65	50% (4 years) P = .007	EFS 49% P = .0001	—
Stewart et al[16]	55	CHOP + DICEP + BEAM auto-HSCT	18–65	79% (4 years)	72% (4 years)	—
Arranz et al[17]	86	MegaCHOP or MegaCHOP + IFE, then BEAM auto-HSCT	—	64% (74%)	PFS 56% (67%)	7%
Radio-immunoconjugates						
Vose et al[24]	38	Iodine-131 tositumomab added to BEAM auto-HSCT	26–65	55% (3 years)	EFS 39% (3 years)	—
Gopal et al[26]	24	Iodine-131 tositumomab added to auto-HSCT	> 60	59% (3 years) (~30% for DLBCL)	51% (3 years)	—
Krishnan et al[25]	41	Yttrium-90 ibritumomab with BEAM	20–79	89% (2 years) (90% DLBCL)	PFS 70% (2 years) (69% DLBCL)	0% (at 100 days)

Abbreviations: BEAC, bischloroethylnitrosourea, etoposide, ara-C, cyclophosphamide; BEAM, bischloroethylnitrosourea, etoposide, ara-C, cyclophosphamide; DHAP, dexamethasone, high-dose cytarabine, cisplatin; DICEP, dose-interactive cyclophosphamide, etoposide, cisplatin; HOVON, Hemato-Oncologie voor Volwassenen Nederland; ICE, ifosfamide, carboplatin, etoposide; IFE, ifosphamide and etoposide; ns, not significant; RCT, randomized, controlled trials, R-DHAP, DHAP with rituximab.
a Number of patients who had a disease that was still responsive to conventional dose chemotherapy.
b Number of patients who underwent transplantation.

to high-dose induction therapy followed by BEAM auto-SCT improved the estimated 4-year OS from 21% to 50%.[15] The use of an intensified induction chemotherapy regimen (CHOP and then dose-interactive cyclophosphamide, etoposide, and cisplatin) followed by BEAM auto-SCT in high-risk aggressive NHL resulted in 4-year OS and EFS rates of 79% and 72%, respectively.[16] A further study in this group of patients used dose-escalated CHOP as intensified first-line chemotherapy followed by BEAM auto-SCT (if response was adequate) or ifosfamide and etoposide and then BEAM auto-SCT (if response was inadequate). At a median follow-up of 34 months, the OS rate was 64%, and the PFS rate was 56%.[17] Although these studies were not randomized, they are encouraging and indicate that auto-SCT following dose-intensified chemotherapy may yet have a role in the first-line treatment of poor-risk, aggressive NHL. An ongoing US Intergroup study (S9704) is being conducted in younger patients who have high-intermediate or high-risk disease comparing eight cycles of CHOP plus rituximab therapy versus five cycles followed by HDT and auto-HSCT.

New Developments with Monoclonal Antibodies

Rituximab

The use of rituximab with CHOP combination chemotherapy now is established as standard first-line therapy for this disease.[18] The use of rituximab in relapsed patients proceeding to auto-HSCT shows promise and may provide benefit through "in vivo purging" with elimination of lymphoma cell contamination at the time of stem cell collection. Continued therapy after auto-HSCT (maintenance therapy) may aid in the elimination of minimal residual disease and so reduce the risk of relapse. The outcome of auto-HSCT in NHL has been demonstrated to be inferior if the contaminating tumor is detected in the infused stem cell collection.[19,20] Consequently, methods that further reduce the risk of harvest contamination by tumor cells may improve long-term outcome following auto-HSCT. OS at 2 years was 80% in a study group of 67 patients who had relapsed aggressive B-cell NHL (B-NHL) and who received standard-dose rituximab 1 day before mobilizing chemotherapy and high-dose rituximab ($1000 mg/m^2$) 7 days after mobilizing chemotherapy and further high-dose rituximab on days 1 and 8 after auto-HSCT. In a historical control group who had received the same conditioning regimen but without the rituximab, the OS was 53%.[21] The ongoing randomized multicenter phase III Collaborative trial in relapsed aggressive lymphoma study assessing rituximab-combination chemotherapy salvage regimens and rituximab therapy as maintenance after BEAM auto-HSCT will provide further information regarding the use of rituximab maintenance to improve the outcome of auto-HSCT in patients who have relapsed DLBCL.[22] Rituximab added to the immune-suppressive effects of auto-HSCT might lead to an increase in infective complications. Although no increased infection was seen in one study[21] a retrospective study has shown that rituximab given before transplantation may be associated with cytomegalovirus infectious complications after auto-HSCT.[23] Further work is required to establish adequately the potential infective complications of rituximab used in the peritransplantation setting.

Radio-immunoconjugates

Anti-CD20 monoclonal antibodies have been combined with radioisotopes as a way of targeting radiation therapy to CD20-expressing lymphomas and have been used with HDT and auto-SCT (see **Table 1**). In a phase I study of 23 cases of chemotherapy-resistant relapsed or refractory B-NHL, the addition of iodine-131 tositumomab to BEAM conditioning with subsequent auto-HSCT produced toxicities similar to those seen with BEAM alone.[24] At a median follow-up of 38 months, the OS and EFS were encouraging at 55% and 39%, respectively. A phase II trial assessed the combination of yttrium-90 ibritumomab with BEAM conditioning chemotherapy and subsequent auto-HSCT in 41 patients who had NHL (20 had DLBCL, and four had transformed NHL). Toxicities were similar to those in historical controls treated with BEAM.[25] Estimated 2-year OS and PFS rates of 88.9% and 69.8%, respectively, were promising. In a study of patients who had relapsed or refractory B-NHL (including nine who had DLBCL), high-dose myeloablative therapy with tositumomab followed by auto-HSCT was safe and effective, achieving estimated 3-year OS and PFS rates of 59% and 51%, respectively, in this heterogeneous group of patients.[26]

Allogeneic Hematopoietic Stem Cell Transplantation in Aggressive Non-Hodgkin's Lymphoma

Allo-HSCT has significantly worse transplantation-related toxicity than auto-HSCT. Myeloablative allo-HSCT usually has been limited to poor-risk patients who have advanced disease. A major potential benefit of allo-HSCT is the potential for a GvL effect mediated by infused donor T-cells present in the stem cell harvest. This effect is demonstrated by the lower relapse rates after allo-HSCT and the response to donor lymphocyte infusion. Frequently, however, the benefit of a lower relapse rate is abrogated by higher TRM. The greater toxicity of allo-HSCT has led to the development of RIC-allo. RIC-allo uses highly immunosuppressive conditioning regimens rather than the more traditional myeloablative conditioning regimens used for allo-HSCT and consequently relies more on GvL than on intensive chemotherapy for anti-lymphoma effect. Concurrent with a GvL effect, donor T cells also mediate GvHD. Ongoing work seeks to modulate the T-cell response to optimize GvL and minimize GvH effects because of the significant morbidity and mortality associated with GvHD. One method of reducing GvHD uses T-cell–depleted grafts. A series of 40 patients, including 11 who had transformed B-cell malignancy, underwent T-cell–depleted allo-HSCT (using CAMPATH-1 G or H) after fully myeloablative conditioning.[27] At 1-year follow-up the TRM was 15%, and 17.5% of patients developed GvHD. At a median of 2.9 years' follow-up 70% of subjects were alive, and 68% were disease free, indicating that this approach may enable patients to tolerate fully myeloablative regimens better.

In aggressive NHL, allo-HSCT typically has been investigated in small studies involving young patients who have very advanced disease, often including various histologies. In these studies allo-HSCT is associated with a high rate of TRM. Auto-HSCT and allo-HSCT have been compared in a case-control study matching 101 patients receiving allo-HSCT and 101 patients receiving auto-HSCT from the registry data of the European Bone Marrow Transplant Registry Group (EBMT).[28] This study revealed that the two approaches had similar outcomes in NHL, with PFS rates of 49% in allo-HSCT and 46% in auto-HSCT. A lower relapse/progression rate was seen in patients who had chronic GvHD, suggesting some GvL effect. The lack of any clear benefit of allo-HSCT over auto-HSCT suggests that auto-HSCT should be offered as the preferred treatment modality when possible.

RIC-allo can increase the number of patients eligible for allogeneic HSCT by reducing toxicities and thereby increasing the age limit of candidates for this procedure (**Table 2**). In one series comparing allo-HSCT versus RIC-allo in 25 patients, the non-relapse mortality (NRM) after a median follow-up of 618 days was 54% in the myeloablative conditioning arm and 17% in the RIC arm.[29] One-year OS was 44% for all patients but was 67% for RIC-allo compared with 23% for allo-HSCT. Aggressive lymphoma needs vigorous debulking before HSCT, and RIC-allo, which limits chemotherapy and relies more on a GvL effect, requires judicious patient selection. In an EBMT study, 188 patients who had lymphoma were treated with RIC-allo. OS

Table 2
Studies of reduced-intensity conditioning allogeneic hematopoietic stem cell transplantation that include patients who have diffuse large B-cell lymphoma

Source	Patients	Intervention	Median Follow-up (Months)	Age Range (Years)	OS	EFS/PFS	Mortality
Bertz et al[29]	25 (12[a])	Allo-HSCT versus RIC-allo	20	20–60	67% (1 year) P <.02	EFS 50% (1 year) P =.04	NRM = 17%
Robinson et al[30]	188 (12[a])	RIC-allo (registry study)	9	2–65	50% (2 years)	PFS 30% (2 years)	NRM (100 days) = 13%
Rodriguez et al[32]	88 (40[a])	Allo-HSCT versus RIC-allo	—	18–67	53% (2 years)	PFS 40% (2 years)	TRM 28% (1 year)
Corradini et al[34]	170	RIC-allo	33	20–69	62% (3 years) (69% for high-grade NHL)	PFS 46% (3 years)	NRM 14% (3 years)
Armand et al[33]	87	RIC-allo	—	—	42% (3 years) (aggressive NHL)	PFS 22% (3 years) (aggressive NHL)	NRM 13% (1 year)
Sorror et al[31]	220 (152[a])	Allo-HSCT versus RIC-allo	44 (RIC-allo)	10–70	53% (3 years)	—	NRM 25% (3 years)

[a] Number of patients receiving RIC-Allo.

was 62% at 1 year and 50% at 2 years.[30] The probability of disease progression at 1 year was worse for chemoresistant disease than for chemosensitive disease (75% and 25%, respectively). Overall PFS was 46% but was significantly worse in patients who had aggressive lymphoma. Interestingly, 10 of 14 patients treated with donor lymphocyte infusion showed response. Furthermore, comparison of allo-HSCT and RIC-allo in 220 patients who had lymphoma (including 91 cases of high-grade NHL) or chronic lymphocytic leukemia showed that NRM, OS, and PFS rates were statistically similar for both approaches in patients who had no comorbitities, but patients who had comorbidities fared better after RIC-allo, showing lower TRM, better survival, and favorable adjusted PFS.[31] In this series the members of the RIC-allo group were older and had more prior therapies and more comorbidities. The proportion of unrelated donors was higher, but patients were more likely to be in remission. Another series retrospectively compared 88 patients treated with either allo-HSCT (n = 48) or RIC-allo (n = 40) and found that 2-year OS and PFS rates were similar but that RIC conditioning and prior auto-HSCT were associated with increased risk of relapse.[32]

The importance of lymphoma subtype on outcome following RIC-allo was demonstrated in a retrospective study in 87 patients.[33] For indolent lymphoma and aggressive NHL, 3-year OS rates were 42% and 81%, respectively, and PFS rates were 22% and 59%, respectively. In addition, the 2-year cumulative incidence of chronic GvHD was 68%, and its presence was associated with a lower risk of progression and improved PFS. Low early donor chimerism did not predict poor outcome, and progression was not associated with loss of chimerism. A prospective, multicenter phase II trial involving 170 cases of relapsed/refractory NHL (including 61 cases of aggressive NHL) showed identical 3-year OS rates of 69% and a 3-year risk of relapse of 31% and 29%, respectively, for aggressive NHL and indolent NHL.[34] NRM was relatively low, at 14% at 3 years. Chemorefractory disease adversely influenced OS on multivariate analysis.

Patients who did not respond to auto-HSCT treatment for aggressive NHL had a very poor prognosis. Studies involving RIC-allo in such patients have shown variable results. A single-center study including 38 patients who had refractory, progressive, or relapsed lymphoid malignancies (aggressive NHL, n = 10) and who received alemtuzumab (anti-CD52 monoclonal antibody) in conditioning showed an actuarial OS rate of 53% and PFS rate of 50% at 14 months, but with relapses continuing to occur.[35] In another study of 20 patients who had low-bulk or chemosensitive disease (10 of whom had DLBCL), the estimated 3-year PFS was 95%.[36]

Burkitt's Lymphoma/Lymphoblastic Lymphoma

Burkitt's lymphoma (BL) and lymphoblastic lymphoma (LL) are highly aggressive diseases. LL responds less well to first-line chemotherapy in adults, analogous to the response in acute lymphoblastic leukemia. Recent work suggests that matched-sibling allo-HSCT in patients at standard risk who have adult acute lymphoblastic leukemia provides the greatest chance of long-term remission.[37] The role of auto-HSCT in first remission was assessed in selected patients who had BL and LL (without central nervous system involvement nor extensive bone marrow involvement) in a multicenter phase II study.[38] Patients received two courses of intensive induction chemotherapy. In responding patients the induction chemotherapy was followed by BEAM and auto-HSCT. Actuarial estimates of 81% and 73% in BL and 46% and 40% in LL were obtained for 5-year OS and EFS, respectively. In a series of 43 patients who had BL, 27 proceeded to first-line HSCT after high-dose chemotherapy. The remaining 16 patients did not receive transplantation, principally because of chemorefractory disease. Those who received transplantation had a 3-year EFS of 51%.[39] Thirty-four patients who had

T- cell lymphoblastic lymphoma were treated with induction chemotherapy followed by HSCT if they showed response. Four patients received allo-HSCT, and 25 received auto-HSCT. On an intention-to-treat analysis, the 4-year OS and EFS rates were 72% and 68%, respectively.[40] The EBMT and the UK Lymphoma Group compared auto-HSCT versus standard consolidation and maintenance chemotherapy as postre-mission therapy in 119 patients who had LL from 37 centers in a prospective, random-ized study.[41] Investigators found no improvement with auto-HSCT as compared with conventional chemotherapy. In patients who had poor-prognosis LL, allo-HSCT showed benefit over auto-HSCT or chemotherapy. In 58 patients in the prospective Leucémie Aigüe Lymphoblastique de l'Adulte-94 study, the patients in CR who had a donor received allo-HSCT, whereas those in CR who did not have a donor were assigned randomly to either auto-HSCT or chemotherapy. Those who underwent allo-HSCT had better disease-free survival (DFS) than those who received auto-HSCT or chemotherapy.[42] Allo-HSCT and auto-HSCT were compared in an EBMT Lymphoma Registry study analyzing 1185 allo-HSCT recipients and 14,687 auto-HSCT recipients, all of whom had lymphoma. The allo-HSCT group included 71 cases of BL and 314 cases of LL. OS was better with auto-HSCT than with allo-HSCT, but the response rate was better with allo-HSCT than with auto-HSCT in LL and was equivalent between these modalities in BL.[43] In view of good responses to first-line (intensive) che-motherapy regimes in BL, the use of HSCT needs optimized in those patients at high risk of treatment failure or whose disease relapses. In LL, better response rates with allo-HSCT (compared with auto-HSCT) support a GvL effect, but improvements are required in TRM.

INDOLENT NON-HODGKIN'S LYMPHOMA

The most common form of indolent NHL is follicular lymphoma (FL), accounting for around one quarter of all NHL cases. It has a median survival of around 10 years, so studying the impact of HSCT in this disease requires long-term follow-up and careful selection of patients, because many will have prolonged survival even without therapy. Most cases occur in older people (median age at diagnosis, 60 years), so many patients are not candidates for intensive chemotherapy. Although FL typically is incurable, many patients who have FL require little or no treatment for the disease, because it often does not cause significant clinical sequelae for many years. Conse-quently, it is critical to select the patients most likely to benefit and to avoid treating patients who might gain no benefit but would be unnecessarily exposed to the risks of HSCT. These risks, particularly for indolent NHL, include an increased risk of secondary malignancy, especially secondary myelodysplastic syndrome and acute myeloid leukemia (MDS/AML). The addition of monoclonal antibody therapy in patients who have untreated, advanced-stage disease has improved in the outcome of FL.[44,45] The low toxicity of this approach may lessen the number of patients for whom HSCT is considered.

Most studies have focused on FL, the most prevalent of the indolent lymphomas. A significant minority of these patients have poor-risk disease, and 28% of patients experience high-grade transformation of their disease to aggressive NHL (typically DLBCL), which carries a very poor prognosis. The median survival time for patients who have transformed FL is only 1.2 years.[46] Major challenges in FL are establishing a way to predict which patients are at high risk of rapid progression or transformation and tailoring risk-adapted therapy appropriately. Continuing work seeks to establish in which patients and at what point in the disease course HSCT may be used optimally in low-grade NHL.

Autologous Hematopoietic Stem Cell Transplantation in Indolent Non-Hodgkin's Lymphoma

First-line therapy

Auto-HSCT might provide prolonged remission in patients who have FL, giving freedom from the relapsing/remitting course including multiple therapies that is typical of the disease and has been examined in a number of studies (**Table 3**). A multicenter Italian study achieved projected 4-year OS and DFS rates of 84% and 67%, respectively, when prospectively assessing intensified chemotherapy with auto-HSCT in 92 patients 60 years of age or younger who had untreated advanced-stage FL.[47] In evaluable patients, 65% achieved CR and molecular remission (MR), and this subgroup was predicted to have a 4-year DFS rate of 85%. In a multicenter prospective, randomized trial, the German Low-Grade Lymphoma Study Group randomly assigned patients up to 60 years old who had previously untreated advanced-stage FL to two courses of chemotherapy (either CHOP or melphalan, cyclophosphamide, and prednisone), and patients who achieved a partial remission (PR) or CR were assigned randomly to receive either HDT and total-body irradiation (TBI) with auto-HSCT or maintenance interferon-alpha (IFN-α) therapy.[48] This study showed a better PFS for the auto-HSCT group. Although there were more toxicities in the auto-HSCT group, the early mortality rates were 2.5% for both groups. The Groupe Ouest Est d'Etude des Leucémies et Autres Maladies du Sang (GOELAMS) study randomly assigned 172 patients who had newly diagnosed advanced-stage FL to CHOP-like chemotherapy with IFN or to HDT with auto-HSCT.[49] The auto-HSCT group had a better EFS, but the OS of 78% at 5 years was no different from that of the chemotherapy arm (at 84%) because of an excess of secondary malignancies in this group. The Groupe d'Etude des Lymphomes Folliculaires-94 trial compared 12 courses of standard CHOP-like chemotherapy with IFN against four courses of standard CHOP-like chemotherapy followed by HDT and TBI with auto-HSCT in previously untreated cases of advanced FL.[50] On an intent-to-treat basis after median follow-up of 7.5 years, the OS and EFS rates were no different between the two groups. In the first study of auto-HSCT in the rituximab era, the Gruppo Italiano Trapianto Midollo Osseo (GITMO) and Intergruppo Italiano Linfoni compared CHOP-R chemotherapy with rituximab-supplemented HDT and auto-HSCT in a prospective, randomized multicenter study of 136 patients who had high-risk FL.[51] This study showed that 4-year OS was no different between the groups, although the auto-HSCT arm had better 4-year EFS. In patients relapsing after CHOP plus rituximab chemotherapy who underwent subsequent auto-HSCT, the 3-year EFS rate was 68%. Importantly, achievement of MR was the biggest predictor of outcome in both groups. Taken together, these studies demonstrate that auto-HSCT should be performed in first remission only in the setting of controlled clinical trials and should not be considered standard of care for patients who have FL.

Relapse

HDT and auto-SCT has been explored more often in relapsed disease (**Table 4**). A clear benefit of auto-HSCT in relapsed FL was shown by the chemotherapy, unpurged, purged trial,[52] a multicenter study in which patients whose disease was responding after three cycles of standard chemotherapy were assigned randomly to three further courses or to auto-HSCT which was either purged or not purged of malignant cells. The PFS rates of 55%, 58%, and 26% at 2 years and OS rates of 77%, 71%, and 46% at 4 years in the patients receiving purged auto-HSCT, unpurged auto-HSCT, and chemotherapy, respectively, demonstrated marked differences between treatment with auto-HSCT and treatment with chemotherapy alone, although there was no difference between patients who received purged or unpurged grafts. There

Table 3
Studies of induction autologous hematopoietic stem cell transplantation in follicular lymphoma

Source	Patients	Intervention	Median Follow-up (Months)	Age Range (Years)	OS	EFS/PFS	Mortality
Ladetto et al[47] (GITMO)	92	Auto-HSCT	43	18–60	84% (4 years)	PFS 60% (4 years)	TRM 2%
Lenz et al[48] (GLSG)	375 (307[a])	Auto-HSCT versus IFN maintenance	50	18–59	84% (overall) (5 years)	PFS (auto-HSCT) = 62% (5 years) P < .0001	—
Deconinck et al[49] (GOELAMS)	172	Auto-HSCT versus CHOP-IFN	60	18–60	78% (5 years) P = ns	EFS (auto-HSCT) = 60% (5 years) P = .05	—
Sebban et al[50] (GELA)	401	Auto-HSCT versus CHOP-like + IFN	92	<61	76% (auto-HSCT) (7 years) P = .53	EFS (auto-HSCT) = 38% (7 years) P = .11	—
Ladetto et al[51] (GITMO and IIL)	134	CHOP + rituximab versus auto-HSCT + rituximab	51	18–60	81% (auto-HSCT) (4 years) P = .96	EFS (auto-HSCT) = 61% (4 years) P < .001	—

[a] Number of patients who have FL.

Table 4
Studies of autologous hematopoietic stem cell transplantation at relapse in follicular lymphoma

Source	Patients	Intervention	Median Follow-up (Months)	Age Range (Years)	OS	EFS/PFS	Mortality
Schouten et al[52] (CUP trial)	140	Purged auto-HSCT (P) versus unpurged auto-HSCT (U) versus chemotherapy (C)	69	29–64	71% (unpurged) (4 years)	EFS (unpurged) 58% (2 years)	—
Sabloff et al[53]	138	Unpurged Auto-HSCT	91	—	57% (10 years) (transformed FL = 56% at 5 years)	PFS 46% (10 years) (transformed FL = 25% at 5 years)	—
Montoto et al[54]	693 (562[a])	123	—	17–63	52% (10 years)	51% (10 years)	NRM (5 years) = 9%

Abbreviation: CUP, chemotherapy, unpurged, purged.
[a] Number of patients not in CR1.

are a number of problems with this study, however, notably the small number of patients enrolled and the poor outcome of the control group.

Single-center studies have demonstrated good outcome in patients who have relapsed FL. One hundred thirty-eight patients who had relapsed FL received salvage therapy and then proceeded to HDT and auto-HSCT.[53] Most had grade 1 nontransformed FL and had received only one prior chemotherapy regimen. The median OS from the diagnosis of the nontransformed FL was 16 years, and there was no difference in OS for patients who had had one, two, or more than two prior chemotherapies. OS rates of 57% and 56% and PFS rates of 46% and 25% for nontransformed FL at 10 years and for transformed FL at 5 years, respectively, compare favorably with historical controls. An EBMT study of 693 patients who underwent auto-HSCT for FL before 1995 assessed their long-term outcome.[54] Median follow-up was 10.3 years for living patients, with a total of 330 deaths. The median OS was 12 years, and OS rates of 64% and 52% were seen at 5 and 10 years, respectively. At 5 years, NRM had occurred in 61 patients (9%) who were age 45 years or older and who had chemoresistant disease at time of auto-HSCT and TBI; both older age and chemoresistant disease were predictive of higher NRM. Significantly, 64 patients developed a second malignancy at a median of 7 years after auto-HSCT with a cumulative incidence at 15 years postprocedure of 21% for patients treated in CR1 and a cumulative incidence of 15% for the other patients. Secondary MDS/AML was the most common second malignancy, developing in 40 patients. A multivariate analysis showed that TBI, age greater than 45 years at time of auto-HSCT, and more than two prior lines of chemotherapy were associated with a greater risk of second malignancy. In a retrospective analysis of long-term follow-up of patients who received cyclophosphamide-TBI followed by auto-HSCT for FL in second or subsequent remission,[55] an increased risk of secondary MDS/AML was observed and accounted for 15 deaths from a study population of 121. This study also showed better survival when transplantation was performed in second rather than subsequent remission and a plateau on the remission duration curve of 48% at 12 years. This finding suggests the possibility of prolonged freedom from recurrence when relapsed FL is treated with auto-HSCT. However, the significant incidence of second malignancy in these patients with the attendant risk of death demonstrated for TBI-containing regimens contrasts with the potential for lower disease recurrence and prolonged EFS associated with this treatment modality. The older age and heavy pretreatment of the FL patient population may predispose them to developing second malignancy after HDT. This risk is unacceptably high in a group whose median OS time is in the region of 10 to 12 years.

Improving autologous hematopoietic stem cell transplantation in follicular lymphoma

Rituximab improves OS and reduces the relapse rate when used as maintenance therapy in FL[56] and will reduce the number of patients proceeding to auto-HSCT. Rituximab also may be beneficial in the transplant setting. In a retrospective study, it appeared that prior rituximab therapy did not reduce the effectiveness of auto-HSCT in FL.[57] Furthermore, in a recent retrospective analysis of 248 patients who had recurrent FL who received HDT and auto-HSCT, those who had a regimen that contained monoclonal antibody had a decreased relative risk of progressive disease.[58] Rituximab "in vivo purging" improves the potential for obtaining a peripheral blood stem cell harvest free of residual disease.[59,60] Radio-immunotherapy with iodine-131 tositumomab and yttrium-90 ibritumomab tiuxetan have been studied with HDT and auto-HSCT and show promise in patients who have NHL (including FL).[25] Myeloablative radio-immunotherapy may allow more patients to receive HDT and auto-HSCT by limiting the exposure of normal organs while delivering curative radiation doses to disease.[26]

The achievement of MR by the eradication of detectable minimal residual disease in FL is important.[47,61–63] The achievement of MR was the biggest predictor of outcome in the GITMO/IIL study.[51] In future studies, failure to achieve MR after auto-HSCT might lead to early intervention to attempt to induce MR before overt clinical relapse (analogous to the current practice in some subtypes of acute leukemia). Efforts to improve the rate of MR achievement postprocedure can be expected to improve outcomes after auto-HSCT and should be addressed further in clinical studies.

Patient selection for autologous hematopoietic stem cell transplantation
In addition to patients who have relapsed FL, patients who have poor-risk FL who are unlikely to achieve durable remission after standard chemoimmunotherapy and maintenance immunotherapy may be candidates for auto-HSCT. Identifying such patients would be an important advance in FL management and would allow the earlier use of this potentially curative technique. Two prognostic indices have been applied to FL. The IPI originally was proposed in 1993, principally with reference to DLBCL,[10] and a modified version tailored to FL, the FLIPI, was produced in 2004.[64] In the GOELAMS study of auto-HSCT in first remission, only patients who had a high-risk FLIPI score showed a superior EFS.[49] In one series of patients who had recurrent FL, the 15% of patients who had high-risk FLIPI scores had worse OS rates.[57]

Allogeneic Hematopoietic Stem Cell Transplantation
Allo-HSCT in indolent lymphoma allows a GvL effect to be used and the risk of graft contamination by residual tumor cells to be avoided (**Table 5**). The high TRM associated with myeloablative allo-HSCT greatly limits the use of this approach, however. Allo-HSCT is associated with a lower risk of relapse, but this reduced risk frequently does not translate to a survival benefit because of the excessive TRM. Allo-HSCT has been used as salvage therapy in patients who have lymphoma that relapsed after previous auto-HSCT;[65] limited success was confined mostly to patients in remission who had good performance status and an HLA-matched sibling donor. The EBMT registry-matched study of allo-HSCT in 1185 patients who had NHL (including 231 who had FL) showed a lower rate of relapse for allo-HSCT in low-grade NHL than in matched auto-HSCT cases.[43] The actuarial 4-year OS rate for patients who had indolent lymphoma receiving allo-HSCT was 51.1%. A high TRM rate of 38% at 4 years was observed for this group. Similarly, an International Bone Marrow Transplant Registry study comparing allo-HSCT and auto-HSCT outcomes in 904 patients who had FL showed a significantly lower relapse rate in the allo-HSCT arm; again, however, a higher TRM meant that the 5-year OS rates in these modalities were similar.[66] In a series of 126 patients who had relapsed, advanced-stage FL, BEAM auto-HSCT and BEAM-alemtuzumab allo-HSCT were compared.[67] The allo-HSCT group had a higher 1-year NRM but a significantly lower relapse rate at 3 years, and this advantage, together with a continual pattern of relapse in the auto-HSCT group, contributed to there being no difference in OS or DFS in the two groups of patients at 3 years. Additionally, donor lymphocyte infusion re-induced remission in certain cases in the allo-HSCT group.

RIC-allo has been used in indolent NHL because of its lower TRM (see **Table 5**). Early work demonstrated impressive DFS and OS rates at 2 years after procedure.[68] Subsequent work showed that this approach may benefit patients who relapse after auto-HSCT for lymphoma who have chemosensitive or stable disease going into RIC-allo.[36] An EBMT study demonstrated that, in a heavily pretreated group of

Table 5
Studies of allogeneic hematopoietic stem cell transplantation and reduced-intensity conditioning allogeneic hematopoietic stem cell transplantation in follicular lymphoma

Source	Patients	Intervention	Median Follow-up (Months)	Age Range (Years)	OS	EFS/PFS/DFS	Mortality
Allo-HSCT							
Peniket et al[43] (EBMT)	1185 (231 low-grade NHL)	Allo-HSCT (matched versus auto HSCT)	—	—	51% (4 years) (low-grade NHL)	—	TRM (4 years) 38% (allo-HSCT/low-grade NHL)
van Besien et al[66] (International Bone Marrow Transplant Registry)	904 (176 allo-HSCT)	Allo-HSCT versus Auto HSCT	36 (allo-HSCT)	18–71 (22–64 for allo-HSCT)	51% (5 years) (allo-HSCT)	DFS P = ns	TRM 30% (allo-HSCT) (5 years)
Ingram et al[67]	126 (relapsed FL)	BEAM auto-HSCT versus BEAM-alemtuzumab allo-HSCT	—	—	(3 years) P = ns	DFS (3 years) P = ns	NRM (allo-HSCT) 20% (1 year)
RIC-allo							
Khouri et al[68]	20 (18 FL)	RIC-allo	21	31–68	—	DFS 84% (2 years)	—
Robinson et al[30]	188 (52 low-grade NHL)	RIC-allo	9	27–65 (low grade NHL)	65% (2 years low-grade NHL)	PFS = 54% (2 years low-grade NHL)	TRM = 22% (1 year)

Morris et al[71]	88 (41 low-grade NHL)	RIC-allo	36	73% (3 years)	65% (3 years low-grade NHL)	TRM 11% (3 years low-grade NHL)
Kusumi et al[91]	112 (45 indolent NHL)	RIC-allo	24	32–61 (indolent NHL)	59% (3 years) (81% for FL)	PFS 57% (3 years)	TRM 25% (3 years)
Vigoroux et al[69]	73	RIC-allo	37	—	66% (3 years) if CR at RIC	PFS = 66% if CR at RIC	32% if CR at RIC
Hari et al[70]	208 (88 RIC)	Allo-HSCT versus RIC-allo	35 (RIC)	—	62% (3 years RIC)	PFS 55% (3 years RIC)	—
Khouri et al[72]	47 (relapsed FL)	RIC-sllo	60	33–68	85% (5 years)	83% (5 years)	—

patients who had lymphoma, almost half of whom had undergone prior auto-HSCT, patients who had low-grade NHL had better PFS than patients who had high-grade NHL, and disease progression was much worse in patients who had chemoresistant disease.[30] A retrospective, multicenter study by the French Society for Bone Marrow Transplantation and Cell Therapy included cases of relapsed or refractory low-grade lymphoma treated by RIC-allo.[69] Patients were heavily pretreated, having had a median of three prior lines of therapy. The median follow-up was 3 years. The 3-year OS was 66% for patients in CR and 64% for patients in PR but was only 32% for patients who had chemoresistant disease. The corresponding 3-year TRM was 32%, 28%, and 63%, respectively. Consequently, although long-term remission could be achieved, high levels of TRM remained.

A further comparison of the use of allo-HSCT and RIC-allo in FL demonstrated that although the 3-year OS and PFS rates were similar, an increased risk of disease progression after RIC-allo was seen on multivariate analysis.[70] GvHD remains a problem, and investigators have attempted to reduce the incidence of GvHD after RIC-allo through the use of alemtuzumab in the conditioning regimens. Low rates of acute GvHD with 3-year OS and TRM rates of 73% and 11% for low-grade NHL have been reported.[71] Excellent results including PFS of 83% at 5 years have been obtained from the MD Anderson Cancer Center in a recent 8-year study of RIC-allo in relapsed FL,[72] which used intensive rituximab therapy peritransplantation. A prospective study from the North American Clinical Trials Network currently is comparing RIC-allo with auto-HSCT in chemosensitive relapsed FL.

MANTLE CELL LYMPHOMA

Mantle cell lymphoma (MCL) is characterized by t(11;14) and overexpression of cyclin D1. Although MCL often is labeled an indolent lymphoma, patients frequently present with advanced-stage disease with median survival in the region of only 3 to 4 years. Variable responses to chemotherapy are achieved including reports of poor response to CHOP-like regimens with the consequent use of more intensive first-line therapy in some studies. In contrast to DLBCL and FL, it is not clear that the addition of rituximab to therapeutic regimens has improved the outcome of this disease.[73,74] Inadequate responses to first-line therapy and the poor prognosis of this condition have led investigators to study intensive first-line therapy in MCL. Studies of HSCT often have included MCL with other forms of NHL. Studies specifically addressing MCL give a better picture of the effect of this intervention on this disease (**Table 6**). One randomized clinical trial compared auto-HSCT and IFN maintenance in patients less than 65 years old who had advanced-stage MCL and who achieved at least PR after CHOP-like induction therapy.[75] PFS rates were better for patients receiving auto-HSCT, but longer follow-up is needed to establish an effect on OS.

In a series of 195 patients in a study by the EBMT and the Autologous Blood and Marrow Transplant Registry, treatment of MCL with auto-HSCT resulted in an OS rate of 76% and a PFS rate of 55% at 2 years, but the OS rate fell to 50% and the PFS rate fell to 33% at 5 years, demonstrating the need for long follow-up in these studies.[76] Patients who underwent transplantation in CR1 fared significantly better than those not in CR1 but who had chemosensitive disease before transplantation. Induction auto-HSCT for patients who had previously untreated MCL gave encouraging results when combined with HDT plus rituximab. Optimal amounts of polymerase chain reaction–negative harvests were obtained from all 20 patients in the series, giving evidence for good "in vivo purging" with the regimen used. At 54 months follow-up, OS and EFS rates were 89% and 79%, respectively.[77] A matched-pair analysis

Table 6
Hematopoietic stem cell transplantation in mantle cell lymphoma

Author	Patients	Intervention	Median Follow-up (Months)	Age Range (Years)	OS	EFS/PFS	Mortality	Reference
Auto-HSCT								
Gianni et al	28	Induction auto-HSCT	35	23–65	89% (54 months)	EFS 79% (54 months)	—	77
Vandenberghe 2003 (EBMT and Autologous Bone Marrow Transplant Registry)	195	Auto-HSCT	47	—	50% (5 years)	33% (5 years)	—	76
Dreyling et al	122 (untreated advanced-stage MCL)	Auto-HSCT versus IFN maintenance	25	35–65	83% (3 years auto-HSCT) P = ns	PFS 54% (3 years auto-HSCT) P = .01	Deaths in remission 5% (3/62)	75
Dreger et al	34	Induction auto-HSCT with rituximab	33	39–67	87% (4 years)	83% (4 years)	—	79
Evens et al	25 (13 auto = HSCT)	Induction auto-HSCT or allo-HSCT	66	< 65 (auto-HSCT)	75%(5 years auto-HSCT)	PFS 54%(5 years auto-HSCT)	TRM 4% overall	92
Allo-HSCT								
Khouri et al	18 (relapsed MCL)	Allo-HSCT	26	46–64	85% (3 years)	EFS 82% (3 years)	NRM at 100 days 0%	80
Maris et al	33 (relapsed/refractory MCL)	Allo-HSCT	25	33–70	65% (2 years)	PFS 60% (2 years)	NRM (2 years) 24%	93
Corradini et al	170 (14 relapsed MCL)	RIC-allo	33 (overall)	20–69	45% (MCL) (3 years)	PFS 33% (MCL) (3 years)	NRM (3 years MCL) 32%	34

comparing rituximab plus auto-HSCT with historical controls treated with chemotherapy showed better PFS and a trend to better OS in the group receiving transplantation[78] and superior EFS in MCL treated with first-line auto-HSCT when rituximab was added.[79] The use of radio-immunotherapy with the addition of yttrium-90 ibritumomab tiuxetan to HDT with auto-HSCT showed encouraging PFS rates in a series of 41 patients (including 13 who had MCL).[25] RIC-allo in 33 patients who had relapsed or refractory MCL showed promising results with 2-year OS and PFS rates of 65% and 60%, respectively, and with a NRM of 24% over this period.[80] Notably, the overall response rate in the patients who had disease at the time of transplantation was 85% (17/20); 15 patients achieved CR, providing evidence for a GvL effect in MCL treated with allo-HSCT. The EBMT previously demonstrated a poor outcome in a study of heavily pretreated patients who had MCL and who received RIC-allo.[30] Promising results were obtained with RIC-allo in a single-center study of 18 patients who had relapsed MCL, 16 of whom had chemosensitive disease.[80] After a median follow-up of 26 months the actuarial probability of 3-year current EFS was 82%. In a prospective, multicenter phase II study of 170 patients who had relapsed lymphomas, a 3-year OS rate of 45% and a relapse incidence of 35% were demonstrated in 14 patients who had relapsed MCL treated with RIC-allo.[34]

Despite these experiences with HSCT, good long-term outcomes can be achieved with less intensive therapy in patients who have MCL, and HSCT should be used judiciously in carefully selected patients to avoid unnecessary overtreatment.

T-CELL NON-HODGKIN'S LYMPHOMA

T-cell NHL (T-NHL) represents only around 5% to 10% of all NHL. Consequently, lower patient numbers make assessing the role of HSCT in these conditions more difficult. Both auto-HSCT and allo-HSCT have been used in various subsets of T-NHL. The Grupo Español de Linfomas/Trasplante Antólogo de Médula Ósea (GELTAMO) assessed 115 patients who had peripheral T-cell lymphoma (PTCL) treated with auto-HSCT who were in CR1 (32%) or who had chemosensitive disease (62%) or refractory disease (5%).[81] With a median of 37 months' follow-up, OS, TTP, and DFS at 3 years were 56%, 51%, and 60%, respectively, presenting results similar to those for patients undergoing salvage auto-HSCT for aggressive B-NHL. Patients undergoing transplantation in CR1 had better OS and DFS. In a prospective phase II trial, the same group assessed auto-HSCT as front-line therapy in high-risk peripheral T-NHL.[82] Included were 26 patients who had high-risk nodal PTCL (anaplastic lymphoma kinase [ALK]-positive cases were not included) who received auto-HSCT if they achieved CR after three courses of mega-CHOP therapy or, if not in CR, they achieved at least PR after subsequent early salvage therapy. With a median follow-up of 35 months OS and PFS rates were 72% and 53%, respectively; in those who received auto-HSCT, OS, PFS, and DFS rates were 84%, 56%, and 63%, respectively. Patients who had advanced-stage PTCL who received auto-HSCT as first-line therapy had encouraging TRM (only 4.8%); the estimated EFS rate was 30% at 12 years after a median follow-up of more than 6 years, although the best long-term CR results after transplantation were in a subgroup of patients who had ALK-positive anaplastic large-cell lymphoma (ALCL).[83] CR before auto-HSCT was predictive of better OS and EFS.

The GELTAMO group assessed 123 patients who had relapsing/refractory PTCL who received auto-HSCT as salvage therapy.[84] Of note, 91% had chemosensitive disease before transplantation. After 5 years' median follow-up, the OS and PFS rates for this were 45% and 34%, respectively. The adjusted IPI and elevated β2-microglobulin predicted outcome after transplantation. In cases of angioimmunoblastic T-cell lymphoma, the GELTAMO group found encouraging results with auto-HSCT: 11 of 19 patients who received transplantation were still alive at a median follow-up of 25 months after the procedure with an actuarial OS rate of 60% at 3 years, indicating encouraging results in a disease that carries a poor prognosis.[85] Patients who had refractory disease did not benefit from transplantation. The subset of T-NHL patients who have ALK-positive ALCL respond well to chemotherapy, so auto-HSCT should be reserved for treatment of relapse in this disease, whereas patients who have ALK-negative ALCL do badly when auto-HSCT is used as salvage for recurrent disease.[86] Allo-HSCT has a high TRM in these conditions, but in a pilot study of 17 patients who had relapsed or refractory PTCL RIC-allo demonstrated 3-year OS and PFS rates of 81% and 64%, respectively,[87] with an estimated 2-year NRM of only 6%. Auto-HSCT has a role in the treatment of relapsed PTCL particularly ALK-positive ALCL.

Consideration should be given to its use in high-risk PTCL as part of induction therapy in clinical trials. RIC-allo shows promise in the treatment of patients who have relapsed PTCL.

HIV-ASSOCIATED NON-HODGKIN'S LYMPHOMA

Previously patients who had HIV and developed NHL had a poor prognosis, but the advent of highly active anti-retroviral therapy (HAART) has made more patients who have HIV able to tolerate standard or only slightly modified chemotherapy regimens because they are less prone to infections and have a more robust hematologic reserve. Encouraging OS and DFS rates were shown in a series of 63 patients who had stage 4 HIV-associated BL treated with intensive chemotherapy.[88] The precise role, if any, of auto-HSCT in HIV-associated NHL is difficult to assess because of the relatively small number of eligible patients previously studied. In a single-center series of 20 patients, HDT with auto-HSCT achieved sustained remissions in patients who had recurrent, chemosensitive HIV-associated NHL.[89] A recent multicenter study of 27 patients who had HIV-associated lymphoma assessed a reduced-dose conditioning regimen before auto-HSCT. Twenty patients received auto-HSCT, and one of these patients died at day 33 after transplantation. Of the remaining patients, 53% remained in CR at 100 days after transplantation, and with 13 of 20 patients alive the median OS had not been reached by the last follow-up.[90] The results, albeit in small studies of selected patients, are encouraging and indicate the ability of at least some patients who have relapsed HIV-associated lymphoma to tolerate intensive chemotherapy and to achieve prolonged remission following auto-HSCT. Case reports indicate some success in the use of allo-HSCT and RIC-allo for HIV-related lymphoma, and in the future there may be a role for these procedures in highly selected patients who have disease with a poor prognosis.

SUMMARY

Auto-HSCT has a clear role in the treatment of patients who have chemosensitive relapsed DLBCL and is a potentially curative option. Auto-HSCT used in second remission of FL may give favorable long-term remission rates from this typically relapsing and remitting disease. The role of auto-HSCT is less established in other NHL subtypes. Although TRM rates have improved in recent years, long-term follow-up of patients who have FL indicates an unacceptably high rate of second malignancy (particularly secondary MDS/AML), especially in those treated with regimens involving TBI. Currently, auto-HSCT cannot be recommended as a front-line therapy in either DLCBL or FL, although improvements in induction and conditioning regimens, including escalated doses and novel combinations of chemotherapeutic regimens, may prove beneficial to patients presenting with high-risk B-NHL. Such patients should continue to be enrolled in clinical studies, when possible, so the effect of early high-dose therapy in patients who have a poor prognosis can be assessed adequately. Patients who have disease that previously was refractory to conventional induction chemotherapy may benefit from intensified salvage regimens followed by auto-HSCT. Fully myeloablative allo-HSCT generally should be avoided in NHL except in carefully selected patients who have not responded to conventional chemotherapy with or without previous auto-HSCT and who are fit enough to be considered for this treatment. Unacceptably high TRM rates preclude the more widespread use of allo-HSCT at present. The advent of RIC-allo shows promise because of its lower TRM with persistent anti-lymphoma activity mediated through a GvL effect. An ongoing study comparing auto-HSCT and RIC-allo in chemosensitive relapsed FL should clarify the role of RIC-allo in FL further. Patients who have MCL seem not to benefit from the addition of rituximab to chemotherapeutic regimens. This lack of benefit, coupled with the reported poor prognosis of this disease, has led to the study of alternative therapies. HSCT shows good responses in selected patients who respond to intensive induction chemotherapy. Of note, rituximab added to auto-HSCT regimens may give better responses. RIC-allo shows some potential in patients who have relapsed chemosensitive disease. Data also show that good long-term outcomes may be obtained with less intensive induction therapy. Consequently, care is needed in selecting the patients who have MCL who are most likely to benefit from HSCT while limiting the exposure of patients who would not benefit from this modality. T-NHL historically has had a poor prognosis, but the relatively small number of patients eligible has made the role of HSCT harder to establish. Auto-HSCT should be reserved for salvage therapy after relapse in patients who have ALCL. Other high-risk T-NHL cases may benefit from induction auto-HSCT in the context of clinical studies. RIC-allo may have a role as part of salvage therapy after disease relapse.

The advent of HAART has allowed more patients who have HIV-associated NHL to be candidates for intensive chemotherapy, and emerging data from several small clinical studies suggest that auto-HSCT may prove to be beneficial in relapsed chemosensitive disease.

In conclusion, HSCT is a valuable tool in the treatment of NHL. Recent advances in peritransplantation regimens, including rituximab as "in vivo graft purging" and for clearance of minimal residual disease after transplantation and the increasing use of radio-immunoconjugates, show promise and seem likely to improve responses to auto-HSCT. By reducing toxicities, RIC-allo increases the number of patients eligible for allogeneic transplantation, although the precise role of this modality in treating NHL remains to be established. The results of ongoing work will further the use of these different approaches in the management of NHL.

REFERENCES

1. Takvorian T, Canellos GP, Ritz J, et al. Prolonged disease-free survival after autologous bone marrow transplantation in patients with non-Hodgkin's lymphoma with a poor prognosis. N Engl J Med 1987;316:1499–505.
2. Gribben JG, Goldstone AH, Linch DC, et al. Effectiveness of high-dose combination chemotherapy and autologous bone marrow transplantation for patients with non-Hodgkin's lymphomas who are still responsive to conventional dose therapy. J Clin Oncol 1989;7:1621–9.

3. Philip T, Guglielmi C, Hagenbeek A, et al. Autologous bone marrow transplantation as compared with salvage chemotherapy in relapses of chemotherapy-sensitive non-Hodgkin's lymphoma. N Engl J Med 1995;333:1540–5.

4. Kewalramani T, Zelenetz AD, Hedrick EE, et al. High-dose chemoradiotherapy and autologous stem cell transplantation for patients with primary refractory aggressive non-Hodgkin lymphoma: an intention-to-treat analysis. Blood 2000; 96:2399–404.

5. Vellenga E, van Putten WL, van't Veer MB, et al. Rituximab improves the treatment results of DHAP-VIM-DHAP and ASCT in relapsed/progressive aggressive CD20+ NHL: a prospective randomized HOVON trial. Blood 2008;111:537–43.

6. Josting A, Sieniawski M, Glossmann JP, et al. High-dose sequential chemotherapy followed by autologous stem cell transplantation in relapsed and refractory aggressive non-Hodgkin's lymphoma: results of a multicenter phase II study. Ann Oncol 2005;16:1359–65.

7. Hamlin PA, Zelenetz AD, Kewalramani T, et al. Age-adjusted international prognostic index predicts autologous stem cell transplantation outcome for patients with relapsed or primary refractory diffuse large B-cell lymphoma. Blood 2003; 102:1989–96.

8. van Imhoff GW, Boerma EJ, van der Holt B, et al. Prognostic impact of germinal center-associated proteins and chromosomal breakpoints in poor-risk diffuse large B-cell lymphoma. J Clin Oncol 2006;24:4135–42.

9. Moskowitz CH, Zelenetz AD, Kewalramani T, et al. Cell of origin, germinal center versus nongerminal center, determined by immunohistochemistry on tissue microarray, does not correlate with outcome in patients with relapsed and refractory DLBCL. Blood 2005;106:3383–5.

10. The International Non-Hodgkin's Lymphoma Prognostic Factors Project. A predictive model for aggressive non-Hodgkin's lymphoma. N Engl J Med 1993;329: 987–94.

11. Kaiser U, Uebelacker I, Abel U, et al. Randomized study to evaluate the use of high-dose therapy as part of primary treatment for "aggressive" lymphoma. J Clin Oncol 2002;20:4413–9.

12. Martelli M, Gherlinzoni F, De Renzo A, et al. Early autologous stem-cell transplantation versus conventional chemotherapy as front-line therapy in high-risk, aggressive non-Hodgkin's lymphoma: an Italian multicenter randomized trial. J Clin Oncol 2003;21:1255–62.

13. Greb A, Bohlius J, Schiefer D, et al. High-dose chemotherapy with autologous stem cell transplantation in the first line treatment of aggressive non-Hodgkin lymphoma (NHL) in adults. Cochrane Database Syst Rev 2008:CD004024.

14. Greb A, Bohlius J, Trelle S, et al. High-dose chemotherapy with autologous stem cell support in first-line treatment of aggressive non-Hodgkin lymphoma—results of a comprehensive meta-analysis. Cancer Treat Rev 2007;33:338–46.

15. van Imhoff GW, van der Holt B, Mackenzie MA, et al. Impact of three courses of intensified CHOP prior to high-dose sequential therapy followed by autologous stem-cell transplantation as first-line treatment in poor-risk, aggressive non-Hodgkin's lymphoma: comparative analysis of Dutch-Belgian Hemato-Oncology Cooperative Group Studies 27 and 40. J Clin Oncol 2005;23:3793–801.

16. Stewart DA, Bahlis N, Valentine K, et al. Upfront double high-dose chemotherapy with DICEP followed by BEAM and autologous stem cell transplantation for poor-prognosis aggressive non-Hodgkin lymphoma. Blood 2006;107: 4623–7.

17. Arranz R, Conde E, Grande C, et al. Dose-escalated CHOP and tailored intensification with IFE according to early response and followed by BEAM/autologous stem-cell transplantation in poor-risk aggressive B-cell lymphoma: a prospective study from the GEL-TAMO Study Group. Eur J Haematol 2008;80:227–35.

18. Coiffier B, Lepage E, Briere J, et al. CHOP chemotherapy plus rituximab compared with CHOP alone in elderly patients with diffuse large-B-cell lymphoma. N Engl J Med 2002;346:235–42.

19. Sharp JG, Kessinger A, Mann S, et al. Outcome of high dose therapy and autologous transplantation based on the presence of tumor in the marrow or infused hematopoietic harvest. J Clin Oncol 1996;14:214–9.

20. Vose JM, Sharp G, Chan WC, et al. Autologous transplantation for aggressive non-Hodgkin's lymphoma: results of a randomized trial evaluating graft source and minimal residual disease. J Clin Oncol 2002;20:2344–52.

21. Khouri IF, Saliba RM, Hosing C, et al. Concurrent administration of high-dose rituximab before and after autologous stem-cell transplantation for relapsed aggressive B-cell non-Hodgkin's lymphomas. J Clin Oncol 2005;23:2240–7.

22. Hagberg H, Gisselbrecht C. Randomised phase III study of R-ICE versus R-DHAP in relapsed patients with CD20 diffuse large B-cell lymphoma (DLBCL) followed by high-dose therapy and a second randomisation to maintenance treatment with rituximab or not: an update of the CORAL study. Ann Oncol 2006; 17(Suppl 4):iv31–2.

23. Lee MY, Chiou TJ, Hsiao LT, et al. Rituximab therapy increased post-transplant cytomegalovirus complications in non-Hodgkin's lymphoma patients receiving autologous hematopoietic stem cell transplantation. Ann Hematol 2008;87:285–9.

24. Vose JM, Bierman PJ, Enke C, et al. Phase I trial of iodine-131 tositumomab with high-dose chemotherapy and autologous stem-cell transplantation for relapsed non-Hodgkin's lymphoma. J Clin Oncol 2005;23:461–7.

25. Krishnan A, Nademanee A, Fung HC, et al. Phase II trial of a transplantation regimen of yttrium-90 ibritumomab tiuxetan and high-dose chemotherapy in patients with non-Hodgkin's lymphoma. J Clin Oncol 2008;26:90–5.

26. Gopal AK, Rajendran JG, Gooley TA, et al. High-dose [131I]tositumomab (anti-CD20) radioimmunotherapy and autologous hematopoietic stem-cell transplantation for adults > or = 60 years old with relapsed or refractory B-cell lymphoma. J Clin Oncol 2007;25:1396–402.

27. Novitzky N, Thomas V. Allogeneic stem cell transplantation with T cell-depleted grafts for lymphoproliferative malignancies. Biol Blood Marrow Transplant 2007; 13:107–15.

28. Chopra R, Goldstone AH, Pearce R, et al. Autologous versus allogeneic bone marrow transplantation for non-Hodgkin's lymphoma: a case-controlled analysis of the European Bone Marrow Transplant Group Registry data. J Clin Oncol 1992;10:1690–5.

29. Bertz H, Illerhaus G, Veelken H, et al. Allogeneic hematopoietic stem-cell transplantation for patients with relapsed or refractory lymphomas: comparison of high-dose conventional conditioning versus fludarabine-based reduced-intensity regimens. Ann Oncol 2002;13:135–9.

30. Robinson SP, Goldstone AH, Mackinnon S, et al. Chemoresistant or aggressive lymphoma predicts for a poor outcome following reduced-intensity allogeneic progenitor cell transplantation: an analysis from the lymphoma working party of the European Group for blood and bone marrow transplantation. Blood 2002; 100:4310–6.

31. Sorror ML, Storer BE, Maloney DG, et al. Outcomes after allogeneic hematopoietic cell transplantation with nonmyeloablative or myeloablative conditioning regimens for treatment of lymphoma and chronic lymphocytic leukemia. Blood 2008; 111:446–52.

32. Rodriguez R, Nademanee A, Ruel N, et al. Comparison of reduced-intensity and conventional myeloablative regimens for allogeneic transplantation in non-Hodgkin's lymphoma. Biol Blood Marrow Transplant 2006;12:1326–34.

33. Armand P, Kim HT, Ho VT, et al. Allogeneic transplantation with reduced-intensity conditioning for Hodgkin and non-Hodgkin lymphoma: importance of histology for outcome. Biol Blood Marrow Transplant 2008;14:418–25.

34. Corradini P, Dodero A, Farina L, et al. Allogeneic stem cell transplantation following reduced-intensity conditioning can induce durable clinical and molecular remissions in relapsed lymphomas: pre-transplant disease status and histotype heavily influence outcome. Leukemia 2007;21:2316–23.

35. Branson K, Chopra R, Kottaridis PD, et al. Role of nonmyeloablative allogeneic stem-cell transplantation after failure of autologous transplantation in patients with lymphoproliferative malignancies. J Clin Oncol 2002;20:4022–31.

36. Escalon MP, Champlin RE, Saliba RM, et al. Nonmyeloablative allogeneic hematopoietic transplantation: a promising salvage therapy for patients with non-Hodgkin's lymphoma whose disease has failed a prior autologous transplantation. J Clin Oncol 2004;22:2419–23.

37. Goldstone AH, Richards SM, Lazarus HM, et al. In adults with standard-risk acute lymphoblastic leukemia, the greatest benefit is achieved from a matched sibling allogeneic transplantation in first complete remission, and an autologous transplantation is less effective than conventional consolidation/maintenance chemotherapy in all patients: final results of the International ALL Trial (MRC UKALL XII/ECOG E2993). Blood 2008;111:1827–33.

38. van Imhoff GW, van der Holt B, MacKenzie MA, et al. Short intensive sequential therapy followed by autologous stem cell transplantation in adult Burkitt, Burkitt-like and lymphoblastic lymphoma. Leukemia 2005;19:945–52.

39. Song KW, Barnett MJ, Gascoyne RD, et al. Haematopoietic stem cell transplantation as primary therapy of sporadic adult Burkitt lymphoma. Br J Haematol 2006;133:634–7.

40. Song KW, Barnett MJ, Gascoyne RD, et al. Primary therapy for adults with T-cell lymphoblastic lymphoma with hematopoietic stem-cell transplantation results in favorable outcomes. Ann Oncol 2007;18:535–40.

41. Sweetenham JW, Santini G, Qian W, et al. High-dose therapy and autologous stem-cell transplantation versus conventional-dose consolidation/maintenance therapy as postremission therapy for adult patients with lymphoblastic lymphoma: results of a randomized trial of the European Group for blood and marrow transplantation and the United Kingdom Lymphoma Group. J Clin Oncol 2001;19: 2927–36.

42. Vey N, Thomas X, Picard C, et al. Allogeneic stem cell transplantation improves the outcome of adults with t(1;19)/E2A-PBX1 and t(4;11)/MLL-AF4 positive B-cell acute lymphoblastic leukemia: results of the prospective multicenter LALA-94 study. Leukemia 2006;20:2155–61.

43. Peniket AJ, Ruiz de Elvira MC, Taghipour G, et al. An EBMT registry matched study of allogeneic stem cell transplants for lymphoma: allogeneic transplantation is associated with a lower relapse rate but a higher procedure-related mortality rate than autologous transplantation. Bone Marrow Transplant 2003;31:667–78.

44. Hiddemann W, Kneba M, Dreyling M, et al. Frontline therapy with rituximab added to the combination of cyclophosphamide, doxorubicin, vincristine, and prednisone (CHOP) significantly improves the outcome for patients with advanced-stage follicular lymphoma compared with therapy with CHOP alone: results of a prospective randomized study of the German Low-Grade Lymphoma Study Group. Blood 2005;106:3725–32.

45. Fisher RI, LeBlanc M, Press OW, et al. New treatment options have changed the survival of patients with follicular lymphoma. J Clin Oncol 2005;23:8447–52.

46. Montoto S, Davies AJ, Matthews J, et al. Risk and clinical implications of transformation of follicular lymphoma to diffuse large B-cell lymphoma. J Clin Oncol 2007; 25:2426–33.

47. Ladetto M, Corradini P, Vallet S, et al. High rate of clinical and molecular remissions in follicular lymphoma patients receiving high-dose sequential chemotherapy and autografting at diagnosis: a multicenter, prospective study by the Gruppo Italiano Trapianto Midollo Osseo (GITMO). Blood 2002;100:1559–65.

48. Lenz G, Dreyling M, Schiegnitz E, et al. Myeloablative radiochemotherapy followed by autologous stem cell transplantation in first remission prolongs progression-free survival in follicular lymphoma: results of a prospective, randomized trial of the German Low-Grade Lymphoma Study Group. Blood 2004;104:2667–74.

49. Deconinck E, Foussard C, Milpied N, et al. High-dose therapy followed by autologous purged stem-cell transplantation and doxorubicin-based chemotherapy in patients with advanced follicular lymphoma: a randomized multicenter study by GOELAMS. Blood 2005;105:3817–23.

50. Sebban C, Mounier N, Brousse N, et al. Standard chemotherapy with interferon compared with CHOP followed by high-dose therapy with autologous stem cell transplantation in untreated patients with advanced follicular lymphoma: the GELF-94 randomized study from the Groupe d'Etude des Lymphomes de l'Adulte (GELA). Blood 2006;108:2540–4.

51. Ladetto M, De Marco F, Benedetti F, et al. Prospective, multicenter randomized GITMO/IIL trial comparing intensive (R-HDS) versus conventional (CHOP-R) chemoimmunotherapy in high-risk follicular lymphoma at diagnosis: the superior disease control of R-HDS does not translate into an overall survival advantage. Blood 2008;111:4004–13.

52. Schouten HC, Qian W, Kvaloy S, et al. High-dose therapy improves progression-free survival and survival in relapsed follicular non-Hodgkin's lymphoma: results from the randomized European CUP trial. J Clin Oncol 2003;21:3918–27.

53. Sabloff M, Atkins HL, Bence-Bruckler I, et al. A 15-year analysis of early and late autologous hematopoietic stem cell transplant in relapsed, aggressive, transformed, and nontransformed follicular lymphoma. Biol Blood Marrow Transplant 2007;13:956–64.

54. Montoto S, Canals C, Rohatiner AZ, et al. Long-term follow-up of high-dose treatment with autologous haematopoietic progenitor cell support in 693 patients with follicular lymphoma: an EBMT registry study. Leukemia 2007;21:2324–31.

55. Rohatiner AZ, Nadler L, Davies AJ, et al. Myeloablative therapy with autologous bone marrow transplantation for follicular lymphoma at the time of second or subsequent remission: long-term follow-up. J Clin Oncol 2007;25:2554–9.

56. van Oers MH, Klasa R, Marcus RE, et al. Rituximab maintenance improves clinical outcome of relapsed/resistant follicular non-Hodgkin's lymphoma, both in patients with and without rituximab during induction: results of a prospective randomized phase III intergroup trial. Blood 2006;108:3295–301.

57. Kang TY, Rybicki LA, Bolwell BJ, et al. Effect of prior rituximab on high-dose therapy and autologous stem cell transplantation in follicular lymphoma. Bone Marrow Transplant 2007;40:973–8.
58. Vose JM, Bierman PJ, Loberiza FR, et al. Long-term outcomes of autologous stem cell transplantation for follicular non-Hodgkin lymphoma: effect of histological grade and follicular international prognostic index. Biol Blood Marrow Transplant 2008;14:36–42.
59. Magni M, Di Nicola M, Devizzi L, et al. Successful in vivo purging of CD34-containing peripheral blood harvests in mantle cell and indolent lymphoma: evidence for a role of both chemotherapy and rituximab infusion. Blood 2000;96:864–9.
60. Belhadj K, Delfau-Larue MH, Elgnaoui T, et al. Efficiency of in vivo purging with rituximab prior to autologous peripheral blood progenitor cell transplantation in B-cell non-Hodgkin's lymphoma: a single institution study. Ann Oncol 2004;15:504–10.
61. Gribben JG, Freedman AS, Neuberg D, et al. Immunologic purging of marrow assessed by PCR before autologous bone marrow transplantation for B-cell lymphoma. N Engl J Med 1991;325:1525–33.
62. Gribben JG, Neuberg D, Freedman AS, et al. Detection by polymerase chain reaction of residual cells with the bcl-2 translocation is associated with increased risk of relapse after autologous bone marrow transplantation for B-cell lymphoma. Blood 1993;81:3449–57.
63. Corradini P, Ladetto M, Zallio F, et al. Long-term follow-up of indolent lymphoma patients treated with high-dose sequential chemotherapy and autografting: evidence that durable molecular and clinical remission frequently can be attained only in follicular subtypes. J Clin Oncol 2004;22:1460–8.
64. Solal-Celigny P, Roy P, Colombat P, et al. Follicular lymphoma international prognostic index. Blood 2004;104:1258–65.
65. Freytes CO, Loberiza FR, Rizzo JD, et al. Myeloablative allogeneic hematopoietic stem cell transplantation in patients who relapse after autologous stem cell transplantation for lymphoma: a report of the International Bone Marrow Transplant Registry. Blood 2004;104:3797–803.
66. van Besien K, Loberiza FR Jr, Bajorunaite R, et al. Comparison of autologous and allogeneic hematopoietic stem cell transplantation for follicular lymphoma. Blood 2003;102:3521–9.
67. Ingram W, Devereux S, Das-Gupta EP, et al. Outcome of BEAM-autologous and BEAM-alemtuzumab allogeneic transplantation in relapsed advanced stage follicular lymphoma. Br J Haematol 2008;141:235–43.
68. Khouri IF, Saliba RM, Giralt SA, et al. Nonablative allogeneic hematopoietic transplantation as adoptive immunotherapy for indolent lymphoma: low incidence of toxicity, acute graft-versus-host disease, and treatment-related mortality. Blood 2001;98:3595–9.
69. Vigouroux S, Michallet M, Porcher R, et al. Long-term outcomes after reduced-intensity conditioning allogeneic stem cell transplantation for low-grade lymphoma: a survey by the French Society of Bone Marrow Graft Transplantation and Cellular Therapy (SFGM-TC). Haematologica 2007;92:627–34.
70. Hari P, Carreras J, Zhang MJ, et al. Allogeneic transplants in follicular lymphoma: higher risk of disease progression after reduced-intensity compared to myeloablative conditioning. Biol Blood Marrow Transplant 2008;14:236–45.
71. Morris E, Thomson K, Craddock C, et al. Outcomes after alemtuzumab-containing reduced-intensity allogeneic transplantation regimen for relapsed and refractory non-Hodgkin lymphoma. Blood 2004;104:3865–71.

72. Khouri IF, McLaughlin P, Saliba RM, et al. Eight-year experience with allogeneic stem cell transplantation for relapsed follicular lymphoma after nonmyeloablative conditioning with fludarabine, cyclophosphamide, and rituximab. Blood 2008; 111:5530–6.

73. Howard OM, Gribben JG, Neuberg DS, et al. Rituximab and CHOP induction therapy for newly diagnosed mantle-cell lymphoma: molecular complete responses are not predictive of progression-free survival. J Clin Oncol 2002;20:1288–94.

74. Lenz G, Dreyling M, Hoster E, et al. Immunochemotherapy with rituximab and cyclophosphamide, doxorubicin, vincristine, and prednisone significantly improves response and time to treatment failure, but not long-term outcome in patients with previously untreated mantle cell lymphoma: results of a prospective randomized trial of the German Low-Grade Lymphoma Study Group (GLSG). J Clin Oncol 2005;23:1984–92.

75. Dreyling M, Lenz G, Hoster E, et al. Early consolidation by myeloablative radiochemotherapy followed by autologous stem cell transplantation in first remission significantly prolongs progression-free survival in mantle-cell lymphoma: results of a prospective randomized trial of the European MCL Network. Blood 2005; 105:2677–84.

76. Vandenberghe E, Ruiz de Elvira C, Loberiza FR, et al. Outcome of autologous transplantation for mantle cell lymphoma: a study by the European Blood And Bone Marrow Transplant and Autologous Blood And Marrow Transplant registries. Br J Haematol 2003;120:793–800.

77. Gianni AM, Magni M, Martelli M, et al. Long-term remission in mantle cell lymphoma following high-dose sequential chemotherapy and in vivo rituximab-purged stem cell autografting (R-HDS regimen). Blood 2003;102:749–55.

78. Mangel J, Leitch HA, Connors JM, et al. Intensive chemotherapy and autologous stem-cell transplantation plus rituximab is superior to conventional chemotherapy for newly diagnosed advanced stage mantle-cell lymphoma: a matched pair analysis. Ann Oncol 2004;15:283–90.

79. Dreger P, Rieger M, Seyfarth B, et al. Rituximab-augmented myeloablation for first-line autologous stem cell transplantation for mantle cell lymphoma: effects on molecular response and clinical outcome. Haematologica 2007;92:42–9.

80. Khouri IF, Lee MS, Saliba RM, et al. Nonablative allogeneic stem-cell transplantation for advanced/recurrent mantle-cell lymphoma. J Clin Oncol 2003;21:4407–12.

81. Rodriguez J, Caballero MD, Gutierrez A, et al. High-dose chemotherapy and autologous stem cell transplantation in peripheral T-cell lymphoma: the GEL-TAMO experience. Ann Oncol 2003;14:1768–75.

82. Rodriguez J, Conde E, Gutierrez A, et al. Frontline autologous stem cell transplantation in high-risk peripheral T-cell lymphoma: a prospective study from The Gel-Tamo Study Group. Eur J Haematol 2007;79:32–8.

83. Corradini P, Tarella C, Zallio F, et al. Long-term follow-up of patients with peripheral T-cell lymphomas treated up-front with high-dose chemotherapy followed by autologous stem cell transplantation. Leukemia 2006;20:1533–8.

84. Rodriguez J, Conde E, Gutierrez A, et al. The adjusted international prognostic index and beta-2-microglobulin predict the outcome after autologous stem cell transplantation in relapsing/refractory peripheral T-cell lymphoma. Haematologica 2007;92:1067–74.

85. Rodriguez J, Conde E, Gutierrez A, et al. Prolonged survival of patients with angioimmunoblastic T-cell lymphoma after high-dose chemotherapy and autologous stem cell transplantation: the GELTAMO experience. Eur J Haematol 2007; 78:290–6.

86. Zamkoff KW, Matulis MD, Mehta AC, et al. High-dose therapy and autologous stem cell transplant does not result in long-term disease-free survival in patients with recurrent chemotherapy-sensitive ALK-negative anaplastic large-cell lymphoma. Bone Marrow Transplant 2004;33:635–8.

87. Corradini P, Dodero A, Zallio F, et al. Graft-versus-lymphoma effect in relapsed peripheral T-cell non-Hodgkin's lymphomas after reduced-intensity conditioning followed by allogeneic transplantation of hematopoietic cells. J Clin Oncol 2004;22:2172–6.

88. Galicier L, Fieschi C, Borie R, et al. Intensive chemotherapy regimen (LMB86) for St Jude stage IV AIDS-related Burkitt lymphoma/leukemia: a prospective study. Blood 2007;110:2846–54.

89. Krishnan A, Molina A, Zaia J, et al. Durable remissions with autologous stem cell transplantation for high-risk HIV-associated lymphomas. Blood 2005;105:874–8.

90. Spitzer TR, Ambinder RF, Lee JY, et al. Dose-reduced busulfan, cyclophosphamide, and autologous stem cell transplantation for human immunodeficiency virus-associated lymphoma: AIDS malignancy consortium study 020. Biol Blood Marrow Transplant 2008;14:59–66.

91. Kusumi E, Kami M, Kanda Y, et al. Reduced-intensity hematopoietic stem-cell transplantation for malignant lymphoma: a retrospective survey of 112 adult patients in Japan. Bone Marrow Transplant 2005;36:205–13.

92. Evens AM, Winter JN, Hou N, et al. A phase II clinical trial of intensive chemotherapy followed by consolidative stem cell transplant: long-term follow-up in newly diagnosed mantle cell lymphoma. Br J Haematol 2008;140:385–93.

93. Maris MB, Sandmaier BM, Storer BE, et al. Allogeneic hematopoietic cell transplantation after Fludarabine and 2 Gy total body irradiation for relapsed and refractory mantle cell lymphoma. Blood 2004;104:3535–42.

Index

Note: Page numbers of article titles are in **boldface** type.

Hematol Oncol Clin N Am 22 (2008) 1081–1097
doi:10.1016/S0889-8588(08)00135-4
0889-8588/08/$ – see front matter © 2008 Elsevier Inc. All rights reserved.

Moving?

Make sure your subscription moves with you!

To notify us of your new address, find your **Clinics Account Number** (located on your mailing label above your name), and contact customer service at:

E-mail: elspcs@elsevier.com

800-654-2452 (subscribers in the U.S. & Canada)
1-407-563-6020 (subscribers outside of the U.S. & Canada)

Fax number: 407-363-9661

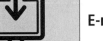

Elsevier Periodicals Customer Service
6277 Sea Harbor Drive
Orlando, FL 32887-4800

*To ensure uninterrupted delivery of your subscription, please notify us at least 4 weeks in advance of move.

United States Postal Service

Statement of Ownership, Management, and Circulation
(All Periodicals Publications Except Requestor Publications)

1. Publication Title	2. Publication Number	3. Filing Date
Hematology/Oncology Clinics of North America	0 0 2 - 4 7 3	9/15/08

4. Issue Frequency	5. Number of Issues Published Annually	6. Annual Subscription Price
Feb, Apr, Jun, Aug, Oct, Dec	6	$262.00

7. Complete Mailing Address of Known Office of Publication (Not printer) (Street, city, county, state, and ZIP+4)

Elsevier Inc.
360 Park Avenue South
New York, NY 10010-1710

Contact Person
Stephen Bushing

Telephone (Include area code)
215-239-3688

8. Complete Mailing Address of Headquarters or General Business Office of Publisher (Not printer)

Elsevier Inc., 360 Park Avenue South, New York, NY 10010-1710

9. Full Names and Complete Mailing Addresses of Publisher, Editor, and Managing Editor (Do not leave blank)

Publisher (Name and complete mailing address)

John Schrefer , Elsevier, Inc., 1600 John F. Kennedy Blvd. Suite 1800, Philadelphia, PA 19103-2899

Editor (Name and complete mailing address)

Kerry Holland, Elsevier, Inc., 1600 John F. Kennedy Blvd. Suite 1800, Philadelphia, PA 19103-2899

Managing Editor (Name and complete mailing address)

Catherine Bewick, Elsevier, Inc., 1600 John F. Kennedy Blvd. Suite 1800, Philadelphia, PA 19103-2899

10. Owner (Do not leave blank. If the publication is owned by a corporation, give the name and address of the corporation immediately followed by the names and addresses of all stockholders owning or holding 1 percent or more of the total amount of stock. If not owned by a corporation, give the names and addresses of the individual owners. If owned by a partnership or other unincorporated firm, give its name and address as well as those of each individual owner. If the publication is published by a nonprofit organization, give its name and address.)

Full Name	Complete Mailing Address
Wholly owned subsidiary of	4520 East-West Highway
Reed/Elsevier, US holdings	Bethesda, MD 20814

11. Known Bondholders, Mortgagees, and Other Security Holders Owning or Holding 1 Percent or More of Total Amount of Bonds, Mortgages, or Other Securities. If none, check box ☐ None

Full Name	Complete Mailing Address
N/A	

12. Tax Status (For completion by nonprofit organizations authorized to mail at nonprofit rates) (Check one)
The purpose, function, and nonprofit status of this organization and the exempt status for federal income tax purposes:
☐ Has Not Changed During Preceding 12 Months
☐ Has Changed During Preceding 12 Months (Publisher must submit explanation of change with this statement)

PS Form 3526, September 2006 (Page 1 of 3 (Instructions Page 3)) PSN 7530-01-000-9931 PRIVACY NOTICE: See our Privacy policy in www.usps.com

---

13. Publication Title	14. Issue Date for Circulation Data Below
Hematology/Oncology Clinics of North America	August 2008

15. Extent and Nature of Circulation		Average No. Copies Each Issue During Preceding 12 Months	No. Copies of Single Issue Published Nearest to Filing Date
a. Total Number of Copies (Net press run)		2300	2300
b. Paid Circulation (By Mail and Outside the Mail)	(1) Mailed Outside-County Paid Subscriptions Stated on PS Form 3541. (Include paid distribution above nominal rate, advertiser's proof copies, and exchange copies)	838	779
	(2) Mailed In-County Paid Subscriptions Stated on PS Form 3541 (Include paid distribution above nominal rate, advertiser's proof copies, and exchange copies)		
	(3) Paid Distribution Outside the Mails Including Sales Through Dealers and Carriers, Street Vendors, Counter Sales, and Other Paid Distribution Outside USPS®	584	566
	(4) Paid Distribution by Other Classes Mailed Through the USPS (e.g. First-Class Mail®)		
c. Total Paid Distribution (Sum of 15b (1), (2), (3), and (4))		1422	1345
d. Free or Nominal Rate Distribution (By Mail and Outside the Mail)	(1) Free or Nominal Rate Outside-County Copies Included on PS Form 3541	118	123
	(2) Free or Nominal Rate In-County Copies Included on PS Form 3541		
	(3) Free or Nominal Rate Copies Mailed at Other Classes Mailed Through the USPS (e.g. First-Class Mail)		
	(4) Free or Nominal Rate Distribution Outside the Mail (Carriers or other means)		
e. Total Free or Nominal Rate Distribution (Sum of 15d (1), (2), (3) and (4))		118	123
f. Total Distribution (Sum of 15c and 15e)		1540	1468
g. Copies not Distributed (See instructions to publishers #4 (page #3))		760	832
h. Total (Sum of 15f and g)		2300	2300
i. Percent Paid (15c divided by 15f times 100)		92.34%	91.62%

16. Publication of Statement of Ownership

If the publication is a general publication, publication of this statement is required. Will be printed in the October 2008 issue of this publication. ☐ Publication not required

17. Signature and Title of Editor, Publisher, Business Manager, or Owner

[signature] Stephen Bushing — Executive Director of Subscription Services

Date September 15, 2008

I certify that all information furnished on this form is true and complete. I understand that anyone who furnishes false or misleading information on this form or who omits material or information requested on the form may be subject to criminal sanctions (including fines and imprisonment) and/or civil sanctions (including civil penalties).

PS Form 3526, September 2006 (Page 2 of 3)